Acute Respiratory Distress Syndrome

Davide Chiumello
Editor

Acute Respiratory Distress Syndrome

Springer

Editor
Davide Chiumello
Director of Anaesthesia and Intensive Care
Services, ASST Santi Paolo e Carlo
Department of Scienze della Salute
University of Milan
Milan
Italy

ISBN 978-3-319-82446-8 ISBN 978-3-319-41852-0 (eBook)
DOI 10.1007/978-3-319-41852-0

Softcover reprint of the hardcover 1st edition 2017

Printed on acid-free paper

This Springer imprint is published by Springer Nature
The registered company is Springer International Publishing AG
The registered company address is: Gewerbestrasse 11, 6330 Cham, Switzerland

Contents

Acute Respiratory Distress Syndrome (ARDS): Definition, Incidence, and Outcome

1

Rémi Coudroy, Florence Boissier, and Arnaud W. Thille

1.1 Definition of ARDS

1.1.1 From the First Clinical Description to the First Consensus Definition of ARDS

In 1967, Ashbaugh and colleagues reported for the first time the clinical and physiological characteristics in 12 patients with sudden respiratory failure that they called "acute respiratory distress syndrome" (ARDS) [1]. None of these patients had past history of cardiac or pulmonary disease, and they rapidly developed acute hypoxemia, stiff lungs, and diffuse bilateral alveolar infiltration on chest X-ray a few days later after a precipitating factor. Their outcome was dramatic as 7 of the 12 patients (58%) died. An autopsy was performed in all deceased patients, and six of them (86%) had a characteristic histological pattern of diffuse alveolar damage including hyaline membranes, edema, cell necrosis, or fibrosis [1].

In 1971, Petty and Ashbaugh described principles of management of ARDS based mainly on mechanical ventilation using high FiO_2 and positive end-expiratory pressure (PEEP) [2]. Whereas cyanosis refractory to oxygen was one of the clinical

R. Coudroy, MD • F. Boissier, MD, PhD
CHU de Poitiers, Réanimation Médicale, Poitiers, France

INSERM CIC 1402 (ALIVE Group), Université de Poitiers, Faculté de Médecine, Poitiers, France

A.W. Thille, MD, PhD (✉)
CHU de Poitiers, Réanimation Médicale, Poitiers, France

INSERM CIC 1402 (ALIVE Group), Université de Poitiers, Faculté de Médecine, Poitiers, France

Réanimation Médicale, CHU de Poitiers,
2 rue la Milétrie, 86021 Poitiers Cedex, France
e-mail: aw.thille@gmail.com

D. Chiumello (ed.), *Acute Respiratory Distress Syndrome (ARDS)*,
DOI 10.1007/978-3-319-41852-0_1

criteria for ARDS, the authors did not specify any hypoxemia threshold. Five years later, Bone and colleagues proposed a threshold of hypoxemia below 70 mmHg despite FiO_2 of at least 0.5 and PEEP [3]. In 1982, Pepe and colleagues added to the definition the presence of new diffuse bilateral infiltrates on chest X-ray and a pulmonary wedge pressure lower than 18 mmHg, thereby excluding cardiogenic pulmonary edema [4]. In 1988, Murray and colleagues proposed the lung injury score (LIS) as a means of assessing the severity of ARDS according to the PaO_2/FiO_2 ratio, the PEEP level, respiratory system compliance, and the number of quadrants with infiltration seen on chest X-ray [5].

Since this original description, the definition of ARDS has considerably evolved over the time, but it was not until 1994 that an international American–European Consensus Conference (AECC) laid the foundations for the first clinical definition of ARDS [6]. This consensus conference aimed to bring uniformity to the definition of ARDS for research, epidemiologic studies, and individual patient care [6]. ARDS was consequently defined using the following four criteria: (1) the acute onset of hypoxemia, (2) a PaO_2 to FiO_2 ratio ≤200 mmHg regardless of PEEP level, (3) the presence of bilateral infiltrates on chest X-ray, and (4) pulmonary artery wedge pressure ≤18 mmHg or no clinical sign of left atrial hypertension [6]. Patients meeting all these criteria but having less severe hypoxemia with a PaO_2 to FiO_2 ratio between 201 and 300 mmHg were considered as having acute lung injury (ALI) and not ARDS. However, this clinical definition has been criticized on each criterion [7] leading to the establishment of a new definition in 2012, the Berlin definition [8].

1.1.2 The Current Berlin Definition

The Berlin definition aimed to provide a better clinical definition and to classify patients according to severity. An expanded rationale was then published by the expert panel to propose treatments and ventilatory management according to the degree of hypoxemia [9]. The changes proposed in the Berlin definition to address the major limitations of AECC definition are the following:

First, the "acute onset" of ARDS has been specified, and respiratory symptoms have to be present within 7 days after a clinical insult (Table 1.1). Timing accuracy enables elimination of mimickers of ARDS who develop respiratory symptoms over several weeks such as idiopathic pulmonary fibrosis, nonspecific interstitial pneumonitis, cryptogenic organizing pneumonia, granulomatosis with polyangiitis, or drug-induced lung disease [10].

Second, patients have been stratified according to their severity in terms of hypoxemia and classified as mild, moderate, and severe ARDS when PaO_2/FiO_2 ratio is between 201 and 300, between 101 and 200, and equal to or below 100 mmHg, respectively [8]. By including patients with a PaO_2/FiO_2 ratio up to 300 mmHg, the Berlin definition now encompasses the patients with mild ARDS that was formerly named acute lung injury. Oxygenation criteria were well correlated to severity with mortality of 27, 32, and 45% in mild, moderate, and severe ARDS, respectively. As a major limitation of the AECC definition was the

Table 1.1 Risk factors of acute respiratory distress syndrome adapted from [9]

Direct lung insult (pulmonary ARDS)
Pneumonia (bacterial, viral, etc.)
Aspiration of gastric content
Inhalation injury
Pulmonary contusion
Pulmonary vasculitis
Near drowning
Indirect lung injury (extrapulmonary ARDS)
Non-pulmonary sepsis
Non-cardiogenic shock
Pancreatitis
Major trauma
Multiple transfusion or transfusion-related acute lung injury
Severe burns
Drug overdose

assessment of PaO_2/FiO_2 ratio regardless of the PEEP level used, the Berlin definition stated that PaO_2/FiO_2 ratio had to be measured with a PEEP level of at least 5 cmH_2O [8].

Third, the AECC definition considered that pulmonary arterial wedge pressure should not exceed 18 mmHg in ARDS [6]. However, high values of pulmonary wedge pressure are commonly observed in patients with ARDS [11, 12], and routine use of pulmonary artery catheter is pointless for hemodynamic management [13]. Therefore, pulmonary artery wedge pressure requirement was removed from the Berlin definition, and it was stated that respiratory failure must not be fully explained by cardiac failure of fluid overload as judged by the clinician or confirmed by echocardiography, if needed, to rule out cardiogenic pulmonary edema [8].

Fourth, the Berlin definition considered radiological findings as bilateral opacities on chest X-ray but also on CT scan, which were not fully explained by effusions, lobar or lung collapse, or nodules [8].

Four ancillary variables were assessed for severe ARDS, including more extensive opacities on chest radiograph, i.e., at least three quadrants, a high PEEP level $\geq$10 cmH_2O, low respiratory system compliance $\leq$40 ml/cm H_2O, and a corrected expired volume $\geq$10 L/min. However, these criteria were not included in the Berlin definition because they did not help to discriminate patients with severe ARDS [8].

1.1.3 What Are the Limitations of the Current Definition?

The major limitation is that ARDS and its severity can be assessed on a single blood gas measurement without prior standardized ventilator settings. However, PEEP may have a major influence on oxygenation, and in the three RCTs that have compared two levels of PEEP (lower vs. higher), oxygenation was always more satisfactory in the higher-PEEP group than in the lower-PEEP group [14–16]. In a meta-analysis including these three trials, survival was better using high PEEP than using low PEEP in patients with a PaO_2 to FiO_2 ratio ≤200 mmHg [17], and therefore, the experts have recommended the use of high PEEP levels in patients with moderate or severe ARDS [9]. After optimizing ventilator settings and by increasing the PEEP level, several studies have shown that a high proportion of patients could have their severity modified based on PaO_2/FiO_2 ratio, from severe to moderate/mild or from moderate to mild [18–20]. FiO_2 variations may also be associated with significant changes in PaO_2/FiO_2 ratio [18, 21], and it has been shown that, for the same PaO_2/FiO_2 ratio, patients ventilated with high FiO_2 had higher mortality than those ventilated with lower FiO_2 [22]. To homogenize disease severity, ventilatory settings should be optimized using low tidal volumes around 6 mL/kg of predicted body weight and high PEEP level. Likewise, the time from ventilator settings to PaO_2/FiO_2 measurement seems crucial. Indeed, Villar and colleagues reported that mortality was more reliably predicted according to the three categories of severity (mild, moderate, and severe) when PaO_2/FiO_2 ratio was measured with a PEEP level at least 10 cmH_2O and FiO_2 at least 0.5 [19, 20]. However, assessment of PaO_2/FiO_2 ratio yielded a more clinically relevant ARDS classification when measured 24 h after ARDS onset than immediately after FiO_2 and PEEP settings [19, 20]. This finding is illustrated by the inclusion criteria used in the PROSEVA trial, which found a significant reduction of mortality in patients treated with prone position for which patients with a PaO_2/FiO_2 below 150 mmHg were eligible if such a high degree of hypoxemia persisted more than 12 h after optimization of ventilator settings [23]. Therefore, standardized ventilator settings with a PEEP level of at least 10 cmH_2O and the persistence of hypoxemia may perhaps help to improve ARDS classification.

The other main limitation is the difficulty in quantifying morphological lung injury. Since it was first reported, diffuse alveolar damage (DAD) has been regarded as the morphological hallmark of the lung in ARDS [24, 25]. However, the incidence of DAD in ARDS is highly variable from one study to another and largely depends on the type of examination (autopsy vs. open lung biopsy) (Table 1.2). In a large database of clinical autopsies including 356 patients with ARDS, overall incidence of DAD was only 45% [42]. However, the incidence of DAD depended on the severity of ARDS and time from ARDS onset to pathological examination. Hyaline membranes may take 2–3 days to appear [24] and this explains why the incidence of DAD was significantly higher (56%) in patients with ARDS for more than 72 h. The proportion of patients with DAD also increased in more severe patients with an incidence of 12, 40, and 58% in mild, moderate, and severe ARDS, respectively. The incidence of DAD was as high as 69% in patients with severe ARDS after 3 days of evolution [42]. In this study, whereas almost all patients with DAD on autopsy examination met the clinical criteria of the Berlin definition for ARDS (high sensitivity), fewer than half of the patients with ARDS had DAD (low specificity). Perhaps the low specificity of the Berlin definition in DAD detection is ascribable to the presence of other processes with a similar clinical picture. Many diseases may mimic ARDS such as alveolar hemorrhage due to vasculitis, drug-induced pulmonary toxic pneumonia with a lymphocytic pattern or acute

Table 1.2 Incidence of diffuse alveolar damage (DAD) on open lung biopsy or autopsy in patients with acute respiratory distress syndrome (ARDS)

Author (year) [Ref]	*N* patients	Time from ARDS onset to examination, days	Overall incidence of DAD, *N* (%)	Mild ARDS	Moderate ARDS	Severe ARDS
Suchyta (1991) [26]	9	<14	6 (67%)	–	–	–
Warner (1988) [27]	80	6 ± 4	0 (0%)	–	–	–
Papazian (1998) [28]	36	10 (5–55)	5 (14%)	–	4/24 (17%)	1/12 (8%)
Patel (2004) [29]	57	3 (0–25)	23 (40%)	–	–	–
Esteban (2004) [30]	127	3 (1–6)	84 (66%)	–	–	–
Cho (2006) [31]	53	–	23 (43%)	–	–	–
Kao (2006) [32]	41	3 ± 2	12 (29%)	–	–	–
Lim (2007) [33]	36	4 (1–23)	0 (0%)	–	–	–
Arabi (2007) [34]	14	9 (1–30)	7 (50%)	–	–	–
Papazian (2007) [35]	100	7 (6–14)	13 (13%)	–	–	–
Baumann (2008) [36]	22	8 (2–76)	2 (9%)	0/4 (0%)	2/15 (13%)	0/3 (0%)
Lin (2009) [37]	60	8 ± 1	16 (27%)	–	–	–
De Hemptinne (2009) [38]	64	6 (0–48)	32 (50%)	–	–	–
Charbonney (2009) [39]	19	5 (2–11)	9 (47%)	–	–	–
Melo (2009) [40]	19	13	7 (37%)	–	–	–
Sarmiento (2011) [41]	49	–	31 (63%)	–	–	–
Thille (2013) [42]	356	5 (2–13)	159 (45%)	6/49 (12%)	56/141 (40%)	97/166 (58%)
Guérin (2015) [43]	83	9 (6–14)	48 (58%)	4/11 (36%)	33/56 (59%)	11/16 (69%)
Kao (2015) [44]	101	7 ± 7	57 (56%)	13/17 (77%)	32/57 (56%)	12/27 (44%)
Total	***N* = 1353**		***N* = 537 (40%)**	**23/81 (28%)**	**127/293 (43%)**	**121/224 (54%)**

eosinophilic pneumonia, organizing or diffuse interstitial pneumonia, cancer infiltration, and at times idiopathic lymphangitis [10, 45]. These ARDS without common risk factors, the so-called ARDS mimickers, represent around 7–8% of patients mechanically ventilated for ARDS and could have higher mortality than the others [45]. For such atypical ARDS cases, a complete diagnostic workup, including bronchoalveolar lavage fluid cytology and chest CT scan patterns, should be performed to identify patients who might benefit from specific therapies, including corticosteroids. A recent study suggests that the presence of DAD is associated with higher mortality as compared to patients without DAD [46]. Unfortunately, no biomarkers exist to diagnose alveolar damage.

1.2 Incidence and Outcome of ARDS

The incidence of ARDS obviously depends on the definition used and will, as expected, be higher using the Berlin definition that includes patients with a PaO_2/FiO_2 up to 300 mmHg. At the beginning of the 2000s, three studies assessed incidence and outcome of ARDS using the AECC definition [47–49]. In these studies, around 7–8% of the patients admitted in the ICU met clinical criteria for ARDS, with mortality ranging from 35 to 50% in patients with a PaO_2/FiO_2 of 200 mmHg or less.

A large international survey performed in 2014 among 459 ICUs in 50 countries and over a 4-week period screened all patients who met clinical criteria for ARDS according to the current Berlin definition [50]. Patients with ARDS represented 10.4% of all ICU admissions, a rate slightly higher than in the abovementioned studies using the previous AECC definition [47–49]. This represented at least 5 patients per bed and per year or at least 100 patients per year in a 20-bed ICU. Among all intubated patients in ICU, 23% had met clinical criteria for ARDS during their ICU stay. Among them, 30% had mild, 47% had moderate, and 23% had severe ARDS. The risk factors triggering ARDS were pneumonia in 59% of cases, aspiration in 14%, extrapulmonary sepsis in 16%, and non-cardiogenic shock in 7.5%. Whereas some patients may have several risk factors, none of the usual risk factors had been identified in around 8% of the cases (ARDS mimickers). This survey also highlighted the fact that many patients with ARDS had not been recognized by the clinician as having this disease. In mild ARDS, this was the case in around half of the patients. Clinical recognition of ARDS was better for severe ARDS but still underdiagnosed since 21% of them were not recognized. Moreover, clinician recognition of ARDS at the time of fulfillment of clinical criteria was only 34%, suggesting that diagnosis of this pathology was frequently delayed. In this survey, overall mortality was 34% in ICU and 40% in hospital [50]. In-hospital mortality was 35% for those with mild, 40% for those with moderate, and 46% for those with severe ARDS.

1.2.1 Has Mortality Decreased Over Time?

One question is whether or not mortality has declined over time. In a systematic review evaluating 89 studies published between 1984 and 2006 and focusing on ARDS, mortality seemed to have decreased from 1984 to 1993 but not from 1993 to 2006 [51]. The use of protective ventilation including low tidal volumes, high PEEP levels, and strict monitoring of plateau pressure to avoid exceeding 30 cmH_2O is the cornerstone of the current recommendation [9]. After the 2000s, several studies have demonstrated that this strategy was associated with better survival [17, 52, 53], and this change in clinical practice should have had an impact on overall mortality. After 2010, several large RCTS have *shown* a reduction in mortality, especially in ARDS patients with PaO_2/FiO_2 ratio below 150 mmHg, using neuromuscular blockers [54] or prone positioning [23]. Despite this, a recent review focusing on the more recent articles suggested that overall mortality did not seem to have changed substantially during the last decade, with a proportion in observational studies greater than 40% in patients with moderate or severe ARDS [55], in keeping with the recent LUNG SAFE study [50].

1.2.2 How Can We Explain the Lack of Improvement in Outcome in ARDS?

The positive results reported in RCTs may not be as efficient when applied to all nonselected patients with ARDS in an ICU. It has been found that mortality in ARDS was lower in RCTs than in observational studies that are closer to real life [51]. Indeed, patients included in RCTs are expressly selected, and those with major comorbidities such as hematological malignancies, cirrhosis, and chronic cardiac or respiratory disease are usually excluded. Among the three studies having compared two levels of PEEP, only one of them has provided a flow chart study. In this study, only 22% of the patients assessed for eligibility were included and randomized (768 of 3429 patients) [15].

In a RCT, after excluding patients with exclusion criteria, a high proportion of patients potentially eligible are not enrolled. The outcome of ARDS patients enrolled in a recent RCT has been compared to that of patients who met inclusion criteria but who were not enrolled in the study due to various reasons such as no consent, physician refusal (24%), missed randomization window, etc. [56]. The patients who were included in the study had lower mortality than those who were potentially eligible but not enrolled, suggesting that enrollment in clinical trials may be associated with improved outcomes. The better outcome reported in patients included in RCTs may be due to optimal management including standardized lung protective ventilation and application of other effective therapies. Indeed, in real-life situations, as reported in the recent LUNG SAFE survey, 35% of patients with ARDS were ventilated with a tidal volume above 8 mL/kg of predicted body weight. The mean PEEP level was only 8 ± 3 cmH_2O in moderate and 10 ± 4 cmH_2O in severe ARDS. Prone positioning was used in only 16% of the patients with severe ARDS. Therefore, in 2014, patients with ARDS were receiving excessively high tidal volumes and excessively low levels of PEEP in "real life," while plateau pressure was measured in only 40% of the cases.

1.2.3 Causes of Death and Subphenotypes in Patients with ARDS

In ARDS, the main cause of death is sepsis complicated by multi-organ failure [42, 57, 58]. In a large database of patients who died of ARDS and had clinical autopsy over a 20-year period from 1990 to 2010, the pattern of death was refractory shock in more than half of the 356 patients analyzed, while refractory hypoxemia did not exceed 20% of the cases [42]. These results are in keeping with previous literature with a rate of death due to refractory hypoxemia of around 20% [57, 58]. Obviously, death due to withdrawal of life support has increased over time [58], and in more recent studies, the vast majority of deaths among patients with ARDS were preceded by a "do not resuscitate" order [59].

Patients with trauma as cause of ARDS have better survival rates than the others [60]. However, the mortality of patients with ARDS of pulmonary origin is similar to that of patients with ARDS of extrapulmonary origin [60]. In a recent study, Calfee and colleagues identified two subphenotypes of ARDS that could have different outcomes [61]. The hyperinflammatory subphenotype was characterized by more severe inflammation with higher plasma concentrations of inflammatory biomarkers and higher prevalence of sepsis. These patients were more likely to have shock and metabolic acidosis, and they had higher mortality than the others. The use of high PEEP levels did not seem beneficial in this subset of patients, while it was beneficial in the other patients.

1.2.4 Long-Term Outcome

ARDS is characterized by specific morphological changes of the lung with an initial exudative and then a proliferative phase. The exudative phase, maximal during the first week after the onset of ARDS, is characterized by capillary congestion and intra-alveolar edema subsequently followed by alveolar type I cell necrosis. The later repair phase is characterized by intense proliferation of alveolar type II cells and interstitial fibroblasts [24, 25]. This phase can either result in normal tissue resolution or progress toward fibrosis if lung injury is persistent. Fibrosis is rare during the first week of evolution of ARDS. However, it can be observed as early as the second week of evolution, and its prevalence markedly increases beyond the third week after the onset of ARDS, especially in ARDS of pulmonary origin [62]. The patients with fibrosis have more altered lung compliance and more frequently interstitial opacities on chest X-ray [63]. After recovery, they may have more long-term residual pulmonary dysfunction than the others [64]. Patients with many radiologic reticulations on chest CT scan 6 months after hospital discharge had altered total lung capacity, forced vital capacity, and carbon monoxide diffusion capacity [65]. In this last study, a chest CT scan performed 14 days after ARDS onset could predict altered quality of life. However, ARDS survivors who have had fibrosis also had more severe disease and more prolonged duration of mechanical ventilation than the others. Moreover, restrictive pulmonary function can be due not only to pulmonary impairment but also to extrapulmonary complications, such as depression and neuromuscular weakness. Herridge and colleagues have followed ARDS survivors discharged from the hospital for 5 years [66, 67]. Among them, 89% were alive at 1 year and 68% at 5 years. They had normal lung volumes and spirometry measurements by 6 months, but carbon monoxide diffusion capacity remained low, and 6-min walk test was abnormal throughout the 12-month follow-up [66]. At 5 years, pulmonary spirometry was normal or near normal, but patients did not return to normal predicted levels of physical function with persistent exercise limitation and decreased physical quality of life [67]. The median 6-min walk distance was 281 m at 3 months, 422 m at 1 year, and 436 m at 5 years (76% of predicted distance), and, although younger patients had a greater rate of recovery than older patients, neither group returned to normal predicted levels of physical function at 5 years. Health-related quality of life was mainly altered due to extrapulmonary complications. Actually, muscle weakness and fatigue were the main reasons for their functional limitation [66–68]. Moreover, 1 or 2 years after ARDS, the majority of survivors present with clinically significant general anxiety, depression, and posttraumatic stress disorder symptoms [69] and even sometimes psychiatric symptoms [70]

Short- and long-term quality of life is markedly altered in ARDS survivors [71] and seems more altered at 12 months than in other critically ill patients with similar severity but without ARDS during their ICU stay [72]. However, in another study, the quality of life was similar between ARDS and non-ARDS patients, and functional status at 6 months after hospitalization could be largely explained by baseline condition [73].

Conclusion

The definition of ARDS is still challenging and problematic, as is improvement of adherence to the "protective bundle" in real life. Indeed, although some RCTs have demonstrated therapeutic strategies that could improve mortality, negative outcome has hardly decreased in the last decade, and survivors still have a markedly altered quality of life.

References

1. Ashbaugh DG, Bigelow DB, Petty TL, Levine BE (1967) Acute respiratory distress in adults. Lancet 2:319–323
2. Petty TL, Ashbaugh DG (1971) The adult respiratory distress syndrome. Clinical features, factors influencing prognosis and principles of management. Chest 60:233–239
3. Bone RC, Francis PB, Pierce AK (1976) Intravascular coagulation associated with the adult respiratory distress syndrome. Am J Med 61:585–589
4. Pepe PE, Potkin RT, Reus DH, Hudson LD, Carrico CJ (1982) Clinical predictors of the adult respiratory distress syndrome. Am J Surg 144:124–130
5. Murray JF, Matthay MA, Luce JM, Flick MR (1988) An expanded definition of the adult respiratory distress syndrome. Am Rev Respir Dis 138:720–723
6. Bernard GR, Artigas A, Brigham KL, Carlet J, Falke K, Hudson L, Lamy M, Legall JR, Morris A, Spragg R (1994) The American-European Consensus Conference on ARDS. Definitions, mechanisms, relevant outcomes, and clinical trial coordination. Am J Respir Crit Care Med 149:818–824
7. Phua J, Stewart TE, Ferguson ND (2008) Acute respiratory distress syndrome 40 years later: time to revisit its definition. Crit Care Med 36:2912–2921
8. Force ADT, Ranieri VM, Rubenfeld GD, Thompson BT, Ferguson ND, Caldwell E, Fan E, Camporota L, Slutsky AS (2012) Acute respiratory distress syndrome: the Berlin Definition. JAMA 307:2526–2533
9. Ferguson ND, Fan E, Camporota L, Antonelli M, Anzueto A, Beale R, Brochard L, Brower R, Esteban A, Gattinoni L, Rhodes A, Slutsky AS, Vincent JL, Rubenfeld GD, Thompson BT, Ranieri VM (2012) The Berlin definition of ARDS: an expanded rationale, justification, and supplementary material. Intensive Care Med 38:1573–1582

10. Guerin C, Thompson T, Brower R (2015) The ten diseases that look like ARDS. Intensive Care Med 41:1099–1102
11. Wheeler AP, Bernard GR, Thompson BT, Schoenfeld D, Wiedemann HP, deBoisblanc B, Connors AF Jr, Hite RD, Harabin AL (2006) Pulmonary-artery versus central venous catheter to guide treatment of acute lung injury. N Engl J Med 354:2213–2224
12. Ferguson ND, Meade MO, Hallett DC, Stewart TE (2002) High values of the pulmonary artery wedge pressure in patients with acute lung injury and acute respiratory distress syndrome. Intensive Care Med 28:1073–1077
13. Richard C, Warszawski J, Anguel N, Deye N, Combes A, Barnoud D, Boulain T, Lefort Y, Fartoukh M, Baud F, Boyer A, Brochard L, Teboul JL (2003) Early use of the pulmonary artery catheter and outcomes in patients with shock and acute respiratory distress syndrome: a randomized controlled trial. JAMA 290:2713–2720
14. Meade MO, Cook DJ, Guyatt GH, Slutsky AS, Arabi YM, Cooper DJ, Davies AR, Hand LE, Zhou Q, Thabane L, Austin P, Lapinsky S, Baxter A, Russell J, Skrobik Y, Ronco JJ, Stewart TE (2008) Ventilation strategy using low tidal volumes, recruitment maneuvers, and high positive end-expiratory pressure for acute lung injury and acute respiratory distress syndrome: a randomized controlled trial. JAMA 299:637–645
15. Mercat A, Richard JC, Vielle B, Jaber S, Osman D, Diehl JL, Lefrant JY, Prat G, Richecoeur J, Nieszkowska A, Gervais C, Baudot J, Bouadma L, Brochard L (2008) Positive end-expiratory pressure setting in adults with acute lung injury and acute respiratory distress syndrome: a randomized controlled trial. JAMA 299:646–655
16. Brower RG, Lanken PN, MacIntyre N, Matthay MA, Morris A, Ancukiewicz M, Schoenfeld D, Thompson BT (2004) Higher versus lower positive end-expiratory pressures in patients with the acute respiratory distress syndrome. N Engl J Med 351:327–336
17. Briel M, Meade M, Mercat A, Brower RG, Talmor D, Walter SD, Slutsky AS, Pullenayegum E, Zhou Q, Cook D, Brochard L, Richard JC, Lamontagne F, Bhatnagar N, Stewart TE, Guyatt G (2010) Higher vs lower positive end-expiratory pressure in patients with acute lung injury and acute respiratory distress syndrome: systematic review and meta-analysis. JAMA 303:865–873
18. Ferguson ND, Kacmarek RM, Chiche JD, Singh JM, Hallett DC, Mehta S, Stewart TE (2004) Screening of ARDS patients using standardized ventilator settings: influence on enrollment in a clinical trial. Intensive Care Med 30:1111–1116
19. Villar J, Perez-Mendez L, Blanco J, Anon JM, Blanch L, Belda J, Santos-Bouza A, Fernandez RL, Kacmarek RM, Spanish Initiative for Epidemiology S, Therapies for AN (2013) A universal definition of ARDS: the PaO_2/FiO_2 ratio under a standard ventilatory setting--a prospective, multicenter validation study. Intensive Care Med 39:583–592
20. Villar J, Perez-Mendez L, Lopez J, Belda J, Blanco J, Saralegui I, Suarez-Sipmann F, Lubillo S, Kacmarek RM (2007) An early PEEP/FiO_2 trial identifies different degrees of lung injury in patients with acute respiratory distress syndrome. Am J Respir Crit Care Med 176:795–804
21. Aboab J, Louis B, Jonson B, Brochard L (2006) Relation between PaO_2/FiO_2 ratio and FiO_2: a mathematical description. Intensive Care Med 32:1494–1497
22. Britos M, Smoot E, Liu KD, Thompson BT, Checkley W, Brower RG (2011) The value of positive end-expiratory pressure and Fio(2) criteria in the definition of the acute respiratory distress syndrome. Crit Care Med 39:2025–2030
23. Guerin C, Reignier J, Richard JC, Beuret P, Gacouin A, Boulain T, Mercier E, Badet M, Mercat A, Baudin O, Clavel M, Chatellier D, Jaber S, Rosselli S, Mancebo J, Sirodot M, Hilbert G, Bengler C, Richecoeur J, Gainnier M, Bayle F, Bourdin G, Leray V, Girard R, Baboi L, Ayzac L (2013) Prone positioning in severe acute respiratory distress syndrome. N Engl J Med 368:2159–2168
24. Katzenstein AL, Bloor CM, Leibow AA (1976) Diffuse alveolar damage--the role of oxygen, shock, and related factors. A review. Am J Pathol 85:209–228
25. Tomashefski JF Jr (2000) Pulmonary pathology of acute respiratory distress syndrome. Clin Chest Med 21:435–466

26. Suchyta MR, Elliott CG, Colby T, Rasmusson BY, Morris AH, Jensen RL (1991) Open lung biopsy does not correlate with pulmonary function after the adult respiratory distress syndrome. Chest 99:1232–1237
27. Warner DO, Warner MA, Divertie MB (1988) Open lung biopsy in patients with diffuse pulmonary infiltrates and acute respiratory failure. Am Rev Respir Dis 137:90–94
28. Papazian L, Thomas P, Bregeon F, Garbe L, Zandotti C, Saux P, Gaillat F, Drancourt M, Auffray JP, Gouin F (1998) Open-lung biopsy in patients with acute respiratory distress syndrome. Anesthesiology 88:935–944
29. Patel SR, Karmpaliotis D, Ayas NT, Mark EJ, Wain J, Thompson BT, Malhotra A (2004) The role of open-lung biopsy in ARDS. Chest 125:197–202
30. Esteban A, Fernandez-Segoviano P, Frutos-Vivar F, Aramburu JA, Najera L, Ferguson ND, Alia I, Gordo F, Rios F (2004) Comparison of clinical criteria for the acute respiratory distress syndrome with autopsy findings. Ann Intern Med 141:440–445
31. Cho MH, Malhotra A, Donahue DM, Wain JC, Harris RS, Karmpaliotis D, Patel SR (2006) Mechanical ventilation and air leaks after lung biopsy for acute respiratory distress syndrome. Ann Thorac Surg 82:261–266
32. Kao KC, Tsai YH, Wu YK, Chen NH, Hsieh MJ, Huang SF, Huang CC (2006) Open lung biopsy in early-stage acute respiratory distress syndrome. Crit Care 10:R106
33. Lim SY, Suh GY, Choi JC, Koh WJ, Lim SY, Han J, Lee KS, Shim YM, Chung MP, Kim H, Kwon OJ (2007) Usefulness of open lung biopsy in mechanically ventilated patients with undiagnosed diffuse pulmonary infiltrates: influence of comorbidities and organ dysfunction. Crit Care 11:R93
34. Arabi Y, Ahmed R, Ahmed Q, Rahman MU, Yamani N (2007) Risks and benefits of open-lung biopsy in the mechanically ventilated critically ill population: a cohort study and literature review. Med Sci Monit 13:CR365–CR371
35. Papazian L, Doddoli C, Chetaille B, Gernez Y, Thirion X, Roch A, Donati Y, Bonnety M, Zandotti C, Thomas P (2007) A contributive result of open-lung biopsy improves survival in acute respiratory distress syndrome patients. Crit Care Med 35:755–762
36. Baumann HJ, Kluge S, Balke L, Yekebas E, Izbicki JR, Amthor M, Kreymann G, Meyer A (2008) Yield and safety of bedside open lung biopsy in mechanically ventilated patients with acute lung injury or acute respiratory distress syndrome. Surgery 143:426–433
37. Lin CY, Kao KC, Tian YC, Jenq CC, Chang MY, Chen YC, Fang JT, Huang CC, Tsai YH, Yang CW (2009) The RIFLE score increases the accuracy of outcome prediction in patients with acute respiratory distress syndrome undergoing open lung biopsy. Respiration 77:398–406
38. de Hemptinne Q, Remmelink M, Brimioulle S, Salmon I, Vincent JL (2009) ARDS: a clinicopathological confrontation. Chest 135:944–949
39. Charbonney E, Robert J, Pache JC, Chevrolet JC, Eggimann P (2009) Impact of bedside open lung biopsies on the management of mechanically ventilated immunocompromised patients with acute respiratory distress syndrome of unknown etiology. J Crit Care 24:122–128
40. Melo N, Figueiredo S, Morais A, Souto Moura C, Pinho P, Bastos P, Oliveira T (2009) Open lung biopsy in patients on mechanical ventilation with suspected diffuse lung disease. Rev Port Pneumol 15:597–611
41. Sarmiento X, Guardiola JJ, Almirall J, Mesalles E, Mate JL, Soler M, Klamburg J (2011) Discrepancy between clinical criteria for diagnosing acute respiratory distress syndrome secondary to community acquired pneumonia with autopsy findings of diffuse alveolar damage. Respir Med 105:1170–1175
42. Thille AW, Esteban A, Fernandez-Segoviano P, Rodriguez JM, Aramburu JA, Penuelas O, Cortes-Puch I, Cardinal-Fernandez P, Lorente JA, Frutos-Vivar F (2013) Comparison of the Berlin definition for acute respiratory distress syndrome with autopsy. Am J Respir Crit Care Med 187:761–767
43. Guerin C, Bayle F, Leray V, Debord S, Stoian A, Yonis H, Roudaut JB, Bourdin G, Devouassoux-Shisheboran M, Bucher E, Ayzac L, Lantuejoul S, Philipponnet C, Kemeny JL, Souweine B, Richard JC (2015) Open lung biopsy in nonresolving ARDS frequently identifies diffuse alve-

olar damage regardless of the severity stage and may have implications for patient management. Intensive Care Med 41:222–230
44. Kao KC, Hu HC, Chang CH, Hung CY, Chiu LC, Li SH, Lin SW, Chuang LP, Wang CW, Li LF, Chen NH, Yang CT, Huang CC, Tsai YH (2015) Diffuse alveolar damage associated mortality in selected acute respiratory distress syndrome patients with open lung biopsy. Crit Care 19:228
45. Gibelin A, Parrot A, Maitre B, Brun-Buisson C, Mekontso Dessap A, Fartoukh M, de Prost N (2016) Acute respiratory distress syndrome mimickers lacking common risk factors of the Berlin definition. Intensive Care Med 42:164–172
46. Cardinal-Fernandez P, Bajwa EK, Dominguez-Calvo A, Menendez JM, Papazian L, Thompson BT (2016) The presence of diffuse alveolar damage on open lung biopsy is associated with mortality in patients with acute respiratory distress syndrome: a systematic review and meta-analysis. Chest 149(5):1155–1164.
47. Bersten AD, Edibam C, Hunt T, Moran J, Australian, New Zealand Intensive Care Society Clinical Trials G (2002) Incidence and mortality of acute lung injury and the acute respiratory distress syndrome in three Australian States. Am J Respir Crit Care Med 165:443–448
48. Brun-Buisson C, Minelli C, Bertolini G, Brazzi L, Pimentel J, Lewandowski K, Bion J, Romand JA, Villar J, Thorsteinsson A, Damas P, Armaganidis A, Lemaire F (2004) Epidemiology and outcome of acute lung injury in European intensive care units. Results from the ALIVE study. Intensive Care Med 30:51–61
49. Rubenfeld GD, Caldwell E, Peabody E, Weaver J, Martin DP, Neff M, Stern EJ, Hudson LD (2005) Incidence and outcomes of acute lung injury. N Engl J Med 353:1685–1693
50. Bellani G, Laffey JG, Pham T, Fan E, Brochard L, Esteban A, Gattinoni L, van Haren F, Larsson A, McAuley DF, Ranieri M, Rubenfeld G, Thompson BT, Wrigge H, Slutsky AS, Pesenti A (2016) Epidemiology, patterns of care, and mortality for patients with acute respiratory distress syndrome in intensive care units in 50 countries. JAMA 315:788–800
51. Phua J, Badia JR, Adhikari NK, Friedrich JO, Fowler RA, Singh JM, Scales DC, Stather DR, Li A, Jones A, Gattas DJ, Hallett D, Tomlinson G, Stewart TE, Ferguson ND (2009) Has mortality from acute respiratory distress syndrome decreased over time?: a systematic review. Am J Respir Crit Care Med 179:220–227
52. Amato MB, Barbas CS, Medeiros DM, Magaldi RB, Schettino GP, Lorenzi-Filho G, Kairalla RA, Deheinzelin D, Munoz C, Oliveira R, Takagaki TY, Carvalho CR (1998) Effect of a protective-ventilation strategy on mortality in the acute respiratory distress syndrome. N Engl J Med 338:347–354
53. Ventilation with lower tidal volumes as compared with traditional tidal volumes for acute lung injury and the acute respiratory distress syndrome. The Acute Respiratory Distress Syndrome Network (2000) N Engl J Med 342:1301–1308
54. Papazian L, Forel JM, Gacouin A, Penot-Ragon C, Perrin G, Loundou A, Jaber S, Arnal JM, Perez D, Seghboyan JM, Constantin JM, Courant P, Lefrant JY, Guerin C, Prat G, Morange S, Roch A, Investigators AS (2010) Neuromuscular blockers in early acute respiratory distress syndrome. N Engl J Med 363:1107–1116
55. Villar J, Blanco J, Kacmarek RM (2016) Current incidence and outcome of the acute respiratory distress syndrome. Curr Opin Crit Care 22:1–6
56. Arabi YM, Cook DJ, Zhou Q, Smith O, Hand L, Turgeon AF, Matte A, Mehta S, Graham R, Brierley K, Adhikari NK, Meade MO, Ferguson ND, Canadian Critical Care Trials G (2015) Characteristics and outcomes of eligible nonenrolled patients in a mechanical ventilation trial of acute respiratory distress syndrome. Am J Respir Crit Care Med 192:1306–1313
57. Montgomery AB, Stager MA, Carrico CJ, Hudson LD (1985) Causes of mortality in patients with the adult respiratory distress syndrome. Am Rev Respir Dis 132:485–489
58. Stapleton RD, Wang BM, Hudson LD, Rubenfeld GD, Caldwell ES, Steinberg KP (2005) Causes and timing of death in patients with ARDS. Chest 128:525–532
59. Mehter HM, Wiener RS, Walkey AJ (2014) "Do not resuscitate" decisions in acute respiratory distress syndrome. A secondary analysis of clinical trial data. Ann Am Thorac Soc 11:1592–1596

60. Eisner MD, Thompson T, Hudson LD, Luce JM, Hayden D, Schoenfeld D, Matthay MA (2001) Efficacy of low tidal volume ventilation in patients with different clinical risk factors for acute lung injury and the acute respiratory distress syndrome. Am J Respir Crit Care Med 164:231–236
61. Calfee CS, Delucchi K, Parsons PE, Thompson BT, Ware LB, Matthay MA (2014) Subphenotypes in acute respiratory distress syndrome: latent class analysis of data from two randomised controlled trials. Lancet Respir Med 2:611–620
62. Thille AW, Esteban A, Fernandez-Segoviano P, Rodriguez JM, Aramburu JA, Vargas-Errazuriz P, Martin-Pellicer A, Lorente JA, Frutos-Vivar F (2013) Chronology of histological lesions in acute respiratory distress syndrome with diffuse alveolar damage: a prospective cohort study of clinical autopsies. Lancet Respir Med 1:395–401
63. Matamis D, Lemaire F, Harf A, Brun-Buisson C, Ansquer JC, Atlan G (1984) Total respiratory pressure-volume curves in the adult respiratory distress syndrome. Chest 86:58–66
64. Burnham EL, Janssen WJ, Riches DW, Moss M, Downey GP (2014) The fibroproliferative response in acute respiratory distress syndrome: mechanisms and clinical significance. Eur Respir J 43:276–285
65. Burnham EL, Hyzy RC, Paine R 3rd, Coley C 2nd, Kelly AM, Quint LE, Lynch D, Janssen WJ, Moss M, Standiford TJ (2013) Chest CT features are associated with poorer quality of life in acute lung injury survivors. Crit Care Med 41:445–456
66. Herridge MS, Cheung AM, Tansey CM, Matte-Martyn A, Diaz-Granados N, Al-Saidi F, Cooper AB, Guest CB, Mazer CD, Mehta S, Stewart TE, Barr A, Cook D, Slutsky AS (2003) One-year outcomes in survivors of the acute respiratory distress syndrome. N Engl J Med 348:683–693
67. Herridge MS, Tansey CM, Matte A, Tomlinson G, Diaz-Granados N, Cooper A, Guest CB, Mazer CD, Mehta S, Stewart TE, Kudlow P, Cook D, Slutsky AS, Cheung AM (2011) Functional disability 5 years after acute respiratory distress syndrome. N Engl J Med 364:1293–1304
68. Fan E, Dowdy DW, Colantuoni E, Mendez-Tellez PA, Sevransky JE, Shanholtz C, Himmelfarb CR, Desai SV, Ciesla N, Herridge MS, Pronovost PJ, Needham DM (2014) Physical complications in acute lung injury survivors: a two-year longitudinal prospective study. Crit Care Med 42:849–859
69. Bienvenu OJ, Colantuoni E, Mendez-Tellez PA, Shanholtz C, Dennison-Himmelfarb CR, Pronovost PJ, Needham DM (2015) Cooccurrence of and remission from general anxiety, depression, and posttraumatic stress disorder symptoms after acute lung injury: a 2-year longitudinal study. Crit Care Med 43:642–653
70. Huang M, Parker AM, Bienvenu OJ, Dinglas VD, Colantuoni E, Hopkins RO, Needham DM (2016) Psychiatric symptoms in acute respiratory distress syndrome survivors: a 1-year national multicenter study. Crit Care Med 44(5):954–965
71. Dowdy DW, Eid MP, Dennison CR, Mendez-Tellez PA, Herridge MS, Guallar E, Pronovost PJ, Needham DM (2006) Quality of life after acute respiratory distress syndrome: a meta-analysis. Intensive Care Med 32:1115–1124
72. Davidson TA, Caldwell ES, Curtis JR, Hudson LD, Steinberg KP (1999) Reduced quality of life in survivors of acute respiratory distress syndrome compared with critically ill control patients. JAMA 281:354–360
73. Biehl M, Kashyap R, Ahmed AH, Reriani MK, Ofoma UR, Wilson GA, Li G, Malinchoc M, Sloan JA, Gajic O (2015) Six-month quality-of-life and functional status of acute respiratory distress syndrome survivors compared to patients at risk: a population-based study. Crit Care 19:356

Pathophysiology of Acute Respiratory Distress Syndrome

2

Pedro Leme Silva and Patricia R.M. Rocco

2.1 Introduction

The acute respiratory distress syndrome (ARDS) is a form of hypoxemic respiratory failure characterized by severe inflammatory damage to the alveolar–capillary barrier. This damage can be triggered by primary injury to the epithelium (pulmonary ARDS), as in cases of pneumonia or bronchial aspiration, or to the endothelium (extrapulmonary ARDS), as in cases of nonpulmonary sepsis [37, 51, 54]. Recently, evidence has emerged showing differences in molecular phenotypes between these two etiologies [8]. In addition, patients who develop ARDS after trauma (trauma-associated lung injury) may exhibit distinct clinical features and biomarker profiles compared to other forms of ARDS [7]. Not only the distinction in severity among ARDS patients seems important, but also discrimination among different ARDS phenotypes and etiologies, i.e., whether associated to trauma, transfusion, cancer, and septic events. Novel therapies targeted specifically at these entities may benefit from this separation by pathophysiology.

2.2 Pathophysiology of Acute Respiratory Distress Syndrome: The Actors

The innate immune response plays a profound role in the pathophysiology of ARDS. Multiple immune processes involving macrophages, neutrophils, and epithelial and endothelial cells are implicated in mediating tissue injury.

P.L. Silva • P.R.M. Rocco, MD, PhD (✉)
Laboratory of Pulmonary Investigation, Carlos Chagas Filho Biophysics Institute, Federal University of Rio de Janeiro, Avenida Carlos Chagas Filho,
373, Bloco G1-014, Ilha do Fundão, 21941-902 Rio de Janeiro, Brazil
e-mail: prmrocco@gmail.com

D. Chiumello (ed.), *Acute Respiratory Distress Syndrome (ARDS)*,
DOI 10.1007/978-3-319-41852-0_2

2.2.1 Alveolar Macrophages

Alveolar macrophages form the first line of defense against airborne particles and microorganisms and use a variety of pattern recognition mechanisms and receptors to sense and phagocytose pathogens [2]. During lung inflammation, two main states of differentiation exist, characterized by classically activated macrophages (CAMs) and alternatively activated macrophages (AAMs). CAMs display the M1 macrophage phenotype and produce high levels of proinflammatory cytokines, such as interleukin (IL)-1β, tumor necrosis factor (TNF)-α, IL-12, and inducible nitric oxide synthase (iNOS), in response to paracrine signaling from the T helper 1 (Th1) cytokine interferon (IFN)-γ and in response to autocrine signaling by IFN-β [28, 62]. AAMs display the M2 macrophage phenotype and produce the anti-inflammatory cytokines IL-10 and IL-1Ra in response to signaling from the Th2 cytokines IL-4 and IL-13. Most studies on detection of macrophage phenotype have been experimental, and, although few studies have been conducted in humans, these investigations are noteworthy. In a comparison of bronchoalveolar lavage fluid (BALF) from patients with ARDS and cardiogenic pulmonary edema, both under mechanical ventilation, and from nonventilated healthy volunteers, Rosseau et al. showed that alveolar macrophages from ARDS patients skewed toward classically activated macrophages, i.e., the M1 phenotype. Persistence of the M1 phenotype is associated with worse outcomes [52]. After exposure of healthy human subjects to intratracheal LPS, an increase was observed in total alveolar macrophages, mainly constituted of pulmonary monocyte-like cells. These cells were recruited to the alveolar space and were $CD16^-$, different from nonresident $CD16^+$ monocytes [71].

2.2.2 Neutrophils

Neutrophils are the first leukocytes to be recruited to sites of inflammation in response to chemotactic factors released by activated macrophages and pulmonary epithelial and endothelial cells [67]. It has been reported that the concentration of neutrophils in the BALF of patients with ARDS correlates with disease severity and with poor outcome [33]. It has been postulated that neutrophils are involved in endothelial–epithelial barrier disruption [16]. On the other hand, neutropenic patients can develop ARDS in the absence of invading neutrophils [44]. This illustrates the heterogeneity of ARDS, since it may involve neutrophil-dependent and neutrophil-independent processes. The chemokine IL-8, also known as CXCL8, is thought to be central to neutrophil recruitment into the lung during ARDS [68]. Important correlations have been drawn from clinical ARDS samples, including pulmonary edema aspirates and BALF, between increased IL-8 concentrations, disease severity [38], and neutrophil migration into airspaces [39]. IL-8 is considered to be the most potent neutrophil chemoattractant in BALF from ARDS patients and is the predominant neutrophilic chemokine released from LPS-stimulated human alveolar macrophages [26]. Not only isolated IL-8 but also its complexes are associated with ARDS pathophysiology. The IL-8 immune complexes are characterized by IL-8 binding to endogenous immunoglobulin G (IgG), mainly the IgG3 and

IgG4 subclasses. Elevated levels of IL-8 immune complexes have been associated with poor clinical outcome in patients with ARDS and in those at risk of developing ARDS [27]. One possible mechanism could be the decrease in neutrophil apoptosis rate, which is associated with an increase in expression of Bcl-xL and a decrease in Bak and Bax [17]. In this line, it is well established that neutrophil apoptosis is delayed in patients with ARDS [29], which may explain the perpetuation of tissue injury by the release of neutrophil products, namely, proteinase-3, cathepsin-G, and several matrix metalloproteinases (MMPs). Another mechanism of neutrophil action is the release of neutrophil extracellular traps (NETs), in a process of cell death known as NETosis [5]. NET formation involves disintegration of the nuclear membrane, chromatin condensation, and release of DNA and granule proteins into the extracellular space [6]. Although NETs have potent antimicrobial properties, they contain histones, enzymes, and peptides that are directly toxic to host cells. NETs have also been observed in sterile transfusion-related acute lung injury (TRALI) in human patients [60], and protection against TRALI has been observed to follow inhibition of extracellular histones [9]. Therefore, in a scenario of uncontrolled NET formation, their inhibition could be an attractive strategy.

2.2.3 Alveolar Epithelium

After a direct insult, the pulmonary epithelium is the primary injured structure. Epithelial damage leads to alveolar flooding [65], reduced removal of edema fluid from the alveolar space [40], decreased production and turnover of surfactant [21], and fibrosis [4]. A recent study with two distinct patient cohorts [8] found that pulmonary ARDS is characterized by more severe lung epithelial injury compared with indirect ARDS and, conversely, that indirect ARDS is characterized by more severe endothelial injury and inflammation. Among the wide range of plasma biomarkers analyzed (surfactant protein [SP]-D, IL-6, IL-8, angiopoietin [Angpt]-2, receptor of advanced glycation end products [RAGE], and von Willebrand factor [vWF]) and their respective prognostic values, the SP-D was the most reliable molecular indicator of the direct lung injury phenotype. SP-D, produced by type II epithelial and club cells, is a large hydrophilic protein that interacts with glycoconjugates and lipids through the carbohydrate recognition domain (CRD) on the surface of microorganisms, including Gram-positive and Gram-negative bacteria [22]. It can cause agglutination of bacteria, hindering their entry into host cells and dissemination, and may lead to bacterial death through permeabilization of the bacterial cell wall, increasing respiratory burst by macrophages and neutrophils and enhancing opsonization by phagocytic cells [25].

2.2.4 Alveolar Endothelium

The vascular endothelium is the first barrier encountered by fluid or inflammatory cells tracking from the vasculature to the alveoli. Endothelial barrier function is an essential and tightly regulated process that ensures proper compartmentalization of the vascular and interstitial spaces while allowing for the diffusive exchange of small molecules and controlled trafficking of macromolecules and immune cells [36]. Failure of endothelial barrier integrity results in excessive leakage of fluid and proteins from the vasculature into the airspace. The loss of barrier integrity can be a consequence of neutrophil activity, in which they accumulate in the microcirculation of the lung, become activated, and subsequently degranulate and release several toxic mediators, including reactive oxygen species (ROS), proteases, proinflammatory cytokines, and procoagulant molecules. Injury done by neutrophils and their intracellular products may increase vascular permeability by altering focal adhesions, transmembrane integrins, and the cytoskeleton of endothelial cells. Further inflammatory mediators, despite neutrophils, can act directly on the lung capillaries, resulting in increased expression of chemokines and cell surface molecules that are important for leukocyte adhesion [35, 49]. Furthermore, injury to the endothelial barrier may be mediated by bacterial or viral products, independently of the effects of activated leukocytes. For example, toxins produced by *Pseudomonas aeruginosa* and *Staphylococcus aureus* break down the endothelial barrier as well as the epithelial barrier [12, 66]. Not only NF-κB pathway inflammatory mediators but also specific transmembrane tyrosine kinases from endothelial cells (Tie-2) play an important role in ARDS pathophysiology. Their ligands Angpt-1 and Angpt-2, with nanomolar affinity, can have opposing effects on endothelial cell function. Angpt-1 is largely synthesized and secreted by periendothelial cells and platelets, whereas Angpt-2 is synthesized in the endothelium, where preformed protein is stored for rapid release in granules called Weibel–Palade bodies [15]. The N-terminal region of Angpt-1 may even promote local adherence to the extracellular matrix [61], leading to a high tissue concentration despite low circulating levels. In sepsis, ARDS, and related conditions, circulating Angpt-1 appears to be suppressed [48]. In addition, the magnitude of Angpt-1 decline tends to be two- to threefold or less, compared with the 5- to 20-fold increase in circulating Angpt-2 observed in sepsis or ARDS. Circulating Angpt-2 concentrations have a much broader dynamic range than Angpt-1. In 2006, Parikh et al. reported 10- to 20-fold elevations of circulating Angpt-2 levels in individuals with severe sepsis at the time of ICU admission as compared with patients with uncomplicated sepsis and hospitalized healthy subjects. The authors noted that subjects with severe sepsis developed higher peak Angpt-2 concentrations than those with uncomplicated sepsis and further observed that individuals with impaired lung gas exchange had higher peak Angpt-2 values than those with normal gas exchange [69]. In single-center and multicenter cohort studies, Angpt-2 was a robust indicator of extrapulmonary ARDS [8]. The induction of Angpt-2 clearly precedes adverse outcomes, a point strongly illustrated in an emergency department-based study of 270 adults with suspected infection in whom circulating Angpt-2 measured within the first hour of hospitalization predicted inpatient mortality, with an area under the receiver operator characteristic (ROC) curve of 0.91 [10]. On comparison of several relevant biomarkers, Angpt-2 was the only one capable of predicting the severity, monitoring the course, and prognosticating the outcome of late-onset ARDS in febrile critically ill patients, irrespective of underlying risk factor [23].

2.3 Pulmonary Versus Extrapulmonary ARDS: The Myth Is a Fact

ARDS was long thought to be a uniform expression of a diffuse, overwhelming inflammatory reaction of the pulmonary parenchyma to a variety of serious underlying diseases. The most frequent causes include sepsis, severe pneumonia, peritonitis, and polytrauma. Since 1999, Gattinoni et al. have highlighted the differential responses of respiratory mechanics in ARDS of pulmonary versus extrapulmonary origin [18]. This could be associated with different underlying pathologies resulting from two different pathogenic pathways: a "direct" insult to the lung parenchyma in ARDS caused by pulmonary diseases, such as diffuse pneumonia, versus an "indirect" insult to the lung parenchyma in ARDS caused by extrapulmonary diseases, such as abdominal sepsis or pancreatitis [45]. One explanation for the differences gathered from this landmark study was that prevalent consolidation is expected in "direct" injury-type ARDS, whereas prevalent interstitial edema and alveolar collapse are seen in "indirect" injury-type ARDS [37, 51, 54]. Sixteen years on, Calfee et al. demonstrated that pulmonary ARDS is characterized by more severe lung epithelial injury compared with extrapulmonary ARDS, while extrapulmonary ARDS is characterized by more severe endothelial injury and inflammation [8]. With few exceptions, these findings were robust to adjustment for differences in severity of illness and of lung injury. These distinct molecular phenotypes of pulmonary versus extrapulmonary lung injury provide strong evidence that the heterogeneity in ARDS pathogenesis observed in experimental models [37] is relevant to human ARDS, a finding that may have important implications for clinical trials of novel therapies. As well as molecular phenotypes, pulmonary permeability also seems to differ between pulmonary and extrapulmonary ARDS. In analyses with the transpulmonary thermodilution method, patients with pulmonary ARDS exhibited a higher pulmonary vascular permeability index compared with extrapulmonary ARDS patients for the first 3 consecutive days of intensive care unit stay [42]. On the other hand, the extravascular lung water index differed only at day 3 (extrapulmonary ARDS, 14.9 ± 6.0; pulmonary ARDS, 17.6 ± 7.8, $p = 0.02$). Although this study had few patients, unbalanced allocation, and SOFA score at baseline measurements, the transpulmonary thermodilution method was able to distinguish between the ARDS etiologies through assessment of pulmonary permeability. In short, there appear to be clear differences in pathophysiology, morphological aspects, respiratory mechanics, and hemodynamic parameters between pulmonary and extrapulmonary ARDS in humans.

2.4 ARDS Phenotypes

The establishment of clear definitions of ARDS has led to significant advances in the standardization of populations in research studies; however, a number of studies have shown significant heterogeneity within the population of patients meeting consensus criteria for ARDS [13, 63]. Heterogeneity has been described on the basis of

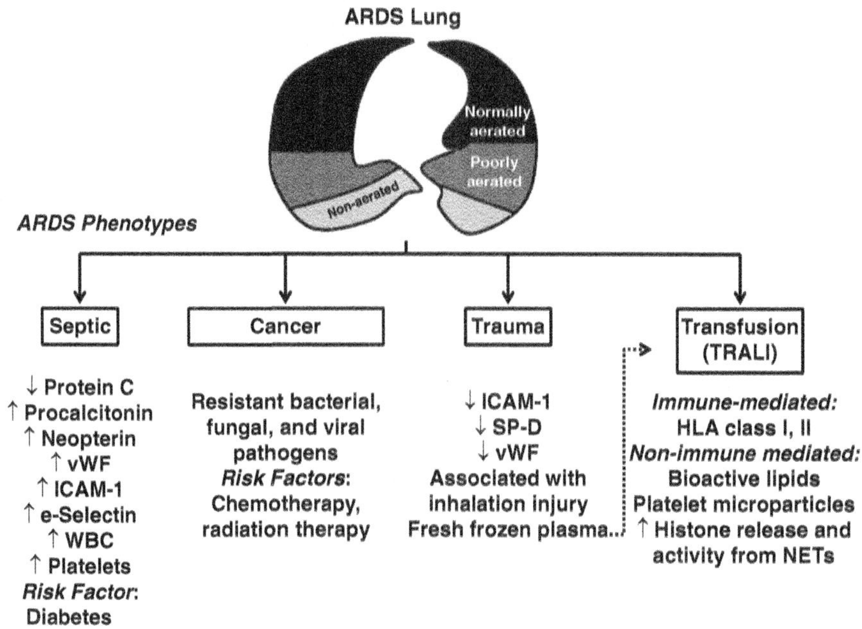

Fig. 2.1 Acute respiratory distress syndrome phenotypes related to sepsis, cancer, trauma, and transfusion. *HLA* human leukocyte antigen, *ICAM-1* intercellular adhesion molecule 1, *NET* neutrophil extracellular traps, *SP-D* surfactant protein D, *TRALI* transfusion-related acute lung injury, *vWF* von Willebrand factor, *WBC* white blood cell

predisposing insult, such as sepsis, cancer, transfusion, and trauma, or by mechanism of injury, such as direct or indirect pulmonary injury [7]. One recent example corroborating the distinction in ARDS phenotypes relates to the presence or absence of diffuse alveolar damage (DAD) on postmortem analysis. Lorente et al. [31] showed that non-survivors of ARDS have different clinical characteristics depending on the underlying histology. Patients with ARDS and DAD at postmortem had a different clinical phenotype than patients with ARDS and other histologic findings without DAD. These findings support the concept that the presence of DAD defines a specific subphenotype within patients with the clinical diagnosis of ARDS. How to detect this or other phenotypes at bedside remains unclear. Figure 2.1 provides an overview of the most common ARDS phenotypes, including expected biomarker levels, likely risk factors, and association with specific injuries.

2.4.1 Septic and Cancer Phenotypes

Studies measuring circulating biomarkers in patients with ARDS showed that protein C levels were lower in patients with sepsis-related ARDS than in those with non-sepsis-related ARDS, whereas procalcitonin, neopterin, von Willebrand factor antigen, soluble intercellular adhesion molecule 1, and soluble E-selectin levels were higher [34]. Among these biomarkers, the levels of IL-6, IL-8, and IL-10 are higher in sepsis-related ARDS, which suggests a higher degree of acute inflammation, endothelial cell activity, and coagulation activation. Sheu et al. [55] found that sepsis-related ARDS is associated with greater overall disease severity, poorer recovery from lung injury, lower successful extubation rate, and higher mortality than non-sepsis-related ARDS. Worse clinical outcomes in sepsis-related ARDS appear to be driven by disease severity and comorbidities. Among the latter, liver cirrhosis was strongly associated with death in ARDS scenarios. In a multivariate Cox regression analysis, the authors showed metastatic cancers as independent predictors of ARDS mortality. Patients with underlying cancer who developed ARDS had a significantly higher risk of 28-day mortality compared to those without cancer, mainly because of the severity of illness at presentation and older age of those with cancer [58]. Likely explanations for this result include severe infectious conditions, such as resistant bacterial, fungal, and viral infections; use of chemotherapeutic agents and radiation exposure; and the delay in ARDS diagnosis. In this study, the delay between onset of respiratory symptoms and ICU admission exceeded 2 days, and this independently contributed to higher 28-day mortality [41].

2.4.2 Trauma and Transfusion Phenotypes

It has been shown that patients with trauma-associated ARDS have markedly different clinical characteristics than patients with other clinical etiologies of ARDS [7]. These differences were associated with lower plasma levels of several biomarkers previously found to be associated with poor clinical outcomes in ARDS, including ICAM-1, SP-D, sTNFr-1, and vWF. Although one previous study [3] focused solely on the prevalence of ARDS based on the Berlin definition among military burn victims, the authors provide important information about the ARDS phenotype. Regardless of trauma, patients were discriminated into mild, moderate, and severe ARDS groups, with mortality rates of 11.1%, 36.1%, and 43.8%, respectively. The following variables were independently associated with moderate or severe ARDS in this population: inhalation injury, injury severity score, pneumonia, and use of fresh frozen plasma. In fact, previous studies have shown a strong link between administration of fresh frozen plasma and development of ARDS in severely injured patients [24, 64]. Transfusion-related acute lung injury (TRALI) could be implicated. Classically, TRALI has been associated with immune-mediated and non-immune-mediated events. The former is caused by human leukocyte antigen (HLA) class I and II and/or less frequent antibodies directed against specific granulocyte antigens, human neutrophil antigen (HNA), which can be present in the serum of the recipient or donor and thus react with donor or recipient leukocytes, respectively [43]. The non-immune-mediated events can be attributed to transfusion of biologically active compounds which accumulate in stored blood components, such as bioactive lipids, proinflammatory cytokines, or platelet microparticles with high procoagulant activity [59]. One further mechanism could be the release of proinflammatory mitochondrial damage-associated molecular patterns (DAMPs), including mitochondrial deoxyribonucleic acid (mtDNA) fragments and mtDNA-associated proteins [30]. Clinically, hemodynamic monitoring helps distinguish TRALI from cardiogenic pulmonary edema. Normal or low pulmonary capillary wedge pressure and central venous pressure values are characteristic of TRALI [56]. Hemodynamic monitoring is needed to exclude other causes of TRALI, because its symptoms are similar to those of other conditions, including anaphylactic reaction, cardiogenic pulmonary edema, ARDS, and bacterial infection. Occasionally, leukopenia, neutropenia, hypoalbuminemia, and hypocomplementemia can be detected. The most prevalent symptom is a transient leukopenia, which arises in 5–35% of patients [14].

The lungs tend to be more frequently affected than any other organ in patients who die of clinical shock or after trauma, a phenomenon associated with neutrophil infiltration, pulmonary edema, hemorrhage, and microvascular thrombosis [32]. The fundamental pathogenic events related to trauma remain incompletely characterized. Studies have shown that nuclear proteins, such as high mobility group box-1 (HMGB-1) [46], and histones [1] are elevated after trauma events related to ARDS scenarios. Histones in particular have demonstrated ability to mediate remote organ damage, particularly in the lungs, and contribute to multiple organ failure. One possible mechanism could be that extracellular histones bind phospholipids, disrupt cell membranes, and cause calcium influx. This indiscriminate activity on all cells tested resulted in sustained elevation of $[Ca^{+2}]i$, causing cell damage and release of cellular stores and content. Furthermore, the increase in histone levels could be associated with NET formation and may become a novel marker reflecting disease activity. In fact, the predominant source of histones in ARDS may be neutrophils that have been activated by C5a to form NETs, which seems to be an ongoing process toward inflammation perpetuation [20]. Extracellular histones are highly proinflammatory and have been shown to cause severe damage to respiratory function. Intratracheal instillation of histones resulted in proinflammatory mediator production, epithelial cell damage, disturbances in alveolar–capillary gas exchange, lung consolidation, and activation of the coagulation cascade [20]. Targeting histones with neutralizing antibody or heparin shows potent protective effects, suggesting a therapeutic strategy [70].

Within trauma populations, different patterns of ARDS onset with distinct ARDS risk factors have been empirically described and may involve different pathogenesis pathways [11]. By using latent class analysis (LCA), a statistical method used to identify unobserved (latent) patterns underlying the observed heterogeneity in a population, one study identified three subgroups of ARDS based on timing of onset and certainty of diagnosis in a cohort of critically ill trauma patients [47]. The model identified a cutoff point of approximately 48 h after presentation separating the early- and late-onset subgroups of ARDS. Early-onset ARDS was associated with increased severity of thoracic trauma, more severe early hypertension, and increased red blood cell transfusion during the initial resuscitation when compared with the later-onset subgroup. In addition, the biomarkers sRAGE and Angpt-2 were significantly higher in the serum of patients with early-onset ARDS, while all other biomarkers, including markers of systemic inflammation, were similar between the two classes of ARDS, suggesting distinct molecular profiles in the early post-trauma period.

2.5 Future Perspectives for Translation of Experimental Models into Therapy

Some pharmacologic treatments proposed or under evaluation for ARDS seek to protect the endothelial cells, thus mitigating fluid extravasation into the alveolar space [35]. These researches are based on physiological foundations but it has not translated to the clinical setting [53]. A recent paper [19, 57] evaluated a new compound, FG-4497, a prolyl hydroxylase domain 2 (PHD2) inhibitor, which has been shown to activate hypoxia-inducible factor-2α (HIF-2α)-mediated transcription in a hypoxia-independent manner in a model of endotoxin-induced ARDS. Once activated, HIF-2α increases the expression of vascular endothelial protein tyrosine phosphatase (VE-PTP), which, in turn, can decrease VE-cadherin phosphorylation, supporting the integrity of adherens junctions (AJs) and preventing loss of endothelial barrier function. FG-4497 may herald a new pharmacologic strategy for ARDS. Also regarding pharmacologic treatment, one recent paper [50] showed that the FDA-approved tyrosine kinase inhibitor imatinib attenuated the inflammation and vascular leak induced by lipopolysaccharide when combined with ventilator-induced lung injury (VILI) and that these protective effects outweigh the deleterious effects of this intervention previously reported in VILI alone. As well as decreasing inflammation, imatinib may act on several vascular leak models, as it inhibits c-Abl, one component of the family of kinases that are critical mediators of vascular function with both protective and disruptive effects.

Conclusion

Different cells play roles in the lung inflammation observed in ARDS. The interplay between resident cells (structural and alveolar macrophages) and nonresident cells (circulating leukocytes, neutrophils) results in lung injury and is implicated in reparative mechanisms in the ARDS lung. Recognition of differences in ARDS manifestations depending on the precipitating insult—whether directed to the epithelium or endothelium, whether related to septic events, to underlying cancer, or to trauma—has enabled elucidation of more phenotypes of this condition. This is an important step; as shown by developments in similar lung diseases such as asthma and chronic obstructive pulmonary disease, phenotyping leads to better elucidation of pathogenesis and discovery of targets for new therapies.

References

1. Abrams ST, Zhang N, Manson J, Liu T, Dart C, Baluwa F et al (2013) Circulating histones are mediators of trauma-associated lung injury. [Research Support, Non-U.S. Gov't]. Am J Respir Crit Care Med 187(2):160–169
2. Aggarwal NR, King LS, D'Alessio FR (2014) Diverse macrophage populations mediate acute lung inflammation and resolution. [Research Support, N.I.H., Extramural Research Support, Non-U.S. Gov't Review]. Am J Physiol Lung Cell Mol Physiol 306(8):L709–L725

3. Belenkiy SM, Buel AR, Cannon JW, Sine CR, Aden JK, Henderson JL et al (2014) Acute respiratory distress syndrome in wartime military burns: application of the Berlin criteria. [Research Support, Non-U.S. Gov't Research Support, U.S. Gov't, Non-P.H.S.]. J Trauma Acute Care Surg 76(3):821–827
4. Bitterman PB (1992) Pathogenesis of fibrosis in acute lung injury. [Review]. Am J Med 92(6A):39S–43S
5. Brinkmann, V., Laube, B., Abu Abed, U., Goosmann, C., & Zychlinsky, A. (2010). Neutrophil extracellular traps: how to generate and visualize them. [Video-Audio Media]. J Visual Exp: JoVE (36).
6. Brinkmann V, Reichard U, Goosmann C, Fauler B, Uhlemann Y, Weiss DS et al (2004) Neutrophil extracellular traps kill bacteria. [Research Support, U.S. Gov't, P.H.S.]. Science 303(5663):1532–1535
7. Calfee CS, Eisner MD, Ware LB, Thompson BT, Parsons PE, Wheeler AP et al (2007) Trauma-associated lung injury differs clinically and biologically from acute lung injury due to other clinical disorders. [Comparative Study]. Crit Care Med 35(10):2243–2250
8. Calfee CS, Janz DR, Bernard GR, May AK, Kangelaris KN, Matthay MA et al (2015) Distinct molecular phenotypes of direct vs indirect ARDS in single-center and multicenter studies. [Comparative Study Multicenter Study Observational Study Randomized Controlled Trial Research Support, N.I.H., Extramural]. Chest 147(6):1539–1548
9. Caudrillier A, Kessenbrock K, Gilliss BM, Nguyen JX, Marques MB, Monestier M et al (2012) Platelets induce neutrophil extracellular traps in transfusion-related acute lung injury. [Research Support, N.I.H., Extramural]. J Clin Invest 122(7):2661–2671
10. David S, Mukherjee A, Ghosh CC, Yano M, Khankin EV, Wenger JB et al (2012) Angiopoietin-2 may contribute to multiple organ dysfunction and death in sepsis*. [Research Support, N.I.H., Extramural]. Crit Care Med 40(11):3034–3041
11. Dicker RA, Morabito DJ, Pittet JF, Campbell AR, Mackersie RC (2004) Acute respiratory distress syndrome criteria in trauma patients: why the definitions do not work. [Research Support, U.S. Gov't, P.H.S.]. J Trauma 57(3):522–526 ; discussion 526–528
12. Diep BA, Chan L, Tattevin P, Kajikawa O, Martin TR, Basuino L et al (2010) Polymorphonuclear leukocytes mediate *Staphylococcus aureus* Panton-Valentine leukocidin-induced lung inflammation and injury. [Research Support, N.I.H., Extramural Research Support, Non-U.S. Gov't]. Proc Natl Acad Sci U S A 107(12):5587–5592
13. Estenssoro E, Dubin A, Laffaire E, Canales H, Saenz G, Moseinco M et al (2002) Incidence, clinical course, and outcome in 217 patients with acute respiratory distress syndrome. [Multicenter Study]. Crit Care Med 30(11):2450–2456
14. Fadeyi EA, De Los Angeles Muniz M, Wayne AS, Klein HG, Leitman SF, Stroncek DF (2007) The transfusion of neutrophil-specific antibodies causes leukopenia and a broad spectrum of pulmonary reactions. [Case Reports Research Support, N.I.H., Intramural Research Support, Non-U.S. Gov't]. Transfusion 47(3):545–550
15. Fiedler U, Scharpfenecker M, Koidl S, Hegen A, Grunow V, Schmidt JM et al (2004) The Tie-2 ligand angiopoietin-2 is stored in and rapidly released upon stimulation from endothelial cell Weibel-Palade bodies. [Research Support, Non-U.S. Gov't]. Blood 103(11):4150–4156
16. Fox ED, Heffernan DS, Cioffi WG, Reichner JS (2013) Neutrophils from critically ill septic patients mediate profound loss of endothelial barrier integrity. [Research Support, N.I.H., Extramural]. Crit Care 17(5):R226
17. Fudala R, Krupa A, Matthay MA, Allen TC, Kurdowska AK (2007) Anti-IL-8 autoantibody: IL-8 immune complexes suppress spontaneous apoptosis of neutrophils. [Research Support, N.I.H., Extramural]. Am J Physiol Lung Cell Mol Physiol 293(2):L364–L374
18. Gattinoni L, Pelosi P, Suter PM, Pedoto A, Vercesi P, Lissoni A (1998) Acute respiratory distress syndrome caused by pulmonary and extrapulmonary disease. Different syndromes? [Research Support, Non-U.S. Gov't]. Am J Respir Crit Care Med 158(1):3–11
19. Gong H, Rehman J, Tang H, Wary K, Mittal M, Chaturvedi P et al (2015) HIF2alpha signaling inhibits adherens junctional disruption in acute lung injury. [Research Support, N.I.H., Extramural Research Support, Non-U.S. Gov't]. J Clin Invest 125(2):652–664

20. Grailer JJ, Ward PA (2014) Lung inflammation and damage induced by extracellular histones. Inflamm Cell Signal 1(4)
21. Greene KE, Wright JR, Steinberg KP, Ruzinski JT, Caldwell E, Wong WB et al (1999) Serial changes in surfactant-associated proteins in lung and serum before and after onset of ARDS. [Research Support, Non-U.S. Gov't Research Support, U.S. Gov't, Non-P.H.S. Research Support, U.S. Gov't, P.H.S.]. Am J Respir Crit Care Med 160(6):1843–1850
22. Hartshorn KL, Crouch E, White MR, Colamussi ML, Kakkanatt A, Tauber B et al (1998) Pulmonary surfactant proteins A and D enhance neutrophil uptake of bacteria. Am J Phys 274(6 Pt 1):L958–L969
23. Hoeboer SH, Groeneveld AB, van der Heijden M, Oudemans-van Straaten HM (2015) Serial inflammatory biomarkers of the severity, course and outcome of late onset acute respiratory distress syndrome in critically ill patients with or at risk for the syndrome after new-onset fever. Biomark Med 9(6):605–616
24. Khan H, Belsher J, Yilmaz M, Afessa B, Winters JL, Moore SB et al (2007) Fresh-frozen plasma and platelet transfusions are associated with development of acute lung injury in critically ill medical patients. [Research Support, N.I.H., Extramural]. Chest 131(5): 1308–1314
25. Kishore U, Greenhough TJ, Waters P, Shrive AK, Ghai R, Kamran MF et al (2006) Surfactant proteins SP-A and SP-D: structure, function and receptors. [Research Support, Non-U.S. Gov't Review]. Mol Immunol 43(9):1293–1315
26. Kurdowska A, Noble JM, Grant IS, Robertson CR, Haslett C, Donnelly SC (2002) Anti-interleukin-8 autoantibodies in patients at risk for acute respiratory distress syndrome. [Research Support, Non-U.S. Gov't Research Support, U.S. Gov't, P.H.S.]. Crit Care Med 30(10):2335–2337
27. Kurdowska AK, Geiser TK, Alden SM, Dziadek BR, Noble JM, Nuckton TJ et al (2002) Activity of pulmonary edema fluid interleukin-8 bound to alpha(2)-macroglobulin in patients with acute lung injury. [Research Support, U.S. Gov't, P.H.S.]. *American journal of physiology*. Lung Cell Mol Physiol 282(5):L1092–L1098
28. Lawrence T, Natoli G (2011) Transcriptional regulation of macrophage polarization: enabling diversity with identity. [Research Support, Non-U.S. Gov't Review]. Nat Rev Immunol 11(11):750–761
29. Lee A, Whyte MK, Haslett C (1993) Inhibition of apoptosis and prolongation of neutrophil functional longevity by inflammatory mediators. [Research Support, Non-U.S. Gov't]. J Leukoc Biol 54(4):283–288
30. Lee YL, King MB, Gonzalez RP, Brevard SB, Frotan MA, Gillespie MN et al (2014) Blood transfusion products contain mitochondrial DNA damage-associated molecular patterns: a potential effector of transfusion-related acute lung injury. [Research Support, N.I.H., Extramural Research Support, Non-U.S. Gov't]. J Surg Res 191(2):286–289
31. Lorente JA, Cardinal-Fernandez P, Munoz D, Frutos-Vivar F, Thille AW, Jaramillo C et al (2015) Acute respiratory distress syndrome in patients with and without diffuse alveolar damage: an autopsy study. Intensive Care Med 41(11):1921–1930
32. Martin AM Jr, Soloway HB, Simmons RL (1968) Pathologic anatomy of the lungs following shock and trauma. J Trauma 8(5):687–699
33. Matthay MA, Eschenbacher WL, Goetzl EJ (1984) Elevated concentrations of leukotriene D4 in pulmonary edema fluid of patients with the adult respiratory distress syndrome. [Comparative Study Research Support, U.S. Gov't, P.H.S.]. J Clin Immunol 4(6): 479–483
34. Matthay MA, Ware LB (2004) Plasma protein C levels in patients with acute lung injury: prognostic significance. [Research Support, U.S. Gov't, P.H.S.]. Crit Care Med 32(5 Suppl):S229–S232
35. Matthay MA, Zimmerman GA (2005) Acute lung injury and the acute respiratory distress syndrome: four decades of inquiry into pathogenesis and rational management. [Research Support, N.I.H., Extramural Research Support, U.S. Gov't, P.H.S. Review]. Am J Respir Cell Mol Biol 33(4):319–327

36. Mehta D, Ravindran K, Kuebler WM (2014) Novel regulators of endothelial barrier function. [Research Support, N.I.H., Extramural Research Support, Non-U.S. Gov't Review]. Am J Physiol Lung Cell Mol Physiol 307(12):L924–L935
37. Menezes SL, Bozza PT, Neto HC, Laranjeira AP, Negri EM, Capelozzi VL et al (2005) Pulmonary and extrapulmonary acute lung injury: inflammatory and ultrastructural analyses. [Comparative Study Research Support, Non-U.S. Gov't]. J Appl Physiol 98(5):1777–1783
38. Miller EJ, Cohen AB, Matthay MA (1996) Increased interleukin-8 concentrations in the pulmonary edema fluid of patients with acute respiratory distress syndrome from sepsis. [Research Support, Non-U.S. Gov't Research Support, U.S. Gov't, P.H.S.]. Crit Care Med 24(9):1448–1454
39. Miller EJ, Cohen AB, Nagao S, Griffith D, Maunder RJ, Martin TR et al (1992) Elevated levels of NAP-1/interleukin-8 are present in the airspaces of patients with the adult respiratory distress syndrome and are associated with increased mortality. [Research Support, Non-U.S. Gov't Research Support, U.S. Gov't, Non-P.H.S. Research Support, U.S. Gov't, P.H.S.]. Am Rev Respir Dis 146(2):427–432
40. Modelska K, Pittet JF, Folkesson HG, Courtney Broaddus V, Matthay MA (1999) Acid-induced lung injury. Protective effect of anti-interleukin-8 pretreatment on alveolar epithelial barrier function in rabbits. [Research Support, U.S. Gov't, P.H.S.]. Am J Respir Crit Care Med 160(5 Pt 1):1450–1456
41. Mokart D, Lambert J, Schnell D, Fouche L, Rabbat A, Kouatchet A et al (2013) Delayed intensive care unit admission is associated with increased mortality in patients with cancer with acute respiratory failure. Leuk Lymphoma 54(8):1724–1729
42. Morisawa K, Fujitani S, Taira Y, Kushimoto S, Kitazawa Y, Okuchi K et al (2014) Difference in pulmonary permeability between indirect and direct acute respiratory distress syndrome assessed by the transpulmonary thermodilution technique: a prospective, observational, multi-institutional study. J Intens Care 2(1):24
43. Muller MC, Juffermans NP (2012) Transfusion-related acute lung injury: a preventable syndrome? [Review]. Expert Rev Hematol 5(1):97–106
44. Ognibene FP, Martin SE, Parker MM, Schlesinger T, Roach P, Burch C et al (1986) Adult respiratory distress syndrome in patients with severe neutropenia. N Engl J Med 315(9):547–551
45. Pelosi P, D'Onofrio D, Chiumello D, Paolo S, Chiara G, Capelozzi VL et al (2003) Pulmonary and extrapulmonary acute respiratory distress syndrome are different. [Review]. Eur Respir J Suppl *42*:48s–56s
46. Peltz ED, Moore EE, Eckels PC, Damle SS, Tsuruta Y, Johnson JL et al (2009) HMGB1 is markedly elevated within 6 hours of mechanical trauma in humans. [Research Support, N.I.H., Extramural]. Shock 32(1):17–22
47. Reilly JP, Bellamy S, Shashaty MG, Gallop R, Meyer NJ, Lanken PN et al (2014) Heterogeneous phenotypes of acute respiratory distress syndrome after major trauma. [Research Support, N.I.H., Extramural]. Ann Am Thorac Soc 11(5):728–736
48. Ricciuto DR, dos Santos CC, Hawkes M, Toltl LJ, Conroy AL, Rajwans N et al (2011) Angiopoietin-1 and angiopoietin-2 as clinically informative prognostic biomarkers of morbidity and mortality in severe sepsis. [Multicenter Study Research Support, Non-U.S. Gov't]. Crit Care Med 39(4):702–710
49. Rittirsch D, Flierl MA, Ward PA (2008) Harmful molecular mechanisms in sepsis. [Research Support, N.I.H., Extramural Review]. Nat Rev Immunol 8(10):776–787
50. Rizzo, A. N., Sammani, S., Esquinca, A. E., Jacobson, J. R., Garcia, J. G., Letsiou, E., et al. (2015). Imatinib attenuates inflammation and vascular leak in a clinically relevant two-hit model of acute lung injury. Am J Physiol Lung Cell Mol Physiol, ajplung 00031 02015
51. Rocco PR, Pelosi P (2008) Pulmonary and extrapulmonary acute respiratory distress syndrome: myth or reality? [Review]. Curr Opin Crit Care 14(1):50–55
52. Rosseau S, Hammerl P, Maus U, Walmrath HD, Schutte H, Grimminger F et al (2000) Phenotypic characterization of alveolar monocyte recruitment in acute respiratory distress syndrome. [Research Support, Non-U.S. Gov't]. Am J Physiol Lung Cell Mol Physiol 279(1):L25–L35

53. Rubenfeld GD (2015) Confronting the frustrations of negative clinical trials in acute respiratory distress syndrome. Ann Am Thorac Soc 12(Suppl 1):S58–S63
54. Santos FB, Nagato LK, Boechem NM, Negri EM, Guimaraes A, Capelozzi VL et al (2006) Time course of lung parenchyma remodeling in pulmonary and extrapulmonary acute lung injury. [Research Support, Non-U.S. Gov't]. J Appl Physiol 100(1):98–106
55. Sheu CC, Gong MN, Zhai R, Chen F, Bajwa EK, Clardy PF et al (2010) Clinical characteristics and outcomes of sepsis-related vs non-sepsis-related ARDS. [Research Support, N.I.H., Extramural]. Chest 138(3):559–567
56. Silliman CC, McLaughlin NJ (2006) Transfusion-related acute lung injury. [Research Support, N.I.H., Extramural Research Support, Non-U.S. Gov't Review]. Blood Rev 20(3):139–159
57. Silva PL, Rocco PR, Pelosi P (2015) FG-4497: a new target for acute respiratory distress syndrome? [Research Support, Non-U.S. Gov't]. Exp Rev Respir Med 9(4):405–409
58. Soubani, A. O., Shehada, E., Chen, W., & Smith, D. (2014). The outcome of cancer patients with acute respiratory distress syndrome. J Crit Care 29(1):183 e187–183 e112
59. Swanson K, Dwyre DM, Krochmal J, Raife TJ (2006) Transfusion-related acute lung injury (TRALI): current clinical and pathophysiologic considerations. [Case Reports Review]. Lung 184(3):177–185
60. Thomas GM, Carbo C, Curtis BR, Martinod K, Mazo IB, Schatzberg D et al (2012) Extracellular DNA traps are associated with the pathogenesis of TRALI in humans and mice. [Research Support, N.I.H., Extramural Research Support, Non-U.S. Gov't]. Blood 119(26):6335–6343
61. Thurston G, Rudge JS, Ioffe E, Zhou H, Ross L, Croll SD et al (2000) Angiopoietin-1 protects the adult vasculature against plasma leakage. [Research Support, U.S. Gov't, P.H.S.]. Nat Med 6(4):460–463
62. Toshchakov V, Jones BW, Perera PY, Thomas K, Cody MJ, Zhang S et al (2002) TLR4, but not TLR2, mediates IFN-beta-induced STAT1alpha/beta-dependent gene expression in macrophages. [Research Support, U.S. Gov't, P.H.S.]. Nat Immunol 3(4):392–398
63. Ware LB, Matthay MA (2000) The acute respiratory distress syndrome. [Historical Article Review]. N Engl J Med 342(18):1334–1349
64. Watson GA, Sperry JL, Rosengart MR, Minei JP, Harbrecht BG, Moore EE et al (2009) Fresh frozen plasma is independently associated with a higher risk of multiple organ failure and acute respiratory distress syndrome. [Multicenter Study Research Support, N.I.H., Extramural]. J Trauma 67(2):221–227 ; discussion 228–230
65. Wiener-Kronish JP, Albertine KH, Matthay MA (1991) Differential responses of the endothelial and epithelial barriers of the lung in sheep to *Escherichia coli* endotoxin. [Research Support, U.S. Gov't, P.H.S.]. J Clin Invest 88(3):864–875
66. Wiener-Kronish JP, Pittet JF (2011) Therapies against virulence products of *Staphylococcus aureus* and Pseudomonas aeruginosa. [Review]. Semin Respir Crit Care Med 32(2):228–235
67. Wilhelmsen K, Mesa KR, Prakash A, Xu F, Hellman J (2012) Activation of endothelial TLR2 by bacterial lipoprotein upregulates proteins specific for the neutrophil response. [Research Support, N.I.H., Extramural Research Support, Non-U.S. Gov't]. Innate Immun 18(4):602–616
68. Williams AE, Chambers RC (2014) The mercurial nature of neutrophils: still an enigma in ARDS? [Research Support, Non-U.S. Gov't Review]. Am J Physiol Lung Cell Mol Physiol 306(3):L217–L230
69. Zhang J, Fukuhara S, Sako K, Takenouchi T, Kitani H, Kume T et al (2011) Angiopoietin-1/Tie2 signal augments basal Notch signal controlling vascular quiescence by inducing delta-like 4 expression through AKT-mediated activation of beta-catenin. [Research Support, Non--U.S. Gov't]. J Biol Chem 286(10):8055–8066
70. Zhang Y, Wen Z, Guan L, Jiang P, Gu T, Zhao J et al (2015) Extracellular histones play an inflammatory role in acid aspiration-induced acute respiratory distress syndrome. [Research Support, Non-U.S. Gov't]. Anesthesiology 122(1):127–139
71. Ziegler-Heitbrock L, Ancuta P, Crowe S, Dalod M, Grau V, Hart DN et al (2010) Nomenclature of monocytes and dendritic cells in blood. [Research Support, Non-U.S. Gov't]. Blood 116(16):e74–e80

Ventilation Strategies: Tidal Volume and PEEP

3

Carmen Sílvia Valente Barbas

3.1 Introduction

Acute respiratory distress syndrome (ARDS), defined as an increment in the lung alveolar-capillary membrane permeability causing a pulmonary edema rich in proteins, has been recently reclassified as mild, moderate, and severe according to Berlin definition [1]. It occurred in 1.8–10% of ICU admissions [1–3] and presents a progressively higher mortality ratio from its mild (34.9%) to the more severe form of presentation (46.1%) [3].

3.2 Respiratory System Structural Dysfunction After ARDS

After the initial lung insult, resulting from the exposition of a genetic predisposing patient to a risk factor (pulmonary infection, sepsis, acid-gastric lung aspiration, etc.), epithelial and endothelial lung barriers can be disrupted liberating, respectively, receptors for advanced glycation end products (RAGE) and angiopoietin-2. The extravasation of plasma inside the alveolar space turns an air-filled lung into a heavy high-osmotic pressure liquid-filled lungs. As a consequence, the higher weight of the lungs under the action of the gravity force predisposes the lowermost lung regions to collapse (Fig. 3.1) provoking a higher intrapulmonary shunt, a refractory hypoxemia, and a decrease in lung compliance. The functional alterations of the respiratory system are expressed by a decrease in the functional residual capacity (FRC) and a shift of the respiratory system pressure-volume curve down and to the right. The clinical manifestations are a dyspneic and hypoxemic patient with a high work of breathing that needs a high nasal flow oxygen system,

C.S.V. Barbas, MD, PhD
Respiratory ICU-University of São Paulo Medical School, Adult ICU Albert Einstein Hospital, São Paulo, Brazil
e-mail: carmen.barbas@gmail.com

D. Chiumello (ed.), *Acute Respiratory Distress Syndrome (ARDS)*,
DOI 10.1007/978-3-319-41852-0_3

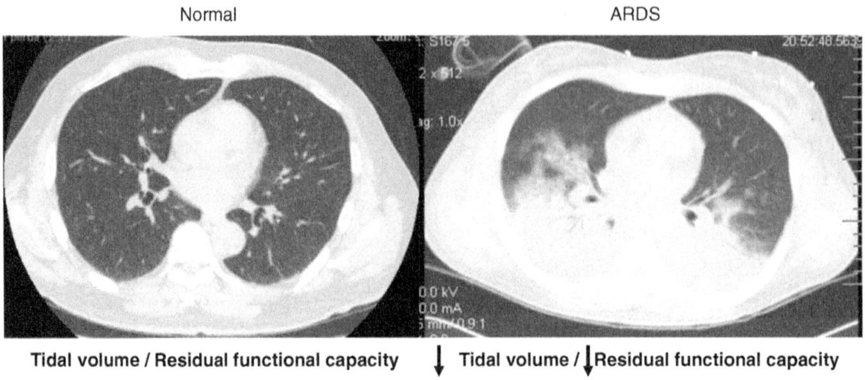

Fig. 3.1 Normal thoracic tomography versus ARDS thoracic tomography (Reprinted with permission from Medical Evidence Percorso Formativo 2015, yr. 8, n. 104, www.ati14.it)

noninvasive ventilation or intubation, and invasive mechanical ventilation to support the patient's gas exchange and respiratory system mechanics while the clinical treatment and avoidance of the risk factors start [4, 5].

3.3 Tidal Volume and PEEP During Spontaneous Ventilatory Support in ARDS Patients

Recently, Frat and colleagues [6] showed that high-flow oxygen through nasal cannula (HFNC= 48 ± 11 L/min) can be used in hypoxemic respiratory failure (PaO_2/FiO_2 ratio less than 300, 79% of these patients with bilateral pulmonary infiltrates) with an intubation rate of 38% in the high-flow oxygen group, 47% in the standard oxygen group, and 50% in the noninvasive ventilation group (p = 0.18; p = 0.17 by the log-rank test). Ventilator-free days at day 28 was significantly lower in high-flow oxygen group as well as crude in ICU and 90-day mortality. One of the hypothesis generated by this study was that the high tidal volume of 9 mL/kg/predicted body weight achieved by the NIV group could be responsible for its poor result. At 1 h after enrollment, the intensity of respiratory discomfort was reduced, and the dyspnea score was improved with the use of high-flow oxygen nasal cannula, as compared with standard oxygen group and NIV generating the hypothesis that HFNC could decrease the patient's inspiratory efforts and their transpulmonary pressures and possibly decreasing their induced lung injury.

Messica and colleagues [7] studied in a 1-year observational study 87 patients with ARDS that received HFNC at least once during their ICU stay. Of those, 45 subjects received HFNC as first-line treatment for respiratory failure, and intubation was needed in 40% of the patients. In the multivariate analysis, SAPS II was significantly associated with intubation requirement.

The role of spontaneous inspiratory effort, intensity of inspiratory muscle activity, and size of tidal volume achieved during spontaneous ventilatory support (Standard oxygen, HFNC or NIV) and their association with ARDS patient outcomes must be better studied in the future. Most of the studies of ARDS patients that needed NIV used low EPAP/PEEP levels (from 0 to 10 cmH_2O). The role of higher PEEP levels or individual PEEP titration in this ARDS population are still not elucidated.

3.4 Invasive Mechanical Ventilation in ARDS Patients: Role of Tidal Volume

It is well documented that lower tidal volumes (6 mL/kg of predicted body weight) compared to higher tidal volumes (12 mL/kg of predicted body weight) associated with PEEP levels titrated by a PEEP/FiO_2 table reduced mortality in a randomized, clinical trial that analyzed 861 ARDS patients (ARMA trial) [8]. In the ARMA trial, lower tidal volumes led to lower levels of plasma IL-6, IL-8 ,and TNFR1 over the subsequent 1–3 days [9].

So, low tidal ventilation (≤6 mL/kg of predicted body weight) must be initiated as soon as the ARDS patient is intubated and mechanically ventilated. The predicted body weight (PBW) can be calculated as follows: for women, PBW= 45.5 + 0.91 (height in centimeters – 152.4) and, for men, PBW = 50.0 + 0.91 (height in centimeters −152.4). It is important to adjust tidal volume to lung size that depends on the height and sex but, more importantly, to adjust the tidal volume to functional lung size that depends on the ARDS severity (lung compliance), sex, height, and chest wall compliance. It also depends where in the pressure-volume curve of the respiratory system the tidal ventilation takes place, even more, the interaction between the FRC (functional residual capacity) and tidal ventilation inside the thoracic cage during controlled ventilation. During assisted ventilation other two factors must be added to the interaction between the FRC and above tidal ventilation inside the thoracic cage: the patient's negative inspiratory efforts, and the pressures that resulted from the desynchronization between the patient and the mechanical ventilator. Recent evidences showed that in severe ARDS, patients' inspiratory efforts during assisted ventilation could worsen ventilator lung injury induced by the mechanical ventilation during the ventilatory support of the ARDS patients [10]. This associated and added injury could explain the results of a phase IV randomized controlled trial in moderate/severe ARDS patients ($PaO_2/FiO_2 < 150$); comparing cisatracurium to placebo for 48 h showed an improved adjusted 90-day survival rate and increased ventilator-free in the cisatracurium group without a significant increase in muscle weakness. Short-term paralysis may facilitate patient-ventilator synchrony in the setting of lung-protective ventilation. Short-term paralysis would eliminate patient triggering and expiratory muscle activity. In combination, these effects may serve to limit regional overdistention and cyclic alveolar collapse. Paralysis may also act to lower metabolism and overall ventilatory demand [11].

At the same time that a low tidal volume is set, an adequate respiratory rate must be concurrently set in order to keep a minute ventilation around 7–8 L/min and a $PaCO_2$ around 40–60 mmHg and a pH above 7.2. In the more severe ARDS patients, sometimes after the adjustment of a minute ventilation around 8 L/min with tidal volumes lesser than 6 mL/kg of predicted body weight, the $PaCO_2$ levels stay above 80 mmHg and pH less than 7.2 (specially patients with septic shock and metabolic acidosis). In these cases, the VCO_2 must be assessed and be kept as least as possible (fever control, low carbohydrate intake), and hemodialysis can be initiated (specially in ARDS patients with concomitant acute renal failure) in order to help control the metabolic acidosis. Efforts must be taken to decrease the pulmonary death space by means of recruitment maneuvers and PEEP titration, tidal volume and respiratory rate adjustments, or even the initiation of prone ventilation. In the most difficult cases, tracheal gas insufflation or extracorporeal CO_2 removal or extracorporeal oxygenation should be started in order to keep the protective low tidal volume ventilation [4].

Potentially harmful consequences of permissive hypercapnia include pulmonary vasoconstriction and pulmonary hypertension, proarrythmic effects of increased discharge of catecholamines, and cerebral vasodilation yielding increased intracranial pressure. Special attention should be given to patients with pulmonary hypertension and right ventricular dysfunction secondary to ARDS that could not tolerate high $PaCO_2$ and low pH levels [4].

Nonetheless, permissive hypercapnia should probably be used with caution in patients with heart disease and is relatively contraindicated in those with elevated intracranial pressure. In ARDS cases with pulmonary hypertension and right ventricular dysfunction, prone position ventilation should be preferred [4].

Recent evidence showed that prolonged prone position ventilation (16 h) must be used in early ARDS with PaO_2/FiO_2 <150 with PEEP levels of or more than 5 cmH_2O in order to significantly improve 90-day mortality compared to supine ventilation [12]. Recent meta-analysis also showed that in the era of low tidal ventilation, the prone position use improved mortality of moderate/severe ARDS patients that needed invasive mechanical ventilatory support [13]. If PEEP titration during prone position ventilation should improve survival of ARDS patients is still a matter of debate [14].

Another recent approach for application of extracorporeal carbon dioxide removal new devices (ECMO-R) in ARDS patients is the demonstration that in severe ARDS, even the low tidal volume ventilation with 6 mL/kg of predicted body weight can cause tidal hyperdistension in the nondependent regions of the lungs accompanied by plateau airway pressures greater than 28 cmH_2O and elevated plasma markers of inflammation. In this group application of ECMO-R could allow the authors to decrease the tidal volume to less than 6 mL/kg with a consequent plateau pressure less than 25 cmH_2O that was associated with a lower radiographic index of lung injury and lower levels of lung-derived inflammatory cytokines [15]. However, prognostic implication of this new ECMO-R devices application in clinical practice is still under investigation [16].

Pumpless interventional lung assist (iLA) is also used in patients with ARDS and is aimed at improving extracorporeal gas exchange with a membrane integrated in a passive arteriovenous shunt. iLA serves as an extracorporeal assist to support mechanical ventilation by enabling low tidal volume and a reduced inspiratory plateau pressure in extremely severe ARDS patients. Zimmermann and colleagues used iLA in 51 severe ARDS patients and observed a decrease in $PaCO_2$ allowing the decrease in tidal volume and plateau pressure (ultraprotective ventilation) with a hospital mortality rate of 49% [17]. Recently, Fanelli and colleagues described the feasibility and safety of use of an ultraprotective strategy using 4 mL/kg of predicted body weight associated with low-flow extracorporeal carbon removal in 15 moderate ARDS patients [18].

3.5 Limiting the Tidal Volumes in ARDS with Modern Ventilators

Recently, Wing and colleagues [19] showed that modern ventilators have an increasing number of optional settings that can change the size of the delivered tidal volume. These settings may increase the delivered tidal volume and disrupt a low tidal volume strategy. Recognizing how each setting within a mode affects the type of breath delivered is critical when caring for ventilator-dependent patients. The AVEA has two options in volume A/C: demand breaths and V-sync. When activated, these options allow the patient to exceed the set tidal volume. When using the Evita XL, the option Auto-Flow can be turned *on* or *off*, and when this option is *on*, the tidal volume may vary. The PB 840 does not have any additional options that affect volume delivery, and it maintains the set tidal volume regardless of patient effort. The SERVO-i's demand valve allows additional flow if the patient's inspiratory flow rate exceeds the set flow rate, increasing the delivered tidal volume; this option can be turned *off* with the latest software upgrade. The continuous monitoring of the low tidal volumes during the ARDS ventlatory support must be implemented in our ICUs in order to guarantee that a protective ventilation is continuously offered to our ARDS patients.

3.6 Low Tidal Volumes Must Generate Low Driving Pressures to Assure It Is Really Protective to ARDS Patients

Recently, Amato and colleagues [20] hypothesized that driving pressure ($\Delta P = VT/CRS$), in which VT is intrinsically normalized to functional lung size (instead of predicted lung size in healthy persons), would be an index more strongly associated with survival than VT or PEEP in patients who are not actively breathing. Using a statistical tool known as multilevel mediation analysis to analyze individual data from 3562 patients with ARDS enrolled in nine previously reported randomized trials, they examined Δp as an independent variable associated with survival. In the mediation analysis, they estimated the isolated effects of changes in Δp resulting from randomized ventilator settings while minimizing confounding due to the baseline severity of lung disease. The authors observed that among ventilation variables, Δp was most strongly associated with survival. A 1-SD increment in Δp (approximately 7 cm of water) was associated with increased mortality (relative risk, 1.41; 95% confidence interval [CI], 1.31–1.51; $p < 0.001$), even in patients receiving "protective" plateau pressures and VT (relative risk, 1.36; 95% CI, 1.17–1.58; $p < 0.001$). Individual changes in VT or PEEP after randomization were not independently associated with survival; they were associated only if they were among the changes that led to reductions in Δp (mediation effects of Δp, $p = 0.004$ and $p = 0.001$, respectively). They concluded that Δp was the ventilation variable that best stratified risk. Decreases in Δp owing to changes in ventilator settings were strongly associated with increased survival.

3.7 Invasive Mechanical Ventilation in ARDS Patients: Role of End-Positive Expiratory Pressure (PEEP) Levels

Recently, three large clinical trials [21–23], including acute lung injury/ARDS patients ventilated with low tidal volume, have compared different PEEP strategies (high vs. low), but none of them could show a significant difference in mortality. Moreover, a recent meta-analysis has pooled those trials [24], revealing some combined benefit of the high PEEP strategy; still, the survival benefit was modest and limited to the subgroup of ARDS patients with $PaO_2/FiO_2 < 200$. Conceptually, one could argue that none of the "high PEEP" strategies was designed to test the "open-lung hypothesis" postulated by Lachmann [25–28], that is, the hypothesis that most of the collapsed lung tissue observed in early ARDS can be reversed at an acceptable clinical cost, potentially resulting in better lung protection. According to a recent study by Borges and colleagues [29], a straight test of the "open-lung hypothesis" would certainly require more aggressive recruiting maneuvers in association with individualized, decremental PEEP titration. Thus, one can speculate that the limited results reported above were related to suboptimal ventilatory strategy. Recently, de Matos and colleagues [30] reported the experience with maximal recruitment rtrategy (MRS) in 51 patients with ARDS. MRS consisted of 2-min steps of tidal ventilation with pressure-controlled ventilation, fixed driving pressure of 15 cmH_2O, respiratory rate of 10 breaths/minute, inspiratory/expiratory ratio of 1:1, and stepwise increments in PEEP levels from 10 to 45 cmH_2O (recruitment phase). After that, PEEP was decreased to 25 cmH_2O and, then, from 25 to 10 cmH_2O (PEEP titration phase) in steps of 5 cmH_2O, each one lasting 4 min. At each of the steps, computer tomography image sequences from the carina to the diaphragm were acquired during an expiratory pause of 6–10 s. Lung collapse was assessed online by visual inspection, for immediate clinical decision, and offline for quantitative measurements.

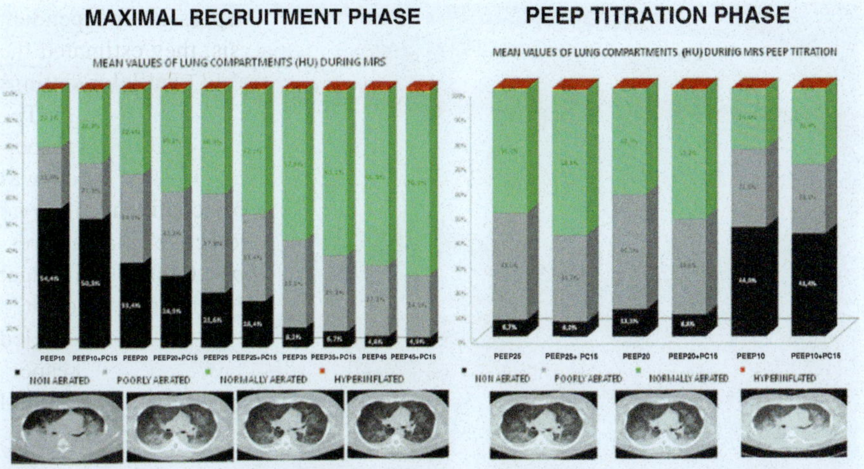

Fig. 3.2 Detailed thoracic Tomographic analysis of nonaerated (HU from −100 to +100U), poorly aerated (HU form −100 to −500 U), normally aerated (HU from −500 to −900U), and hyperinflated (HU more than −900U) in 12 patients with moderate/severe ARDS during maximal recruitment manuevers and PEEP titration (Reprinted with permission from Medical Evidence Percorso Formativo 2015, yr. 8, n. 104, www.ati14.it)

MRS showed a statistically significant decrease in nonaerated areas of the ARDS lungs that was accompanied by a significant increment in oxygenation. The opening plateau pressure observed during the recruitment protocol was 59.6 (±5.9 cmH_2O), and the mean PEEP titrated after MRS was 24.6 (±2.9 cmH_2O). Mean PaO_2/FiO_2 ratio increased from 125 (±43) to 300 (±103; $p < 0.0001$) after MRS and was sustained above 300 throughout 7 days. Nonaerated parenchyma decreased significantly from 53.6% (interquartile range (IQR): 42.5–62.4) to 12.7% (IQR: 4.9–24.2) ($p < 0.0001$) after MRS. The potentially recruitable lung was estimated at 45% (IQR: 25–53). ICU mortality was 28% and hospital mortality was 32%. The independent risk factors associated with mortality were older age and higher driving pressures (or higher delta pressure control). There were no significant clinical complications with MRS or barotrauma. A better evolution of these ARDS patients with less necessity of oxygen supplementation in the recovery phase of the disease and a better quality of life must be tested in prospective, controlled clinical trials. A recent meta-analysis [23] showing beneficial effects on mortality using higher PEEP levels compared with lower PEEP in ARDS patients corroborates the results of our clinical case series of ARDS patients submitted to MRS. A detailed thoracic tomographic analysis performed in 12 of these ARDS patient thoracic computed tomographies during recruitment phase and PEEP titration phase showed a significant increment in normal aerated lungs and decrement of nonaerated during maximal recruitment maneuvers and PEEP titration (Fig. 3.2). These results demonstrated that keep sufficient PEEP levels after recruitment is crucial in ARDS patients (Fig. 3.3).

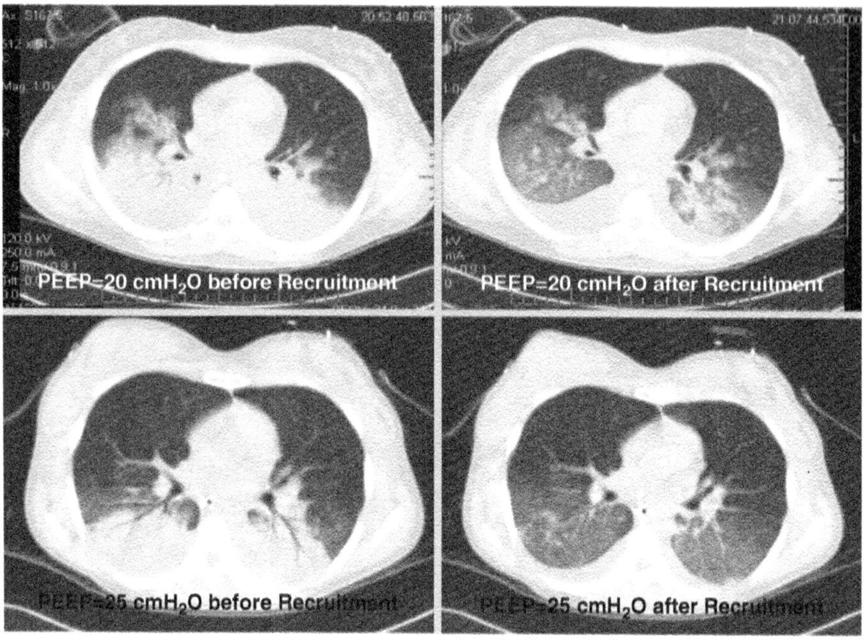

Fig. 3.3 Maximal recruitment manuevers can open up the collapsed lung in ARDS, and high PEEP levels are crucial to keep the lungs open (Reprinted with permission from Medical Evidence Percorso Formativo 2015, yr. 8, n. 104, www.ati14.it)

3.8 Interaction Between Low Tidal Volume and High PEEP Levels During Invasive Mechanical Ventilation in ARDS Patients

Amato and colleagues [31] demonstrated reduction in 28-day mortality in 53 ARDS patients submitted to recruitment maneuver (CPAP 40 cmH_2O) PEEP titrated by static Pressure × Volume ($P \times V$) curve associated with low tidal volume (VT = 6 mL/kg), compared to those ventilated with high VT (12 mL/kg) and low PEEP strategy. Villar and colleagues [32] found congruent results in a similar protocol in 103 ARDS patients. These two clinical, prospective, and control trials showed significant results in improving ARDS mortality with a relatively small number of patients indicating that should be an interaction between high PEEP and low tidal volume during invasive mechanical ventilation in ARDS patients, and static pressure-volume curve of the respiratory system of ARDS patients should be the best window to ventilate our ARDS patients.

Finally, perhaps, it would be important to optimize PEEP in each patient based on the respiratory characteristics. In ARDS, we have to deal with the transpulmonary pressure (airway pressure minus pleural pressure) at both end inspiration and end expiration. If we consider end inspiration, due to the high variability of chest wall to lung elastance ratio across the patients, similar pressure applied to the airway opening can generate different changes in transpulmonary pressure. Consequently, the application of similar tidal volume and PEEP may have harmful or not harmful effects on the lung stress/strain depending on the patient's respiratory characteristics. In addition, for the same tidal volume, different PEEP levels may result in different degrees of ventilator-associated lung injury [33]. Talmor and colleagues [34], in a small single-center randomized controlled trial, individualized PEEP in order to achieve end expiratory transpulmonary pressure between 0 and 10 cmH_2O in ARDS patients for 3 days. They found higher PEEP levels, better oxygenation, and greater compliance of the respiratory system in the esophageal pressure PEEP-guided group as compared to the control group (gas exchange-based PEEP). End inspiratory transpulmonary pressure and mortality rate at 28 days were similar in the two groups.

References

1. Definition Task Force ARDS, Ranieri VM, Rubenfeld GD, Thompson BT, Ferguson ND, Caldwell E, Fan E, Camporota L, Slutsky AS (2012) Acute respiratory distress syndrome: the Berlin Definition. JAMA 307(23):2526–2533
2. Caser EB, Zandonade E, Pereira E, Gama AM, Barbas CS (2014) Impact of distinct definitions of acute lung injury on its incidence and outcomes in Brazilian ICUs: prospective evaluation of 7,133 patients. Crit Care Med 42(3):574–582
3. Bellani G, Laffey JG, Pham T, Fan E, Brochard L, Esteban A, Gattinoni L, van Haren F, Larsson A, DF MA, Ranieri M, Rubenfeld G, Thompson BT, Wrigge H, Slutsky AS, Pesenti A, LUNG SAFE Investigators; ESICM Trials Group (2016) Epidemiology, patterns of care, and mortality for patients with acute respiratory distress syndrome in intensive care units in 50 countries. JAMA 315(8):788–800
4. Barbas CS, Matos GF, Amato MB, Carvalho CR (2012) Goal-oriented respiratory management for critically ill patients with acute respiratory distress syndrome. Crit Care Res Pract 2012:952168
5. Barbas CS, Isola AM, Caser EB (2014) What is the future of acute respiratory distress syndrome after the Berlin definition? Curr Opin Crit Care 20(1):10–16
6. Frat JP, Thille AW, Mercat A, Girault C, Ragot S, Perbet S, Prat G, Boulain T, Morawiec E, Cottereau A, Devaquet J, Nseir S, Razazi K, Mira JP, Argaud L, Chakarian JC, Ricard JD, Wittebole X, Chevalier S, Herbland A, Fartoukh M, Constantin JM, Tonnelier JM, Pierrot M, Mathonnet A, Béduneau G, Delétage-Métreau C, Richard JC, Brochard L, Robert R, FLORALI Study Group; REVA Network (2015) High-flow oxygen through nasal cannula in acute hypoxemic respiratory failure. N Engl J Med 372(23):2185–2196
7. Messika J, Ben Ahmed K, Gaudry S, Miguel-Montanes R, Rafat C, Sztrymf B, Dreyfuss D, Ricard JD (2015) Use of high-flow nasal cannula oxygen therapy in subjects with ARDS: a 1-year observational study. Respir Care 60(2):162–169
8. The Acute Respiratory Distress Syndrome Network (2000) Ventilation with lower tidal volumes as compared with traditional tidal volumes for acute lung injury and the acute respiratory distress syndrome. N Engl J Med 342:1301–1308
9. Parsons PE, Eisner MD, Thompson BT, Matthay MA, Ancukiewicz M, Bernard GR, Wheeler AP (2005) Lower tidal volume ventilation and plasmacytokine markers of inflammation in patients with acute lung injury. Crit Care Med 33:1–6
10. Yoshida T, Torsani V, Gomes S, De Santis RR, Beraldo MA, Costa EL, Tucci MR, Zin WA, Kavanagh BP, Amato MB (2013) Spontaneous effort causes occult pendelluft during mechanical ventilation. Am J Respir Crit Care Med 188(12):1420–1427

11. Papazian L, Forel JM, Gacouin A et al (2010) Neuromuscular blockers in early acute respiratory distress syndrome. N Engl J Med 363(12):1107–1116
12. Guérin C, Reignier J, Richard JC, Beuret P, Gacouin A, Boulain T, Mercier E, Badet M, Mercat A, Baudin O, Clavel M, Chatellier D, Jaber S, Rosselli S, Mancebo J, Sirodot M, Hilbert G, Bengler C, Richecoeur J, Gainnier M, Bayle F, Bourdin G, Leray V, Girard R, Baboi L, Ayzac L, PROSEVA Study Group (2013) Prone positioning in severe acute respiratory distress syndrome. N Engl J Med 368(23):2159–2168
13. Beitler JR, Shaefi S, Montesi SB, Devlin A, Loring SH, Talmor D, Malhotra A (2014) Prone positioning reduces mortality from acute respiratory distress syndrome in the low tidal volume era: a meta-analysis. Intensive Care Med 40(3):332–341
14. Beitler JR, Guérin C, Ayzac L, Mancebo J, Bates DM, Malhotra A, Talmor D (2015) PEEP titration during prone positioning for acute respiratory distress syndrome. Crit Care 19:436
15. Ranieri VM, Terragni PP, Del Sorbo L et al (2009) Tidal volume lower than 6 mL/kg enhances lung protection: role of extracorporeal carbon dioxide removal. Anesthesiology 111(4): 826–835
16. Costa EL, Amato MB (2013) Ultra-protective tidal volume: how low should we go? Crit Care 17(2):127
17. Zimmermann M, Bein T, Arlt M, et al (2009) Pumpless extracorporeal interventional lung assist in patients with acute respiratory distress syndrome: a prospective pilot study. Crit Care 13(1, article no. R10).
18. Fanelli V, Ranieri MV, Mancebo J, Moerer O, Quintel M, Morley S, Moran I, Parrilla F, Costamagna A, Gaudiosi M, Combes A (2016) Feasibility and safety of low-flow extracorporeal carbon dioxide removal to facilitate ultra-protective ventilation in patients with moderate acute respiratory distress syndrome. Crit Care 20(1):36. doi:10.1186/s13054-016-1211-y
19. Wing TJ, Haan L, Ashworth LJ, Anderson J (2015) Limiting volume with modern ventilators. Ther Adv Respir Dis 9(3):75–83
20. Amato MB, Meade MO, Slutsky AS, Brochard L, Costa EL, Schoenfeld DA, Stewart TE, Briel M, Talmor D, Mercat A, Richard JC, Carvalho CR, Brower RG (2015) Driving pressure and survival in the acute respiratory distress syndrome. N Engl J Med 372(8):747–755
21. Brower RG, Lanken PN, MacIntyre N, Matthay MA, Morris A, Ancukiewicz M, Schoenfeld D, Thompson BT (2004) Higher versus lower positive end-expiratory pressures in patients with the acute respiratory distress syndrome. N Engl J Med 351:327–336
22. Mercat A, Richard JC, Vielle B, Jaber S, Osman D, Diehl JL, Lefrant JY, Prat G, Richecoeur J, Nieszkowska A, Gervais C, Baudot J, Bouadma L, Brochard L, Expiratory Pressure (Express) Study Group (2008) Positive end-expiratory pressure setting in adults with acute lung injury and acute respiratory distress syndrome: a randomized controlled trial. JAMA 299:646–655. doi:10.1001/jama.299.6.646
23. Meade MO, Cook DJ, Guyatt GH, Slutsky AS, Arabi YM, Cooper DJ, Davies AR, Hand LE, Zhou Q, Thabane L, Austin P, Lapinsky S, Baxter A, Russell J, Skrobik Y, Ronco JJ, Stewart TE (2008) Lung Open Ventilation Study Investigators. Ventilation strategy using low tidal volumes, recruitment maneuvers, and high positive end-expiratory pressure for acute lung injury and acute respiratory distress syndrome: a randomized controlled trial. JAMA 299:637–645. doi:10.1001/jama.299.6.637
24. Briel M, Meade M, Mercat A, Brower RG, Talmor D, Walter SD, Slutsky AS, Pullenayegum E, Zhou Q, Cook D, Brochard L, Richard JC, Lamontagne F, Bhatnagar N, Stewart TE, Guyatt G (2010) Higher vs lower positive end-expiratory pressure in patients with acute lung injury and acute respiratory distress syndrome: systematic review and meta-analysis. JAMA 303:865–873
25. Bohm SH, Vazquez de Anda GF, Lachmann B. In: Yearbook of intensive care and emergency medicine. Vincent J-L, editor.(1998). Berlin: Springer; The open lung concept; pp. 430–440.
26. Lachmann B (1992) Open up the lung and keep the lung open. Intensive Care Med 18:319–321
27. Barbas CS, de Matos GF, Pincelli MP, da Rosa BE, Antunes T, de Barros JM, Okamoto V, Borges JB, Amato MB, de Carvalho CR (2005) Mechanical ventilation in acute respiratory

failure: recruitment and high positive end-expiratory pressure are necessary. Curr Opin Crit Care 11:18–28

28. Papadakos PJ, Lachmann B (2007) The open lung concept of mechanical ventilation: the role of recruitment and stabilization. Crit Care Clin 23:241–250
29. Borges JB, Okamoto VN, Matos GF, Caramez MP, Arantes PR, Barros F, Souza CE, Victorino JA, Kacmarek RM, Barbas CS, Carvalho CR, Amato MB (2006) Reversibility of lung collapse and hypoxemia in early acute respiratory distress syndrome. Am J Respir Crit Care Med 174:268–278
30. de Matos GF, Stanzani F, Passos RH, Fontana MF, Albaladejo R, Caserta RE, Santos DC, Borges JB, Amato MB, Barbas CS (2012) How large is the lung recruitability in early acute respiratory distress syndrome: a prospective case series of patients monitored by computed tomography. Crit Care 16(1):R4
31. Amato MB, Barbas CS, Medeiros DM, Magaldi RB, Schettino GP, Lorenzi-Filho G, Kairalla RA, Deheinzelin D, Munoz C, Oliveira R, Takagaki TY, Carvalho CR (1998) Effect of a protective-ventilation strategy on mortality in the acute respiratory distress syndrome. N Engl J Med 338(6):347–354
32. Villar J, Kacmarek RM, Pérez-Méndez L, Aguirre-Jaime A (2006) A high positive end-expiratory pressure, low tidal volume ventilatory strategy improves outcome in persistent acute respiratory distress syndrome: a randomized, controlled trial. Crit Care Med 34(5):1311–1318
33. Chiumello D, Guérin C (2015) Understanding the setting of PEEP from esophageal pressure in patients with ARDS. Intensive Care Med 41(8):1465–1467
34. Talmor D, Sarge T, Malhotra A, O'Donnell CR, Ritz R, Lisbon A, Novack V, Loring SH (2008) Mechanical ventilation guided by esophageal pressure in acute lung injury. N Engl J Med 359(20):2095–2104

Ventilation Strategies: High-Frequency Oscillatory Ventilation

4

Spyros D. Mentzelopoulos, George Karlis, Ioannis N. Pantazopoulos, and Charikleia Vrettou

4.1 Introduction

High-frequency oscillatory ventilation (HFOV) is an alternative technique of ventilation in which small tidal volumes (i.e., ≤3.5 mL/kg predicted body weight) are delivered at high frequencies (3–15 Hz) with an oscillatory pump [1]. The technique comprises the application of continuous positive airway pressure and setting of the mean airway pressure (mPaw) through manipulation of bias flow (a continuous fresh gas flow sweeping through the ventilator circuit) and a resistance valve [2]. Oscillations generated by either a piston pump or an electromagnetically driven membrane diaphragm are superimposed on mPaw [2] (Fig.4.1). HFOV frequency and oscillatory pressure amplitude (ΔP; i.e., the transdiaphragmatic pressure swing) can be varied to generate a different tidal volume (V_t). Ventilator circuit pressure swings are substantially attenuated due to tracheal tube impedance and peak-to-trough pressure excursions at tracheal level amount to just 5–16% of circuit pressure excursions. For any given V_t, the dampening of circuit pressure oscillations is inversely proportional to tracheal tube diameter and increases with increasing HFOV frequency [2, 4].

For many years, it was believed that ventilation at V_ts less than the anatomical dead space should be ineffective because inspired air would not reach the alveoli. In 1980, a physiologic study showed that ventilation with V_ts as small as a fraction of the anatomical dead space can maintain adequate ventilation [5]. HFOV combines small pressure oscillations to minimize overdistention with high mPaw to prevent

The contributions of the authors George Karlis and Ioannis N. Pantazopoulos should be considered as equally important.

S.D. Mentzelopoulos, MD, PhD (✉) • G. Karlis, MD, PhD • I.N. Pantazopoulos, MD, PhD
C. Vrettou, MD, PhD
First Department of Intensive Care Medicine, University of Athens Medical School, Evaggelismos General Hospital, 45-47 Ipsilandou Street, GR -10676 Athens, Greece
e-mail: sdmentzelopoulos@yahoo.com; sdm@hol.gr

D. Chiumello (ed.), *Acute Respiratory Distress Syndrome (ARDS)*,
DOI 10.1007/978-3-319-41852-0_4

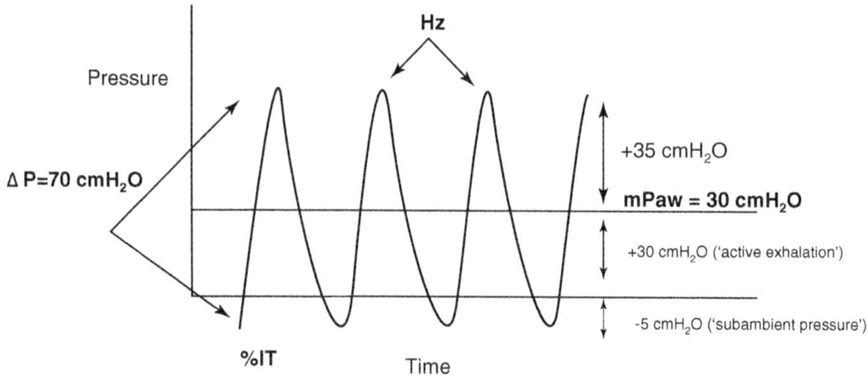

Fig. 4.1 High-frequency pressure wave in the proximal ventilator circuit. Note that both inhalation and exhalation phases are active. The proximal circuit pressure may drop below the ambient pressure if the oscillatory pressure amplitude (ΔP) is more than twice the mean airway pressure (*mPaw*) setting. *IT* inspiratory time (Reproduced with permission from Derdak et al. [3])

atelectrauma (Fig. 4.1). Oxygenation is primarily achieved by increasing mPaw [6]. HFOV became a focus of research, but widespread use was limited by the unavailability of commercial equipment. As the technology gradually evolved and our understanding of the physiology of the acute respiratory distress syndrome (ARDS) improved, HFOV was increasingly used for adult patients with ARDS who did not tolerate conventional ventilation (CV). Currently, its use other than as a "rescue" treatment remains controversial [7, 8].

4.2 Mechanisms of Gas Transport and Exchange

The mechanisms governing gas flow, gas mixing, and pressure transmission during high-frequency oscillatory ventilation (HFOV) are fundamentally different to ventilation at conventional respiratory breathing frequencies. During CV, the main mechanisms of gas exchange are bulk convection and diffusion. During HFOV, there are 5 additional mechanisms of gas exchange, namely, asymmetric velocity profiles, Taylor dispersion and turbulence, cardiogenic mixing, pendelluft effect, and collateral ventilation [4] (Fig. 4.2). A basic understanding of these gas transport mechanisms represents essential background for clinical HFOV use. With the exception of molecular diffusion, all other mechanisms depend on convective fluid motion.

4.2.1 Bulk Convection

Bulk convection is the concerted, collective movement of groups of molecules within fluids. Unlike CV, bulk convection plays a relatively small role in gas transport during HFOV, although it is likely to contribute significantly to ventilatory

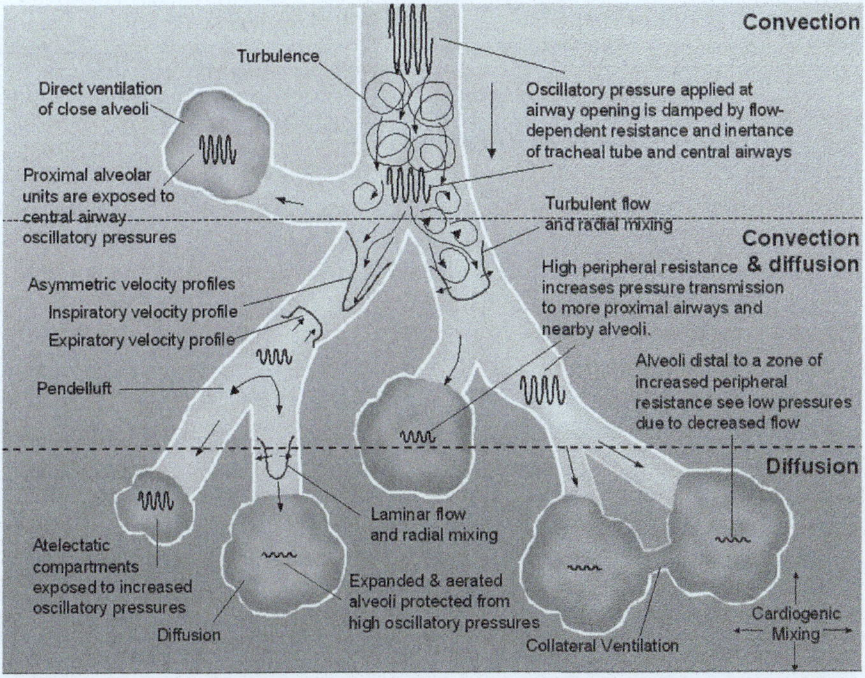

Fig. 4.2 Gas transport mechanisms during high-frequency oscillation. The major gas transport mechanisms that are operative under physiologic conditions within each region are shown (convection, convection and diffusion, diffusion alone). There are seven mechanisms of gas transport during high-frequency oscillation: turbulence in the large airways, causing enhanced mixing; direct ventilation of close alveoli; turbulent flow with lateral convective mixing; pendelluft (asynchronous flow among alveoli due to asymmetries in airflow impedance); gas mixing due to velocity profiles that are axially asymmetric (leading to streaming of gas toward the alveoli along the inner wall of the airway and the streaming of alveolar gas away from the alveoli along the outer wall); laminar flow with lateral transport by diffusion (Taylor dispersion); and collateral ventilation through nonairway connections between neighboring alveoli (Reproduced with permission from Pillow [4])

exchange in the most proximal lung units [4]. Research in animal models showed that decreasing delivered V_t to a level below the HFOV-circuit-related rebreathing volume (as opposed to the larger anatomic dead space) causes a sudden rise in $PaCO_2$. This suggests CO_2 elimination efficiency is dependent on net oscillatory volume and that bulk convection has an essential role during HFOV [9].

4.2.2 Molecular Diffusion

The principal means of gas movement in the alveolar zone is molecular diffusion. In this zone, gas velocities approximate zero as a result of the very high total cross-sectional area, with net gas transport best described by Fick's law. The spontaneous gas particle mixing arising from Brownian motion is likely augmented by the increased turbulence of the gas molecules during HFOV [10].

4.2.3 Asymmetric Velocity Profiles

The gas velocity profile inside large- and middle-size airways is parabolic. The more central particles are propelled faster down the length of the airway, while the peripheral particles diffuse radially, promoting axial gas exchange with expired alveolar gas. This phenomenon is particularly evident at the airway bifurcations. The airway bifurcation phenomenon directs fresh, machine-delivered gas to the alveoli along a cone in the airway center, while exhaled gas moves out of the system along the outer airway wall [11].

4.2.4 Taylor Dispersion

Taylor dispersion is an effect in fluid mechanics in which a shear flow can increase the effective diffusivity of a fluid or gas mixture. In a shearing flow, adjacent layers of fluid move parallel to each other with different speeds. The shear acts to smear out the concentration distribution in the direction of the flow, enhancing the rate at which it spreads in that direction. A semiempiric analysis predicts that the combination of Taylor dispersion and molecular diffusion (augmented dispersion) accounts for almost all gas transport during HFOV [10].

4.2.5 Pendelluft Phenomena

Pendelluft phenomena refer to gas mixing between adjacent alveoli with incongruent time constants. Time-constant inequalities between lung regions may set up bulk convective currents recirculating air between neighboring lung units. In vitro and computational lung models have shown that gas exchange during HFOV may be markedly improved by the interaction of flow between asynchronous neighboring airways resulting from asymmetries in inertance, compliance, or resistance. Asymmetries in inertance and compliance of peripheral airways and lung units are more important determinants of pendelluft than are asymmetries in resistance [12–14].

4.2.6 Cardiogenic Mixing

The superimposition of the rhythmic, strong contractions of the heart may further promote peripheral gas mixing by varying pressure transmission and flow generation within neighboring parenchymal regions. The contribution of cardiogenic oscillation during HFOV has not been quantified. It has been suggested that cardiogenic mixing may account for up to half of the oxygen uptake in the presence of totally apneic respiration [15, 16].

4.2.7 Collateral Ventilation

Collateral ventilation occurring through nonairway connections between neighboring alveoli has also been proposed as an additional mechanism of gas transport during both CV and HFOV. It is thought that this collateral ventilation occurs via the pores of Kohn (discrete holes in walls of adjacent alveoli) and canals of Lambert (accessory connections in the lungs between some bronchioles and their adjacent alveoli). The relatively high resistance of the collateral channels to gas flow is likely to limit the extent to which this mechanism contributes to gas mixing during HFOV [17].

Whereas gas transport is driven by convective fluid motion, the mechanics of the respiratory system are also an important consideration as convective fluid motion is driven by the pressure differences imposed by the chest wall or the ventilator. In this respect, the impedance of the combined ventilator, circuit, tracheal tube, and respiratory system is an important determinant of the efficiency of ventilation during HFOV. Impedance is a global term that encompasses the mechanical properties of elastance (i.e., the reciprocal of compliance), resistance, and the inertance. Although inertance is essentially negligible at conventional breathing frequencies, it assumes a much greater role at higher frequencies and cannot be ignored during HFOV [18].

Studies in both theoretical models and in healthy animals and humans have demonstrated that V_t has a greater effect on gas exchange than frequency during HFOV. As such, ventilation efficiency (Q) may be expressed as:

$$Q = f^a \cdot V_T{}^b$$

The values for a and b in this equation approximate 1 and 2, respectively, although the absolute values may be influenced by other factors such as the shape and complexity of the oscillatory pressure waveform [19, 20].

4.3 Principles of Non-injurious Mechanical Ventilation and HFOV Settings

In ARDS, the principles of any technique of mechanical ventilation should include adequate oxygenation and $PaCO_2$ control, lung protection, and prevention of right ventricular (RV) dysfunction.

4.3.1 Protection of the Lungs

Major mechanisms of ventilator-associated lung injury include increased lung stress and strain [21]. During CV, overall, inspiratory, lung parenchymal stress is reflected by plateau/peak transpulmonary pressure [21, 22]. Strain comprises deformation of the lung parenchyma by the applied distending force and corresponds to the V_t/end-expiratory lung volume ratio [21].

In moderate-to-severe ARDS [23], lung-protective CV with limited lung stress and strain [24, 25] but adequate positive end-expiratory pressure (PEEP) [26] aims at minimizing the probability of barotrauma, volutrauma, atelectrauma, and biotrauma [22]. Barotrauma reflects alveolar overdistention leading to alveolar gas leakage [27]; volutrauma reflects excessive and repetitive mechanical deformation-induced damage to the alveolar capillary membrane, with increased alveolar epithelial and microvascular permeability causing pulmonary edema [28]; atelectrauma reflects distal airway epithelial damage caused by repetitive, expiratory (low-pressure) collapse and inspiratory (high-pressure) reopening [22, 29]; and biotrauma reflects ventilation-induced, lung-parenchymal cell deformation with tissue destruction and amplification of local inflammation being associated with systemic spillover of cytokines and/or bacterial/endotoxin translocation, dysregulation of apoptotic pathways leading to end-organ epithelial cell apoptosis, suppression of the peripheral immune response, and bacterial/endotoxin translocation from the gut [30–32].

During CV, lower V_ts and inspiratory plateau pressures and higher PEEP levels have been associated with improved survival [24–26, 33]. However, the results of a recent mediation analysis suggest that the strongest predictor of survival is the driving pressure defined as V_t/respiratory system compliance, which is equivalent to the difference between plateau pressure and PEEP [34].

Theoretically, HFOV is an ideal mode for lung protection because it may enable ventilation in the "safe," "maximal-respiratory compliance" zone of the volume-pressure curve, thus avoiding both overdistension and derecruitment/atelectasis [35]. Essential prerequisites for this include an "optimal" range of mPaw setting(s) and delivery of small V_ts [2]. Such settings would likely reduce the risk of barotrauma, volutrauma, and atelectrauma.

Current literature lacks randomized clinical trial (RCT) evidence for the superiority of any specific combination of HFOV settings. Theoretically, the risk of HFOV-associated lung injury should increase with increasing HFOV V_t, decreasing frequency, and increasing ΔP and mPaw [3, 36]. HFOV V_t (clinically relevant range, 44–210 mL) increases mainly with decreasing frequency and increasing ΔP, bias flow (from 20 to 30 L/min), and tracheal tube inner diameter [37]. The distal transmission of oscillatory pressure swings (i.e., ΔP) to the alveoli increases with increasing tracheal tube diameter, inspiratory-to-expiratory time ratio, and lung region proximity. Distal ΔP transmission decreases with increasing HFOV frequency, airway resistance, and lung compliance [3, 4, 38]. In the edematous and overdamped, adult ARDS lung, minimal damping of ΔP can be achieved by increasing HFOV frequency above the lung corner frequency [4]. The latter is given by the following equation:

$$\text{Corner frequency} = 1/2\pi \bullet R_L \bullet C_L$$

where R_L = total lung resistance [39] and C_L = lung compliance. In ARDS, the estimated corner frequency level is 3.2 Hz [4].

The placement of a tracheal tube cuff leak augments CO_2 washout around the cuff and may facilitate V_t delivery through the tracheal tube, thus enabling the use of more "protective" settings such as higher frequency and lower ΔP [3]. In the presence of a cuff leak of 3–5 cmH_2O, average mPaw drops of 6 cmH_2O have been observed along tracheal tubes of average inner diameter of 8.0–8.5 mm [39, 40].

Prior RCTs comparing HFOV with CV used initial mPaws of +5 cmH_2O [41–43], or +8–9 cmH_2O relative to pre-HFOV CV [39], or 30 cmH_2O, independently of the mPaw of pre-HFOV CV [44]. Subsequent, protocol-related mPaw adjustments comprised mainly gradual increments or decrements of 2–3 cmH_2O aimed at achieving prespecified oxygenation targets. HFOV frequency, ΔP, use of a tracheal tube cuff leak, and bias flow settings were aimed at maintaining an arterial pH of >7.15 [41], ≥7.20 [39, 42], or ≥7.25 [43, 44]. One study employed additional tracheal gas insufflation (TGI) at a flow rate equal to 50% of the minute ventilation of the pre-HFOV CV [39] to further improve lung recruitment and gas exchange [39, 40, 45–48]; in the same study, HFOV-TGI was used intermittently as extended (i.e., lasting for ≥6 h) and repetitive (according to prespecified oxygenation criteria) lung recruitment sessions aimed at a progressively sustained oxygenation improvement and a rapid reduction of post-intervention CV pressures to non-injurious levels [33]. Two study protocols specified the pre-HFOV use of recruitment maneuvers (RMs) [39, 44], and one study protocol specified the use of frequent RMs, followed by mPaw adjustments titrated according to the achievement of specific oxygenation targets [39]. Lastly, four studies [39, 41, 42, 44] used the Sensormedics 3100B high-frequency ventilator (Sensormedics, Yorba Linda, CA, USA), and one study [43] employed the Novalung R100 ventilator (Metran Co. Ltd., Kawaguchi-shi, Saitama, Japan). Regarding 30-day or in-hospital mortality, three studies did not report any significant differences between HFOV and CV [41–43], one study reported an HFOV-associated harm [44], and the intermittent HFOV-TGI/RMs study reported an experimental intervention-associated benefit [39]. Notably, the control CV strategies differed across the 5 RCTs, mainly with respect to the employed V_t and PEEP settings.

In a randomized study of moderate-to-severe ARDS of mostly pulmonary (i.e., 31/39 patients, 79.5%) etiology, Papazian et al. compared the effects of supine and prone HFOV and prone, lung-protective CV on gas exchange and lung and systemic inflammation [49]. Following an RM, HFOV mPaw was set at +5 cmH_2O relative to baseline, supine CV, and initial HFOV frequency was set at 5 Hz. For $PaCO_2$ control, ΔP could be increased up to 110 cmH_2O, followed by frequency decrease to 4 Hz and placement of a tracheal tube cuff leak. Prone HFOV and prone CV resulted in similar oxygenation improvements relative to baseline CV. However, prone HFOV increased bronchoalveolar lavage fluid (BALF) interleukin (IL)-8 relative to both baseline and prone CV. Supine HFOV did not affect oxygenation relative to baseline CV but increased BALF IL-8 and neutrophil count relative to both baseline and prone CV. The authors attributed their negative for HFOV results to a possible inability of reopening of consolidated lung tissue, in conjunction with higher lung stress, which could be amplified at the boundaries of collapsed and expanding lung units [50]. Notably, in an observational study of supine HFOV employing an initial, slow RM followed by similar settings of mPaw (i.e., +5 cmH_2O relative to pre-HFOV CV) and frequency (i.e., 5 Hz), Camporota et al. reported that an early, favorable oxygenation response to HFOV was the strongest predictor of 30-day survival [51]. The favorable oxygenation response was likely due to lung recruitment and was defined as >38% increase in PaO_2/inspired O_2 fraction (FiO_2) relative to pre-HFOV CV within 72 h of HFOV initiation. $PaCO_2$ control was also improved in survivors vs. non-survivors. Collectively, these results are consistent with the hypothesis that HFOV might confer benefit mainly to moderate-to-severe ARDS patients with a higher percentage of potentially recruitable lung [52]. Such patients also exhibit a favorable response to high CV PEEP levels [52].

A protocol of very high-frequency HFOV (i.e., >6 Hz up to 12 Hz) employing ΔP of ≤90 cmH_2O and/or a 5-cmH_2O tracheal tube cuff leak for $PaCO_2$ control has been previously proposed and applied [53]. While still on lung-protective CV, the 30 studied patients had a pre-HFOV PaO_2/FiO_2 of 78 mmHg at a mean PEEP/FiO_2 level of 13 cmH_2O/0.93 (respectively). Within the first 2 days of HFOV initiation, HFOV frequency could be, respectively, maintained at ≥5 and ≥8 Hz in 25/30 and 22/30 patients, with an arterial pH of ≥7.23 [53]. Administered HFOV V_ts were low (i.e., within ~58–156 mL), but as in CV-treated, severe ARDS subgroups [54], in-hospital mortality exceeded 60% [53].

In a recent review [55], Dreyfuss et al. summarized their concerns about HFOV-induced lung injury in adult ARDS. They argued that:

1. Adult ARDS is more heterogeneous and less recruitable compared to animal models of saline lavage/surfactant deficiency where HFOV has been previously tested [56–62].
2. HFOV-induced static overdistension due to high mPaw may generate lung injury, also through increasing alveolar microvascular and epithelial permeability [63].
3. The high ventilation frequency may potentially raise cell and lung parenchyma stress to injurious levels [64]; in addition, the high-frequency agitation of edema fluid may lead to frequent generation and disruption of foam, which can generate deleterious mechanical forces causing epithelial cell injury [65].
4. High-frequency distal transmission of ΔP may correspond to the delivery of high and potentially "injurious" energy to the lung parenchyma.
5. Energy delivery to the lung parenchyma may be maximized as HFOV frequency approaches lung resonant frequency [66].

In the accompanying editorial [67], Marini agreed with the need to not exceed a lung-distending pressure threshold above which cellular injury, microvascular permeability, and local inflammation exhibit a nonlinear rise [68, 69]. However, he also argued that even for the HFOV RCT that employed the highest mPaw settings [44], it still remains unknown whether tissue tensions, transpulmonary pressures, and distally delivered power were actually injurious to the lungs. Importantly, in both papers [55, 67], major concerns were also expressed about the possibly detrimental effect of combined high mPaw and hypercapnea on the function of the right ventricle (RV; see also below).

Regarding the static overdistension concern, it should be noted that HFOV-TGI with cuff leak employing mPaws of +6–8 cmH_2O relative to preceding, lung-protective CV has resulted in 10% lower extravascular lung water index compared with preceding CV [48]. The rest of the above concerns can be addressed by:

1. Limiting HFOV use to ARDS patients with higher lung recruitability [52] – such patients have poorer oxygenation and in-hospital outcomes compared with patients with lower lung recruitability [52].
2. Using RMs as part of HFOV protocols to expedite lung recruitment and enable the prompt downward titration of an initially relatively high mPaw while still maintaining the recruitment-induced improvements in gas exchange [39].
3. Employing a cuff leak to minimize distal transmission of ΔP [3, 39].
4. Combining cuff leak, high bias flow (i.e., 40–60 L/min), and relatively low frequency (e.g., 3.5–5.0 Hz) with or without superimposed TGI as required to augment $PaCO_2$ clearance and prevent excessive hypercapnia [39, 40, 45–48]; notably, at an inspiratory-to-expiratory ratio of 33%, the associated V_ts of ~150–210 mL [37, 40] should still be considered as lung protective.
5. Avoiding frequencies that are close to 8.6 Hz, i.e., the estimated resonant frequency for the adult ARDS lung [4]; notably, as HFOV frequency approaches lung resonance frequency, gas transport becomes increasingly dependent on resistive [4, 70], inertive [4, 71], and branching angle properties of the central airways [4, 72, 73], and according to theoretical studies, compliant alveoli are spared from excessive oscillatory pressures with the larger alveolar pressure swings being directed to less compliant lung units [4, 38].
6. Considering intermittent HFOV use according to sustained or non-sustained reversal of (solely) severe oxygenation disturbances [39].

4.3.2 Protection of the RV

In 1998, Monchi et al. showed that RV dysfunction is an independent predictor of death in ARDS [74]. The high PEEP of lung-protective conventional ventilation increases RV afterload and can result in leftward shift of the interventricular septum and inversion of the RV to left ventricle (LV) end-systolic gradient [75, 76]. The combination of high PEEP and acute hypercapnia can impair RV function and cause RV dilatation [77] (Fig. 4.3). Acute cor pulmonale (ACP) has been defined as septal dyskinesia with a dilated RV [end-diastolic RV/LV area ratio >0.6, or >0.9–1.0 in severe cases] [79, 80]. The potential clinical significance of ACP has been emphasized by several reviews published within the past decade [76, 81–84]. The association of severe ACP and mortality been confirmed by a recent, large prospective, observational study of lung-protective ventilation in moderate-to-severe ARDS [80]. ACP and severe ACP prevalence, respectively, amounted to 22 and 7%. ACP independent predictors were low V_ts (<7 mL/kg) and respiratory compliance (<30 mL/cmH_2O), high respiratory rates (≥30 breaths/min), plateau pressures (≥27 cmH_2O), driving pressures (≥18 cmH_2O), and moderate-to-severe oxygenation disturbances

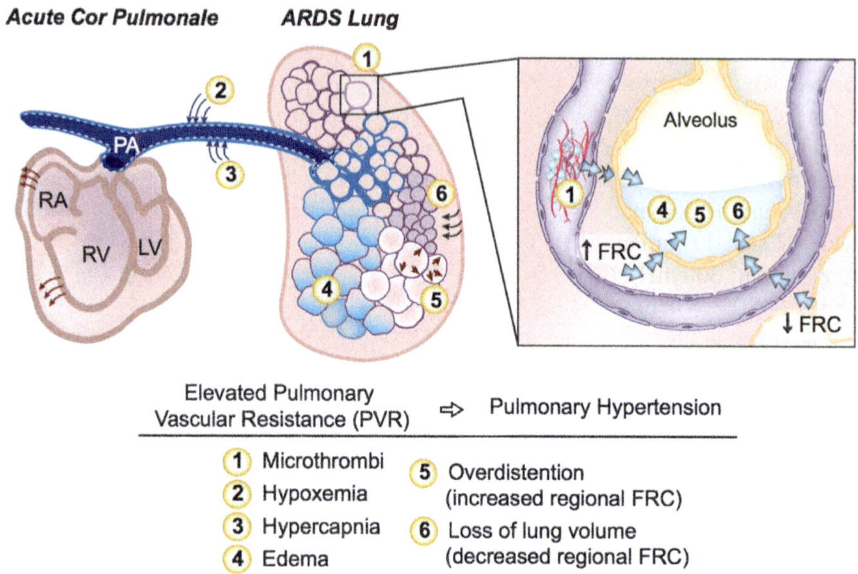

Fig. 4.3 Pathophysiological mechanisms of increased pulmonary vascular resistance (*PVR*) and pulmonary hypertension in moderate-to-severe acute respiratory distress syndrome (*ARDS*). *FRC* functional residual capacity (Reproduced with permission from Guérin and Mattha [78])

(PaO_2/FiO_2 <150 mmHg) and hypercapnia ($PaCO_2$ ≥48 mmHg) [80]. ACP underlying pathophysiology includes pulmonary vascular dysfunction [i.e., >12 mmHg difference between mean pulmonary artery pressure and pulmonary artery occlusion pressure]; pulmonary vascular dysfunction has also been associated with adverse outcomes in ARDS, including mortality [85].

In a transesophageal echocardiographic study of 16 patients with moderate-to-severe and mainly pulmonary ARDS [79], Guervilly et al. evaluated the RV effect of HFOV mPaws of +5, +10, and +15 cmH_2O relative to preceding, lung-protective CV. HFOV frequency of 4–5 Hz and ΔP of ≤110 cmH_2O were adjusted to maintain $PaCO_2$ unchanged throughout the study period. Bias flow was set at 40 L/min and there was no cuff leak use. At baseline CV, 9/16 patients had RV dysfunction [defined as RV end-diastolic area (EDSA)-to LVEDSA ratio of >0.6], and 4/16 patients had RV failure (defined as RVEDSA/LVEDSA ratio of 0.9). HFOV mPaws of +10 and +15 cmH_2O increased the RVEDSA/LVEDSA ratio by 40%, the end-diastolic eccentricity index by 30%, and decreased pulmonary acceleration time [86] by ~25%. Relative to baseline CV, at HFOV mPaws of +10 and +15 cmH_2O, RV dysfunction or failure respectively occurred in an additional 3–6 or 2–5 patients. In patients with RVEDSA/LVEDSA ratio increase of >40%, cardiac index decreased by ~21% and pulmonary vascular resistance index by ~65%. HFOV did not significantly affect oxygenation. However, electrical impedance tomography revealed that in patients without RVEDSA/LVEDSA ratio increase of >40%, HFOV was associated with redistribution of ventilation to the posterior lung while mPaw was increased. The authors concluded that RV function should be monitored during HFOV and that high mPaw-associated overinflation of the anterior lung may predispose to RV dysfunction.

In an observational, physiological study of 24 patients fulfilling prespecified criteria for CV treatment-refractory ARDS [87], Ursulet et al. employed transthoracic echocardiography and pulsatility index continuous cardiac output (PICCO) to study the RV and hemodynamic effects of a 3-h HFOV session. HFOV initial settings were FiO_2 of 1.0, mPaw of +10 cmH_2O relative to preceding, lung-protective CV (upper limit: 30 cmH_2O), frequency of 6 Hz, bias flow of 40 L/min, and oscillator power of 80%. There was no cuff leak use. Frequency and ΔP were subsequently titrated to maintain an arterial pH of >7.25 and a $PaCO_2$ of <55 mmHg. HFOV-induced hemodynamic failure (i.e., >30% decrease in systolic arterial pressure or cardiac index relative to baseline CV) occurred in 3/34 patients. HFOV resulted in an average increase of 14% in the RVEDSA/LVEDSA ratio and an average decrease of 11% in cardiac index. RVEDSA/LVEDSA during baseline CV correlated significantly with HFOV-induced changes in cardiac index ($r = -.78$, $p < 0.001$). Pre-HFOV RV dysfunction (i.e., RVEDSA/LVEDSA >0.6) could predict an HFOV-induced decrease in cardiac index of >15% with a sensitivity of 80% and a specificity of 79%. RV dysfunction was confirmed in 11/24 patients during baseline CV and in an additional 6/24 patients during HFOV. Notably, the high HFOV mPaw had no effect on extravascular lung water index or pulmonary vascular permeability index. During the 3-h study period, PaO_2/FiO_2 improved by >30% in 18/24 patients and by >100% in 11/24 patients. The authors concluded that the RVEDSA/LVEDSA ratio during lung-protective CV may be used as a predictor of hemodynamic intolerance to subsequent HFOV.

In the context of 5 physiological studies [40, 45–48] and an RCT [39], we employed our HFOV-TGI/RMs technique in a total of 137 patients. This ventilatory technique consistently resulted in substantial gas exchange benefit without any evidence of hemodynamic compromise (e.g., cardiac index reduction or hypotension) as compared with lung-protective CV. In the RCT [39], HFOV-TGI/RMs was applied intermittently (average use during days 1–10 postrandomization, 11.2 h) and was interspersed with lung-protective CV; experimental intervention goal comprised reversal of severe oxygenation disturbances (defined as PaO_2/FiO_2 of <150 mmHg at PEEP ≥8 cmH_2O) through lung recruitment and lower/non-injurious ventilation pressures [33] during post-HFOV CV compared with pre-HFOV CV [39]. Lastly, we also successfully applied HFO-TGI/RMs as rescue ventilation in patients with severe ARDS [23] and traumatic brain injury [47].

Possible mechanisms contributing to hemodynamic stability during HFOV-TGI include (1) recruitment of dependent lung units with the addition of TGI to HFO [46] (Fig. 4.4), which may decrease pulmonary vascular resistance and reduce the risk of right ventricular dysfunction [48, 79], and (2) enhanced CO_2 elimination with the use of TGI, cuff leak, and high bias flows of 30–60 L/min, hence further protecting the RV [48, 77]. Moreover, the intermittent use of HFOV-TGI may have prevented long-term HFOV-related adverse effects [39, 40, 45]. In none of our studies was there a need for increasing intravenous fluid and/or vasopressor support [44]

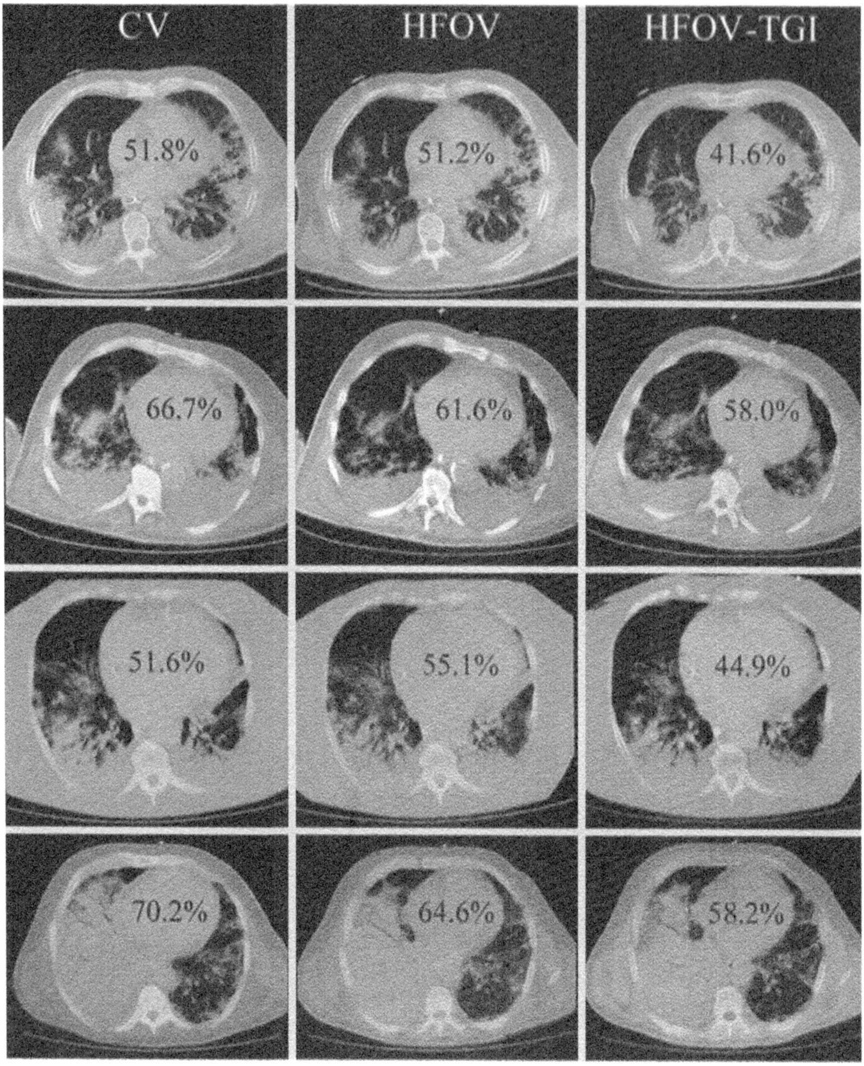

Fig. 4.4 Comparative presentation of scanographic data corresponding to conventional ventilation (*CV*), high-frequency oscillatory ventilation (*HFOV*), and HFOV-tracheal gas insufflations (TGI). Computed tomography (*CT*) sections of the lower lung from four representative patients (1–4). CT sections correspond to approximately 7 cm below the carina. In patients 1 and 3, HFOV preceded HFOV-TGI. In patients 2 and 4, HFOV-TGI preceded HFO. Percentages reflect proportions of nonaerated lung tissue weight (Reproduced with permission from Mentzelopoulos et al. [46])

during HFOV-TGI vs. CV. Nevertheless, we do endorse the recommendation of Vieillard-Baron et al. for echocardiographic monitoring of RV function and adaptation of the mechanical ventilation pressures according to the prevention or reversal of RV dysfunction [88].

4.4 Complications of HFOV

Potential HFOV-induced complications include barotrauma and hemodynamic compromise, i.e., hypotension, increased pulmonary vascular resistance and decreased venous return contributing to RV dysfunction and reduction of cardiac index, desiccation of secretions leading to mucous inspissation and tracheal tube obstruction, increased sedation and/or neuromuscular blockade requirements potentially predisposing to need for prolonged mechanical ventilation and/or critical illness polyneuropathy, and risk of aerosolization of infectious droplets due to lack of an approved expiratory filter for the high-frequency ventilator [3, 39, 41–44, 79, 87–93].

The cumulative, RCT-reported incidence of frequent and serious complications such as barotrauma and hemodynamic compromise does not significantly differ between HFOV and CV. Indeed, in recent meta-analyses of RCTs that compared HFOV to CV, the reported risk ratios for barotraumas during HFOV vs. CV ranged within 1.17–1.21, and the corresponding 95% confidence intervals ranged within 0.83–1.74 [94–97]. Accordingly, the reported risk ratios for hypotension during HFOV vs. CV ranged within 1.16–1.33, and corresponding 95% confidence intervals ranged within 0.27–6.48 [94–97].

Regarding tension pneumothorax, clinicians should keep in mind that its recognition is challenging during HFOV [89]. Auscultation of breath sounds is not helpful [89]. Initial clinical signs may include hypotension or hypoxemia, without concurrent change in ventilator-displayed mPaw and ΔP, or alarm activation [3, 55, 89]; a new or worsening air leak may actually cause a drop in mPaw, without concurrent change in ΔP [3]. Subsequently, a reduction or asymmetry in the body wiggle, in response to HFOV pressure waves, or a rise in ΔP may be noted [89]. Mucous plugging of the tracheal tube may also manifest as hypoxemia and/or acute hypercapnia and concurrent ΔP rise [3, 89]; adequate humidification of inspired gases is essential for the prevention of this relatively rare complication [89]. An acute rise in ΔP can also be caused by an inadvertent tracheal tube migration into the right main stem bronchus or a rise in airway resistance [3].

4.5 Adjunctive Therapies to HFOV

The addition of a continuous, forward thrust TGI flow of 6–7 L/min to "low (i.e., 3.5–5.5 Hz)"-frequency HFOV with a cuff leak has been associated with improved gas exchange vs. both standard HFOV and lung-protective CV without any concurrent, adverse hemodynamic effect [39, 40, 45–48]. Daily 12-h sessions of "low (i.e., 3.5 Hz)"-frequency HFOV-TGI have been successfully used for rescue oxygenation of patients with severe ARDS and traumatic brain injury [23, 47]. When added to HFOV with a cuff leak, continuous, forward thrust TGI augments the washout of anatomic dead space, generates an additional expiratory flow resistance or "PEEP-like effect," promotes recruitment of dependent lung regions, and may also enhance molecular diffusion of oxygen to distal lung units [39, 40, 45–48, 98]. Limitations of long-term TGI include lack of commercially available equipment and possible tracheal mucosal damage, retention and inspissation of secretions, hemodynamic compromise, pneumothorax, and gas embolism [39, 40, 45, 99]. Humidification of TGI gas and cuff leak during HFO-TGI are essential [40].

Other adjunctive therapies previously combined with HFOV to improve gas exchange include prone positioning and inhaled nitric oxide. In a randomized, physiological study of moderate-to-severe ARDS [23], supine HFOV after prone positioning resulted in maintenance of pronation-induced improvements in PaO_2/FiO_2 and shunt fraction; this was not achieved when pronation was followed by supine CV [100]. Effective prevention of elsewhere-detailed complications of prone position [101] requires specific personnel experience and training [102]. In an uncontrolled, physiological study of severe ARDS [23], the administration of 5–20 parts per million of inhaled nitric oxide during HFOV resulted in a PaO_2/FiO_2 rise of ≥20% (average rise, 38%) [103]. Limitations of inhaled nitric oxide pertain to the formation of reactive nitrogen species [104].

4.6 Clinical Evidence for the Use of HFOV

A meta-analysis of eight RCTs of HFOV vs. CV performed either in children (n = 2) or in adults (n = 6) with acute lung injury/ARDS suggested that HFOV is unlikely to cause harm and may improve survival [105]. Notably, in 3 of the included adult RCTs, control patients were not treated with low V_t, lung-protective CV [2, 44]. The results of this meta-analysis were refuted by the 2 recent, large, multicenter RCTs that showed either neutral results [43] or HFOV-associated harm [44]. However, it should also be recognized that the latter study's control arm may have actually received a very effective high-PEEP, low-V_t CV treatment based on decades of extensive, pertinent laboratory and clinical research, including 9 RCTs of "protective" vs. "non-protective" CV settings in ARDS [34]. In contrast, the employed, "lung-protective" but potentially "RV stressing" HFOV protocol [55, 67, 79, 87] was based (at least partly) on an expert consensus [36] reached according to the results of mainly laboratory HFOV data, uncontrolled clinical HFOV studies, and just 2 small (one completed and one prematurely stopped) RCTs of HFOV vs. CV in ARDS [36, 41, 42, 89].

Our favorable RCT results on the intermittent use of "low"-frequency HFOV-TGI with cuff leak and RMs are encouraging [39]. However, our study's sample size was small (n = 125), the study was unblinded, results originated from just 2 centers, the study was conducted in 2 periods for reasons of feasibility, and CV group mortality of 64.1% was high [39]; the latter was justifiable by baseline disease severity which was similar in the control and intervention groups and was also comparable to contemporarily reported outcomes of severe ARDS [39, 54]. Nevertheless, according to these arguments, the external validity of these results [39] still requires further multicenter and multinational confirmation.

Recently published meta-analyses of RCTs comparing HFOV with CV in ARDS have reported inconclusive results [93–97]. The publication of the results of an individual patient data-based meta-analysis of the 4 prior RCTs of continuous HFOV vs. CV [41–44] is awaited. The main objective of this methodologically advantageous [106] meta-analysis is to identify ARDS patient subgroup(s) that could benefit from HFOV.

Conclusions Despite a strong physiological background suggesting prevention of ventilator-associated lung injury, current clinical evidence does not support the routine use of standard and continuous (as opposed to intermittent) HFOV in ARDS. HFOV may be associated with concurrent high intrathoracic pressures and hypercapnia, and this may cause RV dysfunction and impact patient outcomes. Therefore, it may be prudent to adjust HFOV settings according to echocardiographic monitoring data. The potential clinical usefulness of intermittent HFOV-TGI warrants further RCT confirmation. However, even if any supine HFOV/adjunct strategy ultimately proves superior to supine, high-PEEP, low-V_t CV [44], it may still be unlikely to prove superior to prone, lung-protective CV [102]. Nevertheless, progress might still be achievable through an optimal combination [100] of these physiologically sound [39, 107] strategies.

References

1. Slutsky AS, Drazen JM (2002) Ventilation with small tidal volumes. N Engl J Med 347:630–631
2. Goffi A, Ferguson ND (2014) High-frequency oscillatory ventilation for early acute respiratory distress syndrome in adults. Curr Opin Crit Care 20:77–85
3. Derdak S (2003) High-frequency oscillatory ventilation for acute respiratory distress syndrome in adult patients. Crit Care Med 31(Suppl):S317–S323
4. Pillow JJ (2005) High frequency oscillatory ventilation: Mechanisms of gas exchange and lung mechanics. Crit Care Med 33(suppl):S135–S141
5. Bohn DJ, Miyasaka K, Marchak BE, Thompson WK, Froese AB, Bryan AC (1980) Ventilation by high frequency oscillation. J Appl Physiol 48:710–716
6. Brazelton TV, Watson WF, Murphy M, Al-Khandra E, Thompson JE, Arnold JH (2001) Identification of optimal lung volume during high-frequency oscillatory ventilation using respiratory inductive plethysmography. Crit Care Med 29:2349–2359
7. Mehta S, Granton J, MacDonald RJ, Bowman D, Matte-Martyn A, Bachman T, Smith T, Stewart TE (2004) High-frequency oscillatory ventilation in adults: the Toronto experience. Chest 126:518–527
8. Malhotra A, Drazen JM (2013) High-frequency oscillatory ventilation on shaky ground. N Engl J Med 368:863–865
9. Spahn DR, Leuthold R, Schmid ER, Niederer PF (1991) Significance of bulk convection during high frequency oscillation. Respir Physiol 84:1–11
10. Fredberg JJ (1980) Augmented diffusion in the airways can support pulmonary gas exchange. J Appl Physiol 49:446–448
11. Haselton FR, Scherer PW (1980) Bronchial bifurcations and respiratory mass transport. Science 208:69–71
12. Ultman JS, Shaw RG, Fabiano DC, Cooke KA (1988) Pendelluft and mixing in a single bifurcation lung model during high-frequency oscillation. J Appl Physiol 65:146–155
13. Tanida Y (1990) Analysis of gas transport in high frequency ventilation. Front Med Biol Eng 2:181–185

14. High KC, Ultman JS, Karl SR (1991) Mechanically induced pendelluft flow in a model airway bifurcation during high frequency oscillation. J Biomech Eng 113:342–347
15. Slutsky AS (1981) Gas mixing by cardiogenic oscillations: a theoretical quantitative analysis. J Appl Physiol 51:1287–1293
16. Slutsky AS, Brown R (1982) Cardiogenic oscillations: a potential mechanism enhancing oxygenation during apneic respiration. Med Hypotheses 8:393–400
17. Armengol J, Jones RL, King EG (1985) Collateral ventilation during high-frequency oscillation in dogs. J Appl Physiol 58:173–179
18. Venegas JG, Fredberg JJ (1994) Understanding the pressure cost of ventilation: why does high frequency ventilation work? Crit Care Med 22:S49–S57
19. Rossing TH, Slutsky AS, Lehr JL, Drinker PA, Kamm R, Drazen JM (1981) Tidal volume and frequency dependence of carbon dioxide elimination by high-frequency ventilation. N Engl J Med 305:1375–1379
20. Jaeger MJ, Kurzweg UH, Banner MJ (1984) Transport of gases in high-frequency ventilation. Crit Care Med 12:708–710
21. Gattinoni L, Carlesso E, Cadringher P, Valenza F, Vagginelli F, Chiumello D (2003) Physical and biological triggers of ventilator-induced lung injury and its prevention. Eur Respir J 47(Suppl):15s–25s
22. Slutsky AS (1999) Lung injury caused by mechanical ventilation. Chest 116(1 Suppl):9S–15S
23. Definition Task Force ARDS, Ranieri VM, Rubenfeld GD, Thompson BT, Ferguson ND, Caldwell E, Fan E, Camporota L, Slutsky AS (2012) Acute respiratory distress syndrome: the Berlin Definition. JAMA 307:2526–2533
24. Amato MB, Barbas CS, Medeiros DM, Magaldi RB, Schettino GP, Lorenzi-Filho G, Kairalla RA, Deheinzelin D, Munoz C, Oliveira R, Takagaki TY, Carvalho CR (1998) Effect of a protective-ventilation strategy on mortality in the acute respiratory distress syndrome. N Engl J Med 338:347–354
25. [No authors listed] (2000) Ventilation with lower tidal volumes as compared with traditional tidal volumes for acute lung injury and the acute respiratory distress syndrome. The Acute Respiratory Distress Syndrome Network. N Engl J Med 342:1301–1318
26. Briel M, Meade M, Mercat A, Brower RG, Talmor D, Walter SD, Slutsky AS, Pullenayegum E, Zhou Q, Cook D, Brochard L, Richard JC, Lamontagne F, Bhatnagar N, Stewart TE, Guyatt G (2010) Higher vs lower positive end-expiratory pressure in patients with acute lung injury and acute respiratory distress syndrome: systematic review and meta-analysis. JAMA 303:865–873
27. Macklin CC (1939) Transport of air along sheaths of pulmonic blood vessels from alveoli to mediastinum. Arch Intern Med 64:913–926
28. Dreyfuss D, Soler P, Basset G, Saumon G (1988) High inflation pressure pulmonary edema: respective effects of high airway pressure, high tidal volume, and positive end-expiratory pressure. Am Rev Respir Dis 137:1159–1164
29. Yalcin HC, Perry SF, Ghadiali SN (2007) Influence of airway diameter and cell confluence on epithelial cell injury in an in vitro model of airway reopening. J Appl Physiol 103:1796–1807
30. Ranieri VM, Suter PM, Tortorella C, De Tullio R, Dayer JM, Brienza A, Bruno F, Slutsky AS (1999) Effect of mechanical ventilation on inflammatory mediators in patients with acute respiratory distress syndrome: a randomized controlled trial. JAMA 282:54–61
31. Imai Y, Parodo J, Kajikawa O, de Perrot M, Fischer S, Edwards V, Cutz E, Liu M, Keshavjee S, Martin TR, Marshall JC, Ranieri VM, Slutsky AS (2003) Injurious mechanical ventilation and end-organ epithelial cell apoptosis and organ dysfunction in an experimental model of acute respiratory distress syndrome. JAMA 289:2104–2112
32. Plötz FB, Slutsky AS, van Vught AJ, Heijnen CJ (2004) Ventilator-induced lung injury and multiple system organ failure: a critical review of facts and hypotheses. Intensive Care Med 30:1865–1872

33. Hager DN, Krishnan JA, Hayden DL, Brower RG, Clinical Trials Network ARDS (2005) Tidal volume reduction in patients with acute lung injury when plateau pressures are not high. Am J Respir Crit Care Med 172:1241–1245
34. Amato MB, Meade MO, Slutsky AS, Brochard L, Costa EL, Schoenfeld DA, Stewart TE, Briel M, Talmor D, Mercat A, Richard JC, Carvalho CR, Brower RG (2015) Driving pressure and survival in the acute respiratory distress syndrome. N Engl J Med 372:747–755
35. Froese AB (1997) High-frequency oscillatory ventilation for adult respiratory distress syndrome: let's get it right this time! Crit Care Med 25:906–908
36. Fessler HE, Derdak S, Ferguson ND, Hager DN, Kacmarek RM, Thompson BT, Brower RG (2007) A protocol for high-frequency oscillatory ventilation in adults: results from a roundtable discussion. Crit Care Med 35:1649–1654
37. Hager DN, Fessler HE, Kaczka DW, Shanholtz CB, Fuld MK, Simon BA, Brower RG (2007) Tidal volume delivery during high-frequency oscillatory ventilation in adults with acute respiratory distress syndrome. Crit Care Med 35:1522–1529
38. Pillow JJ, Sly PD, Hantos Z, Bates JH (2002) Dependence of intrapulmonary pressure amplitudes on respiratory mechanics during high-frequency oscillatory ventilation in preterm lambs. Pediatr Res 52:538–544
39. Mentzelopoulos SD, Malachias S, Zintzaras E, Kokkoris S, Zakynthinos E, Makris D, Magira E, Markaki V, Roussos C, Zakynthinos SG (2012) Intermittent recruitment with high-frequency oscillation/tracheal gas insufflation in acute respiratory distress syndrome. Eur Respir J 39:635–647
40. Mentzelopoulos SD, Malachias S, Kokkoris S, Roussos C, Zakynthinos SG (2010) Comparison of high-frequency oscillation and tracheal gas insufflation versus standard high-frequency oscillation at two levels of tracheal pressure. Intensive Care Med 36:810–816
41. Derdak S, Mehta S, Stewart TE, Smith T, Rogers M, Buchman TG, Carlin B, Lowson S, Granton J, Multicenter Oscillatory Ventilation For Acute Respiratory Distress Syndrome Trial (MOAT) Study Investigators (2002) High-frequency oscillatory ventilation for acute respiratory distress syndrome in adults: a randomized, controlled trial. Am J Respir Crit Care Med 166:801–808
42. Bollen CW, van Well GT, Sherry T, Beale RJ, Shah S, Findlay G, Monchi M, Chiche JD, Weiler N, Uiterwaal CS, van Vught AJ (2005) High frequency oscillatory ventilation compared with conventional mechanical ventilation in adult respiratory distress syndrome: a randomized controlled trial [ISRCTN24242669]. Crit Care 9:R430–R439
43. Young D, Lamb SE, Shah S, MacKenzie I, Tunnicliffe W, Lall R, Rowan K, Cuthbertson BH, OSCAR Study Group (2013) High-frequency oscillation for acute respiratory distress syndrome. N Engl J Med 368:806–813
44. Ferguson ND, Cook DJ, Guyatt GH, Mehta S, Hand L, Austin P, Zhou Q, Matte A, Walter SD, Lamontagne F, Granton JT, Arabi YM, Arroliga AC, Stewart TE, Slutsky AS, Meade MO, OSCILLATE Trial Investigators; Canadian Critical Care Trials Group (2013) High-frequency oscillation in early acute respiratory distress syndrome. N Engl J Med 368:795–805
45. Mentzelopoulos SD, Roussos C, Koutsoukou A, Sourlas S, Malachias S, Lachana A, Zakynthinos SG (2007) Acute effects of combined high-frequency oscillation and tracheal gas insufflation in severe acute respiratory distress syndrome. Crit Care Med 35:1500–1508
46. Mentzelopoulos SD, Theodoridou M, Malachias S, Sourlas S, Exarchos DN, Chondros D, Roussos C, Zakynthinos SG (2011) Scanographic comparison of high frequency oscillation with versus without tracheal gas insufflation in acute respiratory distress syndrome. Intensive Care Med 37:990–999
47. Vrettou CS, Zakynthinos SG, Malachias S, Mentzelopoulos SD (2013) High-frequency oscillation and tracheal gas insufflation in patients with severe acute respiratory distress syndrome and traumatic brain injury: an interventional physiological study. Crit Care 17:R136
48. Vrettou CS, Zakynthinos SG, Malachias S, Mentzelopoulos SD (2014) The effect of high-frequency oscillatory ventilation combined with tracheal gas insufflation on extravascular

lung water in patients with acute respiratory distress syndrome: a randomized, crossover, physiologic study. J Crit Care 29:568–573

49. Papazian L, Gainnier M, Marin V, Donati S, Arnal JM, Demory D, Roch A, Forel JM, Bongrand P, Brégeon F, Sainty JM (2005) Comparison of prone positioning and high-frequency oscillatory ventilation in patients with acute respiratory distress syndrome. Crit Care Med 33:2162–2171
50. Mead J, Takishima T, Leith D (1970) Stress distribution in lungs: a model of pulmonary elasticity. J Appl Physiol 28:596–608
51. Camporota L, Sherry T, Smith J, Lei K, McLuckie A, Beale R (2013) Physiological predictors of survival during high-frequency oscillatory ventilation in adults with acute respiratory distress syndrome. Crit Care 17:R40
52. Gattinoni L, Caironi P, Cressoni M, Chiumello D, Ranieri VM, Quintel M, Russo S, Patroniti N, Cornejo R, Bugedo G (2006) Lung recruitment in patients with the acute respiratory distress syndrome. N Engl J Med 354:1775–1786
53. Fessler HE, Hager DN, Brower RG (2008) Feasibility of very high-frequency ventilation in adults with acute respiratory distress syndrome. Crit Care Med 36:1043–1048
54. Taccone P, Pesenti A, Latini R, Polli F, Vagginelli F, Mietto C, Caspani L, Raimondi F, Bordone G, Iapichino G, Mancebo J, Guérin C, Ayzac L, Blanch L, Fumagalli R, Tognoni G, Gattinoni L, Prone-Supine II Study Group (2009) Prone positioning in patients with moderate and severe acute respiratory distress syndrome: a randomized controlled trial. JAMA 302:1977–1984
55. Dreyfuss D, Ricard JD, Gaudry S (2015) Did studies on HFOV fail to improve ARDS survival because they did not decrease VILI? On the potential validity of a physiological concept enounced several decades ago. Intensive Care Med 41:2076–2086
56. Hamilton PP, Onayemi A, Smyth JA, Gillan JE, Cutz E, Froese AB, Bryan AC (1983) Comparison of conventional and high frequency ventilation. J Appl Physiol 55:131–138
57. McCulloch PR, Forkert PG, Froese AB (1988) Lung volume maintenance prevents lung injury during high-frequency ventilation in surfactant-depleted rabbits. Am Rev Respir Dis 137:1185–1192
58. Meredith KS, deLemos RA, Coalson JJ, King RJ, Gerstmann DR, Kumar R, Kuehl TJ, Winter DC, Taylor A, Clark RH et al (1989) Role of lung injury in the pathogenesis of hyaline membrane disease in premature baboons. J Appl Physiol 66:2150–2158
59. Matsuoka T, Kawano T, Miyasaka K (1994) Role of high-frequency ventilation in surfactant-depleted lung injury as measured by granulocytes. J Appl Physiol 79:539–544
60. Imai Y, Kawano T, Miyasaka K, Takata M, Imai T, Okuyama K (1994) Inflammatory chemical mediators during conventional ventilation and high frequency oscillatory ventilation. Am J Respir Crit Care Med 150:1550–1554
61. Takata M, Abe J, Tanaka H, Kitano Y, Doi S, Kohsaka T, Miyasaka K (1997) Intraalveolar expression of tumor necrosis factor-alpha gene during conventional and high frequency ventilation. Am J Respir Crit Care Med 156:272–279
62. von der Hardt K, Kandler MA, Fink L, Schoof E, Dötsch J, Brandenstein O, Bohle RM, Rascher W (2004). High frequency ventilation suppresses inflammatory response in lung tissue and microdissected alveolar macrophages in surfactant depleted piglets. Pediatr Res 55:339–346
63. de Prost N, Dreyfuss D, Saumon G (2007) Evaluation of two-way protein fluxes across the alveolo-capillary membrane by scintigraphy in rats: effect of lung inflation. J Appl Physiol 102:794–802
64. Fabry B, Maksym GN, Butler JP, Glogauer M, Navajas D, Fredberg JJ (2001) Scaling the microrheology of living cells. Phys Rev Lett 87:148102
65. Huh D, Fujioka H, Tung YC, Futai N, Paine R 3rd, Grotberg JB, Takayama S (2007) Acoustically detectable cellular-level lung injury induced by fluid mechanical stresses in microfluidic airway systems. Proc Natl Acad Sci U S A 104:18886–188891
66. Brusasco V, Beck KC, Crawford M, Rehder K (1986) Resonant amplification of delivered volume during high-frequency ventilation. J Appl Physiol 60:885–892
67. Marini JJ (2015) Does high-pressure, high-frequency oscillation shake the foundations of lung protection? Intensive Care Med 41:2210–2212

68. Vlahakis NE, Hubmayr RD (2005) Cellular stress failure in ventilator-injured lungs. Am J Respir Crit Care Med 171:1328–1342
69. Protti A, Cressoni M, Santini A, Langer T, Mietto C, Febres D, Chierichetti M, Coppola S, Conte G, Gatti S, Leopardi O, Masson S, Lombardi L, Lazzerini M, Rampoldi E, Cadringher P, Gattinoni L (2011) Lung stress and strain during mechanical ventilation: any safe threshold? Am J Respir Crit Care Med 183:1354–1362
70. Simon BA, Weinmann GG, Mitzner W (1984) Mean airway pressure and alveolar pressure during high-frequency ventilation. J Appl Physiol Respir Environ Exerc Physiol 57:1069–1078
71. Allen JL, Frantz ID 3rd, Fredberg JJ (1985) Regional alveolar pressure during periodic flow. Dual manifestations of gas inertia. J Clin Invest 76:620–629
72. Tsuda A, Kamm R, Fredberg JJ (1990) Periodic flow at airway bifurcations. II. Flow partitioning. J Appl Physiol 69:553–561
73. Tsuda A, Fredberg JJ (1990) Periodic flow at airway bifurcations. I. Development of steady pressure differences. J Appl Physiol 69:546–552
74. Monchi M, Bellenfant F, Cariou A, Joly LM, Thebert D, Laurent I, Dhainaut JF, Brunet F (1998) Early predictive factors of survival in the acute respiratory distress syndrome. A multivariate analysis. Am J Respir Crit Care Med 158:1076–1081
75. Jardin F, Farcot JC, Boisante L, Curien N, Margairaz A, Bourdarias JP (1981) Influence of positive end-expiratory pressure on left ventricular performance. N Engl J Med 304:387–892
76. Bouferrache K, Vieillard-Baron A (2011) Acute respiratory distress syndrome, mechanical ventilation, and right ventricular function. Curr Opin Crit Care 17:30–35
77. Mekontso Dessap A, Charron C, Devaquet J, Aboab J, Jardin F, Brochard L, Vieillard-Baron A (2009) Impact of acute hypercapnia and augmented positive end-expiratory pressure on right ventricle function in severe acute respiratory distress syndrome. Intensive Care Med 35:1850–1858
78. Guérin C, Matthay MA (2016) Acute cor pulmonale and the acute respiratory distress syndrome. Intensive Care Med. [Epub ahead of print]. doi:10.1007/s00134-015-4197-z
79. Guervilly C, Forel JM, Hraiech S, Demory D, Allardet-Servent J, Adda M, Barreau-Baumstark K, Castanier M, Papazian L, Roch A (2012) Right ventricular function during high-frequency oscillatory ventilation in adults with acute respiratory distress syndrome. Crit Care Med 40:1539–1545
80. Mekontso Dessap A, Boissier F, Charron C, Bégot E, Repessé X, Legras A, Brun-Buisson C, Vignon P, Vieillard-Baron A (2016). Acute cor pulmonale during protective ventilation for acute respiratory distress syndrome: prevalence, predictors, and clinical impact. Intensive Care Med 42:862-870
81. Vieillard-Baron A, Jardin F (2003) Why protect the right ventricle in patients with acute respiratory distress syndrome? Curr Opin Crit Care 9:15–21
82. Jardin F, Vieillard-Baron A (2005) Monitoring of right-sided heart function. Curr Opin Crit Care 11:271–279
83. Woods J, Monteiro P, Rhodes A (2007) Right ventricular dysfunction. Curr Opin Crit Care 13:532–540
84. Jardin F, Vieillard-Baron A (2009) Acute cor pulmonale. Curr Opin Crit Care 15:67–70
85. Bull TM, Clark B, McFann K, Moss M, National Institutes of Health/National Heart, Lung, and Blood Institute ARDS Network (2010) Pulmonary vascular dysfunction is associated with poor outcomes in patients with acute lung injury. Am J Respir Crit Care Med 182:1123–1128
86. Granstam SO, Björklund E, Wikström G, Roos MW (2013) Use of echocardiographic pulmonary acceleration time and estimated vascular resistance for the evaluation of possible pulmonary hypertension. Cardiovasc Ultrasound 11:7
87. Ursulet L, Roussiaux A, Belcour D, Ferdynus C, Gauzere BA, Vandroux D, Jabot J (2015) Right over left ventricular end-diastolic area relevance to predict hemodynamic intolerance of high-frequency oscillatory ventilation in patients with severe ARDS. Ann Intensive Care 5:25
88. Vieillard-Baron A, Price LC, Matthay MA (2013) Acute cor pulmonale in ARDS. Intensive Care Med 39:1836–1838

89. Chan KPW, Stewart TE, Mehta S (2007) High frequency oscillatory ventilation for adult patients with ARDS. Chest 131:1907–1916
90. Latronico N, Peli E, Botteri M (2005) Critical illness myopathy and neuropathy. Curr Opin Crit Care 11:126–132
91. Sweeney AM, Lyle J, Ferguson ND (2005) Nursing and infection control issues during high-frequency oscillatory ventilation. Crit Care Med 33(Suppl):S204–S208
92. David M, von Bardeleben RS, Weiler N, Markstaller K, Scholz A, Karmrodt J, Eberle B (2004) Cardiac function and haemodynamics during transition to high-frequency oscillatory ventilation. Eur J Anaesthesiol 21:944–952
93. Adhikari NK, Bashir A, Lamontagne F, Mehta S, Ferguson ND, Zhou Q, Hand L, Czarnecka K, Cook DJ, Granton JT, Friedrich JO, Freitag A, Watpool I, Meade MO (2011) High-frequency oscillation in adults: a utilization review. Crit Care Med 39:2631–2644
94. Maitra S, Bhattacharjee S, Khanna P, Baidya DK (2015) High-frequency ventilation does not provide mortality benefit in comparison with conventional lung-protective ventilation in acute respiratory distress syndrome: a meta-analysis of the randomized controlled trials. Anesthesiology 122:841–851
95. Mentzelopoulos SD, Malachias S, Vrettou C, Zakynthinos SG (2016) Meta-analysis of High-frequency Oscillation in Acute Respiratory Distress Syndrome and Accuracy of Results. Anesthesiology 124:246–247
96. Huang CT, Lin HH, Ruan SY, Lee MS, Tsai YJ, Yu CJ (2014) Efficacy and adverse events of high-frequency oscillatory ventilation in adult patients with acute respiratory distress syndrome: a meta-analysis. Crit Care 18:R102
97. Gu XL, Wu GN, Yao YW, Shi DH, Song Y (2014) Is high-frequency oscillatory ventilation more effective and safer than conventional protective ventilation in adult acute respiratory distress syndrome patients? A meta-analysis of randomized controlled trials. Crit Care 18:R111
98. Pelosi P, Sutherasan Y (2013) High-frequency oscillatory ventilation with tracheal gas insufflation: the rescue strategy for brain-lung interaction. Crit Care 17:R179
99. Nahum A (1998) Equipment review: tracheal gas insufflation. Crit Care 2:43–47
100. Demory D, Michelet P, Arnal JM, Donati S, Forel JM, Gainnier M, Brégeon F, Papazian L (2007) High-frequency oscillatory ventilation following prone positioning prevents a further impairment in oxygenation. Crit Care Med 35:106–111
101. Gattinoni L, Tognoni G, Pesenti A, Taccone P, Mascheroni D, Labarta V, Malacrida R, Di Giulio P, Fumagalli R, Pelosi P, Brazzi L, Latini R, Prone-Supine Study Group (2001) Effect of prone positioning on the survival of patients with acute respiratory failure. N Engl J Med 345:568–573
102. Guérin C, Reignier J, Richard JC, Beuret P, Gacouin A, Boulain T, Mercier E, Badet M, Mercat A, Baudin O, Clavel M, Chatellier D, Jaber S, Rosselli S, Mancebo J, Sirodot M, Hilbert G, Bengler C, Richecoeur J, Gainnier M, Bayle F, Bourdin G, Leray V, Girard R, Baboi L, Ayzac L, PROSEVA Study Group (2013) Prone positioning in severe acute respiratory distress syndrome. N Engl J Med 368:2159–2168
103. Mehta S, MacDonald R, Hallett DC, Lapinsky SE, Aubin M, Stewart TE (2003) Acute oxygenation response to inhaled nitric oxide when combined with high-frequency oscillatory ventilation in adults with acute respiratory distress syndrome. Crit Care Med 31:383–389
104. Ricciardolo FL, Di Stefano A, Sabatini F, Folkerts G (2006) Reactive nitrogen species in the respiratory tract. Eur J Pharmacol 533:240–252
105. Sud S, Sud M, Friedrich JO, Meade MO, Ferguson ND, Wunsch H, Adhikari NK (2010) High frequency oscillation in patients with acute lung injury and acute respiratory distress syndrome (ARDS): systematic review and meta-analysis. BMJ 340:c2327
106. Simmonds MC, Higgins JP, Stewart LA, Tierney JF, Clarke MJ, Thompson SG (2005) Meta-analysis of individual patient data from randomized trials: a review of methods used in practice. Clin Trials 2:209–207
107. Mentzelopoulos SD, Roussos C, Zakynthinos SG (2005) Prone position reduces lung stress and strain in severe acute respiratory distress syndrome. Eur Respir J 25:534–544

Ventilation Strategies: Recruitment Maneuvers

5

Lorenzo Ball and Paolo Pelosi

5.1 Introduction

Acute respiratory distress syndrome (ARDS) is characterized by refractory hypoxemia, reduced lung compliance [1], and increased lung inhomogeneity [2]. After the landmark studies carried out in the early 2000s, the so-called protective ventilation, comprising a low tidal volume (V_T) titrated to 6 mL/kg of predicted body weight and positive end-expiratory pressure (PEEP), has gained wide acceptance in the management of patients with ARDS, as it showed an improvement in mortality [3]. However, low tidal volumes are associated with cyclic opening and closing of collapsed lung regions, in a potentially harmful mechanism referred to as atelectrauma [4]. The use of PEEP is currently recommended to prevent this phenomenon and maintain patency of alveoli, but the use of high pressures can be associated with barotrauma. Both atelectrauma and volutrauma are putative mechanisms of ventilator-induced lung injury (VILI) [5]; therefore the clinician should balance between these two conditions while ensuring an acceptable gas exchange to the patient [6].

Recruitment maneuvers (RMs) are transient procedures that increase the transpulmonary pressure, with the aim of obtaining a mechanical reopening of collapsed lung units [7]. The first assessment of these techniques dates back to two decades ago, when the concept of lung recruitment has been studied. There are several arguments that provide a pathophysiological rationale supporting the implementation of RMs as part of the ventilatory setting in ARDS, as sedation, neuromuscular blockade, and the absence of sigh reflex facilitate the alveolar collapse. RMs have been implemented in protocols for ventilation in ARDS and constitute a common but debated part of the management of these patients. In a recent meta-analysis, the

L. Ball, MD • P. Pelosi, MD, FERS (✉)
IRCCS AOU San Martino-IST, Department of Surgical Sciences and Integrated Diagnostics, University of Genoa, Largo Rosanna Benzi 8, 16131 Genoa, Italy
e-mail: lorenzo.loryball@gmail.com; ppelosi@hotmail.com

D. Chiumello (ed.), *Acute Respiratory Distress Syndrome (ARDS)*,
DOI 10.1007/978-3-319-41852-0_5

contribution to mortality reduction in moderate/severe ARDS of RMs was estimated around 6% [8]. This improvement in outcome is relatively small, contributing to a high degree of variability in the techniques, timing, and protocols implementing RMs in the clinical and research practice.

In fact, there are several unclear aspects that hinder a widely accepted approach to RMs. The techniques and timings are still under investigation, and it is not clear which subgroups of patients are more likely to take benefit from RMs. Already opened alveoli are at risk of overinflation, and the result of a RM in some case only consists in the achievement of an anatomical rather than functional recruitment, without improvement of gas exchange and potentially worsening hypoxia in the longer term [7]. Nonetheless, safety concerns must be taken into account, as the airway pressure increase can lead to a hemodynamic impairment and hypotension, due to an increased workload for right ventricle, left ventricle underfilling, or worsening of a pre-existing diastolic dysfunction [9, 10]. In addition to this, the optimal ventilatory settings and PEEP titration after RMs are still controversial. For all these reasons, guidelines for the use of RMs are still lacking.

The aim of this chapter is to illustrate the physiologic rationale and mechanism of RMs, the different techniques to perform RMs, their clinical effects and safety, as well as clinical tools to assess the efficacy of RMs.

5.2 Physiology of Recruitment Maneuvers

5.2.1 Definition and Rationale

The transpulmonary pressure, calculated as difference between airway pressure and pleural pressure, is the mediator of lung recruitment and represents the distending force of the lung. A RM is a transient increase of the transpulmonary pressure, sufficient to overcome the chest wall elastance and to open collapsed alveoli [11]. In ARDS, the loss of aeration is due to alveolar flooding, as well as resorption and compression atelectasis. In most of the cases, moderate-high airway pressures, between 30 and 40 cmH_2O, are able to recruit most of the compression atelectasis, while loss of aeration due to resorption mechanisms may require higher pressures, especially when a rigid chest wall coexists, such as in obese patients [12]. The potential of lung recruitment can be defined as the increase in end-expiratory lung volume or as a decrease in the non-aerated lung regions as a consequence of an increase of the transpulmonary pressure and has huge heterogeneity in ARDS patients [13]. Most of the studies investigated the use of RMs in patients with injured lungs; however they might have a role also in patients with healthy lungs both in the ICU and in the operating room, and their efficacy in those settings is under investigation [14–16]. Moreover, it must be underlined that even if the transpulmonary pressure is the real mediator of RMs, in most of the patients, its actual value is not known, because pleural pressure estimation with esophageal pressure monitoring is not often implemented in the clinical practice. Therefore in most cases the clinician sets the airway pressure on the ventilator rather than the transpulmonary pressure.

5.2.2 Consequences and Safety

For two decades, the paradigm has been that of opening the lung through RMs and maintaining it open with PEEP [17]. However, recent investigation showed conflicting results as an excessive lung inflation has been related to higher inflammation in experimental models, compared to that due to cyclic opening and closing of alveoli [5]. Moreover, a distinction must be made between RMs resulting in a functional and a merely anatomical recruitment [7]. In an effective alveolar reaeration maneuver, pressure results in alveolar reopening, without hyperinflation and with an acceptable blood vessel compression, contributing to an improvement of gas exchange as shown by an increase in the PaO_2/FiO_2 ratio. On the other hand, when a RM reaches higher pressures, alveolar reopening is achieved at the price of hyperinflation and blood vessel compression: therefore, despite an observed increase in lung aeration, the worsening of the ventilation-perfusion matching frustrates the improvement of aeration, leading to a potential decrease in the PaO_2/FiO_2 ratio. Once a successful RM is performed, PEEP can maintain the achieved improvements. Several studies are testing protocols and techniques to titrate PEEP after RMs [18–20]. Details on the different PEEP titration techniques can be found in Chap. 3. However, in some other patients, the benefits of RMs are only transient, and in these cases they should be omitted, as the increase in pressures increases the risk of barotrauma and VILI, while temporary improvements in gas exchange have a merely cosmetic value, without long-term benefits [21]. Recent findings concerning the role of driving pressure ($P_{Driving} = P_{Plateau} - PEEP$) in the management of patients with ARDS [22] suggest that a RM should have the goal to improve gas exchange and possibly reduce the driving pressure needed to maintain an adequate tidal volume. The reduction of the driving pressure can be seen as a direct preventive measure against VILI, as it is proportional to the energy load delivered from the ventilator to the respiratory system [23].

RMs usually have a big impact in the first few seconds from the start of the maneuver, but often the duration of these positive effects on gas exchange are limited in time. Some authors suggest that the short duration of the beneficial effects could be related to an incorrect PEEP titration after the RMs. PEEP after the RMs maintains the alveoli opened and prevents de-recruitment: it is advisable to set at least the same level of PEEP titrated before the RMs [21].

A safe pressure threshold for RMs applicable to all patients cannot be determined, and it is likely to be a consequence of the patient characteristics, in particular the type and extension of lung injury. For instance, in one of the first studies investigating the effect of repetitive RMs in ARDS, a higher improvement in gas exchange was observed in patients with ARDS due to extrapulmonary causes, compared to those with pulmonary ARDS [24]. RMs can cause hemodynamic instability, and prolonged and abrupt maneuvers tend to be more prone to these side effects [11].

While this instability is almost always temporary and reversible, the long-term effects on VILI are still unclear [21].

5.3 Techniques of Recruitment Maneuvers

Different techniques have been proposed to perform RMs, with different magnitudes of increase in transpulmonary pressure, rise time, duration of the maneuver, and timing of implementation [7, 11]. The findings of the most recent studies are conflicting. Most of the reaeration occurs in the first seconds after the increase of airway pressure [25], and therefore several authors conclude that longer RMs are unlikely to be more beneficial while increasing the risk of hemodynamic impairment. Moreover, there is evidence that RMs consisting in an abrupt rise of pressure might result in an increased lung inflammation and VILI [26]; therefore slower RMs consisting in stepwise changes in airway pressure are often advocated [7, 11, 21]. Despite several efforts in building a consistent amount of evidence, the role of RMs is still debated, as is the technique that should be used and the timing during the course of illness. Often seen as a rescue measure to overcome gas exchange impairment resulting in life-threatening hypoxemia, their potential as part of the ventilatory strategy of ARDS is more controversial [21]. Figure 5.1 summarizes the different types of RMs described in this paragraph.

5.3.1 Sigh

A RM consisting in interleaving uninterrupted mechanical ventilation with a certain number of breaths with a higher plateau pressure is referred to as ‘sigh’ RM and was the first technique proposed [24]. Such maneuver has been showed to improve oxygenation, lung compliance, and increase EELV, but these benefits are transient, and the sigh has to be performed frequently in order to maintain the patency of recruited lung units [27]. In animal models, patterns of sigh RMs with high frequency, e.g., 180/h as proposed in the first studies, were associated with elevated inflammation markers compared to ventilation without RMs and to CPAP maneuvers [28]. However, the clinical relevance of these aspects remains to be clarified. With the increased availability of more sophisticated ICU ventilators, sighs can be delivered with a predetermined frequency. Due to the lack of evidence concerning their safety and long-term efficacy, their routine cannot be recommended.

5.3.2 Sustained Inflation

Sustained inflation is the most described RM. It is performed increasing abruptly the airway pressure to a certain level and maintaining it constant for several seconds. A common sustained inflation maneuver consists in the application of a constant airway pressure of 40 cmH_2O for 40s [29, 30]. These RMs can rapidly revert

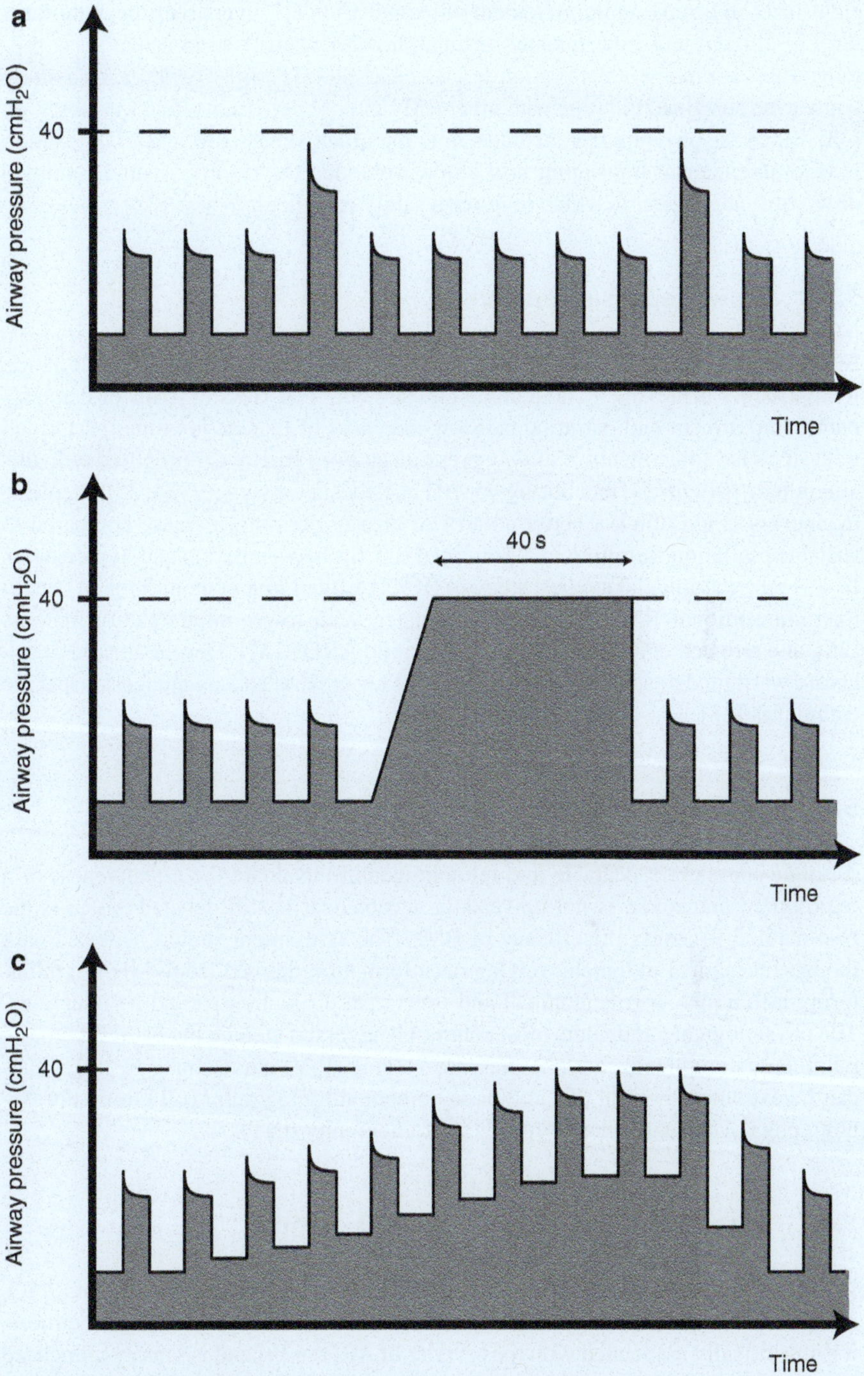

Fig. 5.1 Types of recruitment maneuvers. Sigh maneuver (**a**), typical sustained inflation maneuver (**b**), slow stepwise maneuver based on step-by-step changes in PEEP (**c**)

atelectasis and cause an improvement of oxygenation and lung function in the short term in clinical and experimental settings; however their role in achieving a prolonged gas exchange amelioration is less clear [20, 31, 32]. However, in a study comparing sustained inflation with other RMs, a more persistent effect was observed [33]. Since the pressure rise mediates both the effectiveness RM and VILI, caution is recommended in translating into clinical practice the results of small sampled observational studies, in which long-term safety is difficult to assess.

5.3.3 Slow Stepwise Maneuvers

Efforts were made by the researchers to find alternatives to the sustained inflation RM, possibly achieving a comparable efficacy with less risks in terms of hemodynamic impairment and barotrauma. Slow increases of plateau pressure, performed with stepwise adjustments of airway pressure and/or PEEP, were proposed with this aim in ICU patients [7] and during general anesthesia for surgery [34, 35]. Stepwise maneuvers could allow a better control of airway pressure increase compared to sustained inflation, resulting in a decreased risk for hyperinflation and hypotension. In several experimental studies, stepwise RMs resulted in a more prolonged benefit than conventional RMs [36], were associated with lower inflammatory markers [26], and reduced epithelial cell damage in mild ARDS [37]. Despite this, large trials are warranted to assess the safety and efficacy of RMs and advantages of specific techniques [38].

5.4 Evaluation of Recruitment Maneuver Effects

A single standard, repeatable and reliable mean to evaluate the effectiveness of a recruitment maneuver, is not universally accepted: it is still debated which is the best method to assess the efficacy of RMs. The assessment should be based on a thoughtful clinical judgment, relying on information derived from different monitoring techniques, and anatomical and functional evaluation should be integrated. The physiological parameters most commonly assessed include the PaO_2/FiO_2 ratio, pulmonary compliance, and the pressure-volume (P-V) curve. Imaging techniques can be extremely helpful and comprise computed tomography (CT), lung ultrasonography (LUS), and electric impedance tomography (EIT).

5.4.1 Blood Gas Analysis and PaO_2/FiO_2 Ratio

In the clinical practice, one of the most evaluated clinical outcome is the PaO_2/FiO_2 ratio, for its low cost, widespread availability, and ease of interpretation. Furthermore, it is intrinsically associated with the severity of ARDS [39] and is rapidly influenced by an effective RM. Transcutaneous SpO_2 is a rough estimate of PaO_2 and can be used to monitor in real time the modifications of gas exchange, and to verify that during the apnea phase of the RM, the oxygenation remains within a safety range. After the RM, a decrease of $PaCO_2$ is usually observed consensually to the increase of the SpO_2 and PaO_2/FiO_2 ratio, adding completeness to the overall evaluation. The major limit of blood gas analysis parameters is that they are strongly influenced by other variables. Before a RM, the baseline intrinsic recruitability of the lung and gas exchange are both related to the severity of ARDS [13, 40]: the PaO_2/FiO_2 ratio could show greater improvement in the most severe ARDS forms, compared to the mild ones [40]. Moreover, a transient improvement of gas exchange does not necessarily translate in improved outcome, as it might be achieved at the price of a higher risk for barotrauma and VILI. The ventilatory settings, including PEEP level and the cardiac output, can influence the PaO_2/FiO_2 ratio, leading to a misinterpretation of the evaluation of RMs [20]. Therefore, the PaO_2/FiO_2 ratio assessed by blood gas analysis and the SpO_2 represent the two most widely available parameters used to evaluate RMs but, assessing the efficacy of the RM only on oxygenation, does not give a complete description of the recruitment and should be a part of an integrated evaluation.

5.4.2 Compliance and Pressure-Volume Curve

The lung (C_L) is a measure of its ability to increase volume in response to an increase of the distending force, i.e., the transpulmonary pressure (P_{tp}), and is calculated as $C_L = \Delta V / \Delta P_{tp}$. This parameter is the slope of the pressure-volume (P-V) curve. As already mentioned, P_{tp} is the mediator of the mechanical effects of a RM and reflects in magnitude the elastic recoil pressure of the lungs. P_{tp} can be estimated at the bedside as $P_{tp} = P_{aw} - P_{es}$, where P_{aw} is the airway pressure and P_{es} is the esophageal pressure, approximating the pleural pressure. Despite recommendations to increase its implementation in the clinical practice, the measurement of esophageal pressure is not often monitored in the ICU [41]. As a surrogate, most clinicians perform RMs relying on the respiratory system compliance (C_{rs}), calculated as $C_{rs} = V_T / (P_{Plateau} - PEEP)$. Nowadays, all the ICU ventilators can calculate the C_{rs}, helping to titrate the PEEP and to monitor the effectiveness of a RM. This approximation is often considered acceptable, but it must be stressed that in several cases such as in severe ARDS and morbid obesity [33], monitoring C_{rs} can lead to a misinterpretation of the respiratory system mechanics and to an inappropriate setting of ventilatory parameters, including PEEP. Therefore, monitoring the transpulmonary pressure should be considered in patients with severe ARDS or in the obese [21, 33, 41]. The evaluation of a RM based on the ventilator P-V curve calculation relies on the assumption that the increase of the volume at a certain pressure is caused by the recruitment of non-aerated lung areas and has been demonstrated that this physiological property could be used to define the level of pulmonary recruitment because it tightly correlates with CT scan evaluation [42]. Likewise PaO_2/FiO_2, both C_L and C_{rs} tend to reflect the baseline severity of the patient's lung condition, and, paradoxically, a greater improvement can often be seen in most severe patients, while this does not necessarily imply an improvement in outcome.

As the PaO_2/FiO_2 ratio assessment alone only reflects the transient improvement of gas exchange due to a RM, conversely a clinical evaluation limited to the observation of the P-V curve could only take into account changes in respiratory mechanics: a balance between the two should be achieved. Simple parameters such as the PaO_2/FiO_2 ratio, SpO_2, and the C_{rs} are easy-to-use tools, but they might not give a complete overview of the effects of RMs in all patients.

5.4.3 Computed Tomography

The quantitative analysis of lung CT scan allows to obtain useful information about the lung tissue aeration and, when performed at different pressure levels, can assess the potential recruitability. Historically, the concept of lung recruitability and PEEP titration in ARDS was investigated by means of CT analysis [13] that represents the most informative tool to assess lung aeration. CT can be considered as the gold standard to estimate lung recruitability, but it has several pitfalls that hamper its clinical application: the patients have to move to the ICU to the CT facility, the acquisition involves a high exposure to ionizing radiations, and the image post-processing is time-consuming. Several solutions are under investigation, including the possibility to assess visually images to avoid manual image segmentation [43], to extrapolate the information from a reduced number of CT slices [44], and to use low-dose protocols to reduce radiation exposure [45, 46]. While its role has been established to assess lung recruitability, CT cannot be used for the assessment of a single RM. Further studies are necessary to clarify whether RMs should be the included in the standard ventilatory approach to patients showing a high recruitability at the CT scan.

In conclusion, CT is fundamental for diagnosis, to evaluate the lung recruitability at the admission, to assess the best ventilatory settings, and to titrate the initial PEEP [47], but more versatile tools are warranted to assess reliably recruitability, possibly at the bedside [48, 49].

5.4.4 Lung Ultrasound

Lung ultrasound at the bedside is an increasingly popular technique in the ICU: it is an easy, cheap, repeatable, real-time, and noninvasive method to assess several lung conditions [50]. It has been also proposed as a tool to assess the efficacy of lung recruitment [19, 51]. The exam is performed scoring visually different pulmonary regions, in order to obtain a global score that correlates with the degree of lung aeration [51]. This application of lung ultrasound has not yet been completely standardized: its operator dependence raises concerns among some authors, and for this reason automated computer-based image analysis is under investigation [52, 53]. Moreover, lung ultrasound is not able so far to discriminate normal aeration from hyperaeration.

5.4.5 Electrical Impedance Tomography

Electrical impedance tomography (EIT) is a real-time imaging technique, which shows dynamically the lung aeration changes. It is based on the principle that changes in lung aeration modify the chest conductivity, and electrical signals recorded with electrodes placed on the skin are analyzed to produce a real-time lung aeration map. EIT is an emerging technique, but needs technical improvements to enhance resolution and clinical trials to clarify its role in decision making [54, 55].

Conclusions

While often useful as a rescue measure to overcome an acute gas exchange impairment in ARDS, there is still not univocal evidence that recruitment maneuvers can improve patient's outcome. Alveolar recruitment can be achieved in many patients, but efforts must be made to balance between an acceptable oxygenation and the risk to deliver harmful pressures to the patient. Gas exchange, ventilator-derived parameters, esophageal pressure, and imaging techniques should be integrated to assess the efficacy and safety of recruitment maneuvers. After recruitment, a sufficient PEEP is mandatory to maintain the improvement. Stepwise slow recruitment maneuvers should be preferred to abrupt sustained inflation. Transient hypotension or desaturation are common during the procedure, but serious immediate adverse reactions are infrequent. However, long-term positive or negative effects are unknown.

At the moment, no evidence is available to support the use of recruitment maneuvers as a routine measure in all ARDS patients, but their indication should be tailored individually, as a part of a lung protective ventilatory strategy.

Bibliography

1. Ashbaugh DG, Bigelow DB, Petty TL, Levine BE (1967) Acute respiratory distress in adults. Lancet Lond Engl 2:319–323
2. Cressoni M, Cadringher P, Chiurazzi C et al (2014) Lung inhomogeneity in patients with acute respiratory distress syndrome. Am J Respir Crit Care Med 189:149–158. doi:10.1164/rccm.201308-1567OC
3. The ARDS Clinical Trials Network, National Heart, Lung, and Blood Institute, National Institutes of Health (2000) Ventilation with lower tidal volumes as compared with traditional tidal volumes for acute lung injury and the acute respiratory distress syndrome. The Acute Respiratory Distress Syndrome Network. N Engl J Med 342:1301–1308. doi:10.1056/NEJM200005043421801
4. Treschan TA, Beiderlinden M (2015) Role of recruitment maneuvers for lung-protective ventilation in the operating room remains unclear. Anesthesiology 122:472–473. doi:10.1097/ALN.0000000000000549
5. Güldner A, Braune A, Ball L et al (2016) Comparative effects of volutrauma and atelectrauma on lung inflammation in experimental acute respiratory distress syndrome. Crit Care Med. doi:10.1097/CCM.0000000000001721

6. Slutsky AS, Ranieri VM (2014) Ventilator-induced lung injury. N Engl J Med 370:980. doi:10.1056/NEJMc1400293
7. Santos RS (2015) Recruitment maneuvers in acute respiratory distress syndrome: the safe way is the best way. World J Crit Care Med 4:278. doi:10.5492/wjccm.v4.i4.278
8. Suzumura EA, Figueiró M, Normilio-Silva K et al (2014) Effects of alveolar recruitment maneuvers on clinical outcomes in patients with acute respiratory distress syndrome: a systematic review and meta-analysis. Intensive Care Med 40:1227–1240. doi:10.1007/s00134-014-3413-6
9. Chin JH, Lee EH, Kim WJ et al (2013) Positive end-expiratory pressure aggravates left ventricular diastolic relaxation further in patients with pre-existing relaxation abnormality. Br J Anaesth 111:368–373. doi:10.1093/bja/aet061
10. Fan E, Wilcox ME, Brower RG et al (2008) Recruitment maneuvers for acute lung injury: a systematic review. Am J Respir Crit Care Med 178:1156–1163. doi:10.1164/rccm.200802-335OC
11. Keenan JC, Formenti P, Marini JJ (2014) Lung recruitment in acute respiratory distress syndrome: what is the best strategy? Curr Opin Crit Care 20:63–68. doi:10.1097/MCC.0000000000000054
12. Marini JJ (2001) Recruitment maneuvers to achieve an "open lung" – whether and how? Crit Care Med 29:1647–1648
13. Gattinoni L, Caironi P, Cressoni M et al (2006) Lung recruitment in patients with the acute respiratory distress syndrome. N Engl J Med 354:1775–1786. doi:10.1056/NEJMoa052052
14. Neto AS, Simonis FD, Barbas CSV et al (2015) Lung-protective ventilation with low tidal volumes and the occurrence of pulmonary complications in patients without acute respiratory distress syndrome: a systematic review and individual patient data analysis. Crit Care Med 43:2155–2163. doi:10.1097/CCM.0000000000001189
15. Serpa Neto A, Hemmes SNT, Barbas CSV et al (2015) Protective versus conventional ventilation for surgery: a systematic review and individual patient data meta-analysis. Anesthesiology 123:66–78. doi:10.1097/ALN.0000000000000706
16. PROVE Network Investigators for the Clinical Trial Network of the European Society of Anaesthesiology, SNT H, Gama de Abreu M et al (2014) High versus low positive end-expiratory pressure during general anaesthesia for open abdominal surgery (PROVHILO trial): a multicentre randomised controlled trial. Lancet Lond Engl 384:495–503. doi:10.1016/S0140-6736(14)60416-5
17. Lachmann B (1992) Open up the lung and keep the lung open. Intensive Care Med 18:319–321
18. Lu Q, Constantin J-M, Nieszkowska A et al (2006) Measurement of alveolar derecruitment in patients with acute lung injury: computerized tomography versus pressure–volume curve. Crit Care 10:R95
19. Rouby J-J, Arbelot C, Brisson H et al (2013) Measurement of alveolar recruitment at the bedside: the beginning of a new era in respiratory monitoring? Respir Care 58:539–542
20. Chiumello D, Algieri I, Grasso S et al (2016) Recruitment maneuvers in acute respiratory distress syndrome and during general anesthesia. Minerva Anestesiol 82:210–220
21. Hess DR (2015) Recruitment maneuvers and PEEP titration. Respir Care 60:1688–1704
22. Amato MBP, Meade MO, Slutsky AS et al (2015) Driving pressure and survival in the acute respiratory distress syndrome. N Engl J Med 372:747–755. doi:10.1056/NEJMsa1410639
23. Protti A, Andreis DT, Milesi M et al (2015) Lung anatomy, energy load, and ventilator-induced lung injury. Intensive Care Med Exp 3:34. doi:10.1186/s40635-015-0070-1
24. Pelosi P, Cadringher P, Bottino N et al (1999) Sigh in acute respiratory distress syndrome. Am J Respir Crit Care Med 159:872–880
25. Garnero A, Tuxen D, Corno G et al (2015) Dynamics of end expiratory lung volume after changing positive end-expiratory pressure in acute respiratory distress syndrome patients. Crit Care. doi:10.1186/s13054-015-1044-0
26. Santos RS, Moraes L, Samary CS et al (2016) Fast versus slow recruitment maneuver at different degrees of acute lung inflammation induced by experimental sepsis. Anesth Analg. doi:10.1213/ANE.0000000000001173

27. Fujino Y, Goddon S, Dolhnikoff M et al (2001) Repetitive high-pressure recruitment maneuvers required to maximally recruit lung in a sheep model of acute respiratory distress syndrome. Crit Care Med 29:1579–1586
28. Steimback PW, Oliveira GP, Rzezinski AF et al (2009) Effects of frequency and inspiratory plateau pressure during recruitment manoeuvres on lung and distal organs in acute lung injury. Intensive Care Med 35:1120–1128
29. Oczenski W, Hörmann C, Keller C et al (2004) Recruitment maneuvers after a positive end-expiratory pressure trial do not induce sustained effects in early adult respiratory distress syndrome. Anesthesiology 101:620–625
30. Grasso S, Mascia L, Del Turco M et al (2002) Effects of recruiting maneuvers in patients with acute respiratory distress syndrome ventilated with protective ventilatory strategy. Anesthesiology 96:795–802
31. Arnal J-M, Paquet J, Wysocki M et al (2011) Optimal duration of a sustained inflation recruitment maneuver in ARDS patients. Intensive Care Med 37:1588–1594. doi:10.1007/s00134-011-2323-0
32. Spieth PM, de Abreu MG (2012) Lung recruitment in ARDS: we are still confused, but on a higher PEEP level. Crit Care 16:1–2
33. Katsiari M, Koulouris NG, Orfanos SE et al (2012) Intercomparison of three recruitment maneuvers in acute respiratory distress syndrome: the role of body mass index. Minerva Anestesiol 78:675–683
34. Güldner A, Kiss T, Serpa Neto A et al (2015) Intraoperative protective mechanical ventilation for prevention of postoperative pulmonary complications: a comprehensive review of the role of tidal volume, positive end-expiratory pressure, and lung recruitment maneuvers. Anesthesiology 123:692–713. doi:10.1097/ALN.0000000000000754
35. Ball L, Dameri M, Pelosi P (2015) Modes of mechanical ventilation for the operating room. Best Pract Res Clin Anaesthesiol 29:285–299. doi:10.1016/j.bpa.2015.08.003
36. Riva DR, Contador RS, Baez-Garcia CSN et al (2009) Recruitment maneuver: RAMP versus CPAP pressure profile in a model of acute lung injury. Respir Physiol Neurobiol 169:62–68. doi:10.1016/j.resp.2009.08.010
37. Morán I, Blanch L, Fernández R et al (2011) Acute physiologic effects of a stepwise recruitment maneuver in acute respiratory distress syndrome. Minerva Anestesiol 77:1167–1175
38. Investigators ART et al (2012) Rationale, study design, and analysis plan of the Alveolar Recruitment for ARDS Trial (ART): study protocol for a randomized controlled trial. Trials 13:1–14
39. Definition Task Force ARDS, Ranieri VM, Rubenfeld GD et al (2012) Acute respiratory distress syndrome: the Berlin Definition. JAMA 307:2526–2533. doi:10.1001/jama.2012.5669
40. Constantin J-M, Grasso S, Chanques G et al (2010) Lung morphology predicts response to recruitment maneuver in patients with acute respiratory distress syndrome. Crit Care Med 38:1108–1117. doi:10.1097/CCM.0b013e3181d451ec
41. Akoumianaki E, Maggiore SM, Valenza F et al (2014) The application of esophageal pressure measurement in patients with respiratory failure. Am J Respir Crit Care Med 189:520–531. doi:10.1164/rccm.201312-2193CI
42. Ranieri VM, Giuliani R, Fiore T et al (1994) Volume-pressure curve of the respiratory system predicts effects of PEEP in ARDS: "occlusion" versus "constant flow" technique. Am J Respir Crit Care Med 149:19–27
43. Chiumello D, Marino A, Brioni M et al (2013) Visual anatomical lung CT scan assessment of lung recruitability. Intensive Care Med 39:66–73. doi:10.1007/s00134-012-2707-9
44. Reske AW, Reske AP, Gast HA et al (2010) Extrapolation from ten sections can make CT-based quantification of lung aeration more practicable. Intensive Care Med 36:1836–1844. doi:10.1007/s00134-010-2014-2
45. Chiumello D, Langer T, Vecchi V et al (2014) Low-dose chest computed tomography for quantitative and visual anatomical analysis in patients with acute respiratory distress syndrome. Intensive Care Med 40:691–699. doi:10.1007/s00134-014-3264-1
46. Vecchi V, Langer T, Bellomi M et al (2013) Low-dose CT for quantitative analysis in acute respiratory distress syndrome. Crit Care Lond Engl 17:R183. doi:10.1186/cc12866

47. Chiumello D, Marino A, Brioni M et al (2015) Lung recruitment assessed by respiratory mechanics and by CT scan: what is the relationship? Am J Respir Crit Care Med. doi:10.1164/rccm.201507-1413OC
48. Luecke T, Corradi F, Pelosi P (2012) Lung imaging for titration of mechanical ventilation. Curr Opin Anaesthesiol 25:131–140. doi:10.1097/ACO.0b013e32835003fb
49. Ball L, Sutherasan Y, Pelosi P (2013) Monitoring respiration: what the clinician needs to know. Best Pract Res Clin Anaesthesiol 27:209–223. doi:10.1016/j.bpa.2013.06.004
50. Volpicelli G, Elbarbary M, Blaivas M et al (2012) International evidence-based recommendations for point-of-care lung ultrasound. Intensive Care Med 38:577–591. doi:10.1007/s00134-012-2513-4
51. Bouhemad B, Brisson H, Le-Guen M et al (2011) Bedside ultrasound assessment of positive end-expiratory pressure–induced lung recruitment. Am J Respir Crit Care Med 183:341–347. doi:10.1164/rccm.201003-0369OC
52. Corradi F, Ball L, Brusasco C et al (2013) Assessment of extravascular lung water by quantitative ultrasound and CT in isolated bovine lung. Respir Physiol Neurobiol 187:244–249. doi:10.1016/j.resp.2013.04.002
53. Corradi F, Brusasco C, Garlaschi A et al (2015) Quantitative analysis of lung ultrasonography for the detection of community-acquired pneumonia: a pilot study. Biomed Res Int 2015:868707. doi:10.1155/2015/868707
54. Long Y, Liu D-W, He H-W et al (2015) Positive end-expiratory pressure titration after alveolar recruitment directed by electrical impedance tomography. Chin Med J 128:1421
55. Cinnella G, Grasso S, Raimondo P et al (2015) Physiological effects of the open lung approach in patients with early, mild, diffuse acute respiratory distress syndrome: an electrical impedance tomography study. Anesthesiology 123:1113–1121. doi:10.1097/ALN.0000000000000862

Prone Position

6

Claude Guérin

6.1 Introduction

In an editorial in 1974, A.C. Bryan [1], the inventor of the high-frequency oscillation ventilation device, suggested to try prone positioning in children with acute respiratory failure still hypoxemic under this ventilator strategy. He anticipated an improvement in oxygenation from the reaeration of the dorsal lung regions, which would be no longer compressed by the gravity. As we shall see later, for such an oxygenation improvement to occur, the blood should continue to flow predominantly toward these regions, a finding that is not so intuitive. Over the subsequent years, a large amount of evidence confirmed that oxygenation was frequently improved, sometimes dramatically, with the proning session. Therefore, the attention was turned toward the mechanisms of oxygenation improvement and then the prevention of ventilator-induced lung injury (VILI) [2]. Several large trials were then performed to test the effect of prone position as compared to the maintenance in the supine position on patient outcome. It came out that prone position can improve survival in patients with ARDS and severity criteria based on oxygenation. Actually, the story of prone position was a continuous refinement of the clinical trials fed from the continuous improvement in our knowledge in ARDS and VILI [3]. The goal of this chapter is to cover the physiological and clinical effects of prone position in ARDS and to update the readership on the last data available.

C. Guérin
Service de Réanimation Médicale, Hôpital de la Croix Rousse, Lyon, France

Université de Lyon, Lyon, France

IMRB INSERM, 955 Equipe 13, Créteil, France
e-mail: claude.guerin@chu-lyon.fr

D. Chiumello (ed.), *Acute Respiratory Distress Syndrome (ARDS)*,
DOI 10.1007/978-3-319-41852-0_6

6.2 Physiological Effects

6.2.1 Oxygenation

From an historical point of view, improving oxygenation was the primary goal of any ventilator intervention directed to ARDS. Up to the end of the 1990s, studies concentrated on the effects of prone position sessions on oxygenation and largely confirmed that oxygenation frequently and markedly improved [4–8]. Further, the meta-analysis of trials on prone versus supine position found significant higher risk for better oxygenation in the prone than in the supine arm [9]. However, the mechanisms by which this effect comes from are important to consider. Indeed, in the landmark ARMA trial comparing lower and higher tidal volume in ARDS patients [10], oxygenation was better in the higher tidal volume group in which the survival was worse. With higher tidal volume, both alveolar ventilation and lung recruitment increase and oxygenation improves. At the very end, VILI follows with its resulting higher death rate from the decompartmentalization of lung inflammation outside the lung to the distant end organs [11].

The primary mechanism of better oxygenation with the prone position is the reduction in shunt [12]. Reduction of shunt may result from either more perfusion in ventilated areas or more ventilation in perfused areas. The former mechanism is likely not prevalent because blood flow continues to predominate in the dorsal regions in the prone position [13] (Fig. 6.1 panels e, f). Therefore, the second mechanism is the most important. Reaeration in dorsal lung regions has been demonstrated in animals [13] and humans [14] with ARDS (Fig. 6.1 panels a–d). A typical scenario in prone position involves lung recruitment in dorsal regions, which continue to receive most of the blood flow, a situation that has been called functional recruitment and results in marked oxygenation improvement (Fig. 6.1 panels a–d).

The prediction of oxygenation improvement with prone position is difficult. CT scan studies failed to demonstrate a correlation between the improvement in oxygenation in prone and the amount of consolidated areas [15] or the potential of lung recruitment [16] in the supine position. One of the single predictors of oxygenation improvement with proning has been shown as the chest wall compliance (C_{CW}) in the supine position and its reduction in the prone position [17].

6.2.2 Respiratory Mechanics

The increase in C_{CW} in the prone position [17], which has also been documented by other authors [8, 18], partly results from an increase in abdominal pressure [17]. However, whether or not abdomen is supported in the prone position does not change the effect on either oxygenation or end-expiratory lung volume [19]. If we assume a decrease in C_{CW} in the prone position from the supine position, the absence of change in the compliance of the respiratory system (C_{RS}) should indicate a concomitant increase in lung compliance (C_L). By contrast a decrease in C_{RS} should herald an increase in C_L and, hence, a net lung recruitment. Interestingly,

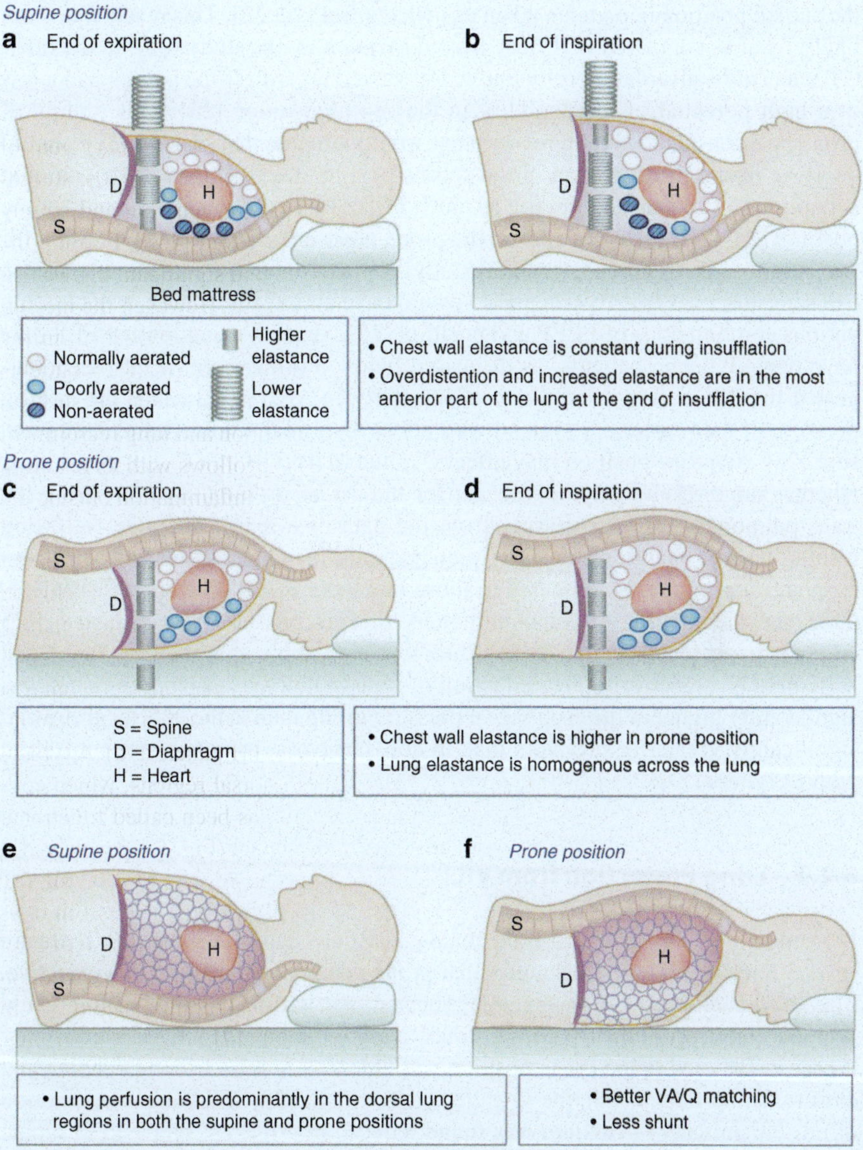

Fig. 6.1 Distribution of aerated, poorly aerated, and non-aerated lung regions at end expiration (**a** and **c**) and end inspiration (**b** and **d**) in supine and in prone position. The springs are the elastance shown for the lung and the chest wall. Panels (**e** and **f**) display the distribution of lung perfusion in supine and in prone position. See text for further explanation

across the trials the impact of the prone positioning on C_{RS} was not similar. In the trial by Mancebo et al. [20], C_{RS} has been found decreasing with proning, while no significant change has been observed in the PROSEVA trial [21]. Two CT scan studies demonstrated alveolar recruitment in the prone position as compared to the supine position in patients taken as own control [22, 23]. This result was more likely focal as compared to diffuse loss of aeration in one study [22]. In the other CT scan study, alveolar recruitment was observed regardless the patient had a low or a high potential of recruitability in the supine position [23]. This finding of prone position-induced lung recruitment would indicate that higher PEEP should be set in prone position than in the supine position. A recent study showed that actually the clinicians did not use as much PEEP as they should have in the prone position [24]. The level of PEEP in the prone position is still an open question for two reasons. First, an experimental study in pigs concluded that prone position had same effect as PEEP of 7 cmH_2O would have on oxygenation by investigating various combinations of PEEP and position [25]. Second, using lower PEEP may have hemodynamic benefits, as discussed below. Furthermore, it has been suggested that the strongest predictor of mortality in ARDS patients is the driving pressure of the respiratory system, well above C_{RS}, tidal volume, or plateau pressure [26]. As prone position may affect C_{RS} due to its effect on C_{CW}, it is not clear whether same results may be relevant for the use of proning. By computing the trans-pulmonary driving pressure from the data of a recent trial, the following results deserve mention [27]. Between patients in whom PEEP was set from esophageal pressure as compared to those receiving PEEP set from a PEEP/FiO_2 table, the mean value of trans-pulmonary driving pressure was 10.6 and 10.5 cmH_2O, respectively. At day 3 after randomization, these values averaged 7.3 and 8.7 cmH_2O, respectively. The reduction of trans-pulmonary driving pressure was significantly higher in the esophageal pressure group than in the control group and significantly greater in survivors than in non-survivors (personal communication with D Talmor).

6.2.3 Lung Protection from VILI

Protecting the lung from VILI is the main goal of mechanical ventilation. There are several lines of evidence to support that prone position can achieve this objective. The abovementioned CT scan studies showed that not only prone position could promote lung recruitment but also reduce hyperinflation [22, 23]. However, only higher PEEP used in the prone position was able to minimize cycling opening and closure during tidal breath, the so-called atelectrauma [23]. The lung concentration of pro-inflammatory cytokines was found reduced in prone as compared to supine position in ARDS patients [28]. The overall stress and strain is reduced in prone position in ARDS patients [18]. Experimental studies found that prone position reduced VILI due to high tidal volume and made it more homogeneously distributed throughout the lung in dogs [29], increased the time required to double elastance of the respiratory system as compared to supine position in rats [30], modulated the expression of a kinase strongly involved in VILI in rats [31], and attenuated VILI due to injurious ventilation in mice deficient for this kinase [31]. Therefore, there is a strong background for VILI prevention by using prone position. The likely mechanism for this to occur is by making the lung distribution of tidal volume, and hence the strain more homogenous, and by minimizing the compression of the lung by its own weight and also that of the heart. It should be made clear from the onset that VILI was not assessed in the trials that investigated the effect of prone position on patient outcome as we shall discuss below. That means that the mechanics by which prone position improves survival in ARDS patients should stem from these beneficial physiological effects.

6.3 Patient Outcome

6.3.1 Survival

Five large trials (Table 6.1) have been performed over the last 15 years comparing prone position to supine position, and the results on patient survival can be summarized as follows. First, the mortality was significantly only reduced in patients with the highest severity of hypoxemia (PaO_2/FiO_2 <100 mmHg) as demonstrated in a patients' data meta-analysis [9]. Second, this was confirmed in a single trial in select ARDS patients with moderate to severe ARDS (PaO_2/FiO_2 <150 mmHg and PEEP of 5 cmH_2O or more and FiO_2 of 0.6 or more at the time of inclusion) after a 12–24-h stabilization period. Third, subsequent meta-analysis suggested that

Table 6.1 Main characteristics of five large multicenter prospective randomized trials comparing prone to supine position in ARDS patients

Trial (first author and acronym)	Gattinoni PS I [32]	Guérin DDDV [33]	Mancebo [20]	Taccone PS II [34]	Guérin PROSEVA [21]
n patients (SP/PP groups)	152/152	378/413	60/76	174/168	229/237
% of ARDS (SP/PP groups)	93.3/94.7	28/33.9	100/100	100/100	100/100
PaO_2/FiO_2 (mmHg) at the time of randomization	127	150	147	113	100
Tidal volume (mL/kg) at the time of randomization	10.3 MBW	8 MBW	8.4 PBW	8 PBW	6.1 PBW
PEEP at the time of randomization (cmH_2O)	10	8	12	10	10
PP session duration (average hours per session)	7	8	17	18	17
Mortality (SP/PP groups) (%)	25.0/21.1	31.5/32.4	58.0/43.0	32.8/31.0	32.8/16.0[a]

SP Supine position, *PP* Prone position, *PEEP* Positive end-expiratory pressure, *MBW* Measured body weight, *PBW* Predicted body weight from gender and height
[a]$P < 0.001$

benefit of proning on survival was associated with length of proning sessions, lung protective ventilation, and intensity of hypoxemia [35].

6.3.2 Why Survival Goes Up with the Prone Position in the Most Severely Hypoxemic Patients?

As discussed previously, the physiologic beneficial effects of prone positioning should explain its effect on survival. However, the cause to effect relationship between them is not so clear in particular regarding oxygenation.

Even though there is no doubt that oxygenation was found better in the prone as compared to the supine group, the fact that better survival results from better oxygenation is not supported by the analysis of the data. In the PROSEVA trial [21], the patients in each group were split into four quartiles of PaO_2/FiO_2 ratio at the time of randomization. The benefit of proning was present at every quartile. Furthermore, the magnitude of change in oxygenation during the first proning session was not associated with a better survival [36]. This result is in line with previous studies [37, 38]. Therefore, even though prone positioning may prevent death from life-threatening hypoxemia, and in this way proning can be seen as a rescue therapy, this mechanism is not the main factor to explain survival improvement with this procedure.

VILI prevention is the second candidate for explaining survival improvement with prone. Even though it is highly likely, it has not been directly demonstrated in the trials because these did not include any assessment of VILI.

The hemodynamic effects may be a mechanism of better survival with prone that has not receive much attention. The use of proning in the early experience regularly showed lack of hemodynamic worsening contrary to the well-known deleterious effects of higher PEEP. In the PROSEVA trial, there was a greater number of days where patient was not in shock, i.e., 2 days greater for the prone group as compared to the supine group [21]. Recently, prone position was associated with an even increase in cardiac output in those patients who were preload dependent in the supine position [39]. By increasing abdominal pressure, prone position may push the stressed intravascular volume into the right atrium in patients with reserve of preload. Interestingly in this study, the improvement of oxygenation in prone was less important in those patients with the increased cardiac index than in those with no change (with no preload reserve). This may be explained by the increased intrapulmonary shunt resulting from the increased cardiac index as originally demonstrated by Dantzker [40]. As important, proning has a beneficial impact on the right ventricle function [41], and this may explain survival benefit with this strategy. The right ventricle function can be impaired as a result from an acute increase in afterload due to different contributing factors that are working in ARDS, like hypoxemia, hypercapnia, overdistension [42]. This culminates into the acute cor pulmonale (ACP) and acute right ventricle failure. ACP has been found to occur in 22% of ARDS patients and is a predictor of worst outcome [43]. Earlier, Vieillard-Baron by using transesophageal echocardiography found that prone position reverted acute cor pulmonale in ARDS patients [44]. Very recently a multicenter observational study in ICUs in France over a large cohort of ARDS patients confirmed these findings and found that ACP was an independent predictor of death [45]. Interestingly in this cohort, prone position was an independent factor associated with better survival. By allowing lower PEEP, and hence minimizing the risk of overdisetnsion as previously discussed, and by improving oxygenation, prone position could prevent ACP occurrence and could be a strategy for the clinicians facing ACP in association with inhaled nitric oxide and dobutamine [41, 42]. This real preventive and curative effect of ACP by using prone position should be tested prospectively in trials, and, as a whole, the hemodynamic effects of prone position deserve further studies.

Finally, prevention of ventilator-associated pneumonia (VAP) could be a mechanism by which prone position reduces mortality. Prone position may reduce VAP by enhancing respiratory secretion removal. However, the attributable mortality of VAP is low, in particular in ARDS patients [46]. Indeed, a post hoc analysis of the PROSEVA trial found that prone position was not associated with a reduction in VAP [47].

6.4 Clinical Practice

In daily practice the rate of use of prone position is still limited (Table 6.2). The most recent data, not published as yet, from the large observational international Large Observational Study to Understand the Global Impact of Severe Acute Respiratory Failure (LUNG SAFE) study found that prone position was used in 7% of ARDS patients and in 14% of those with severe ARDS. It is likely that the risk of complications, like vascular line kinking or withdrawal and endotracheal tube obstruction or removal, are barriers that restraint the caregivers from performing prone positioning more frequently. It should be noted that in the PROSEVA trial, the rate of these complications was not significantly different between the two groups contrary to previous trials. This may reflect the fact that centers that participated in

Table 6.2 Rate of use of prone position in ARDS patients

Trial acronym or first author	Experimental group	Control group	All patients
Randomized controlled trials			
LOVS [48]	1.42	2.1	3.6
EXPRESS [49]	8.8	18.8	13.8
CESAR [50]	35.6	42.2	38.9
ACURASYS [51]	28.0	29.0	28.6
OSCILLATE [52]	2.6	3.7	3.1
OSCAR [53]	10.1	19.9	15.0
Observational studies			
Esteban [54]			9.0
Esteban [55]			5.0
Esteban [56]			7.0
LUNG SAFE (unpublished results)			7.0

Values are percentage points in each group

this trial have used prone positioning for many years and were able to provide with a safe procedure. Another concern is the pressure sores that occurred more frequently in the prone than in the supine position [57], which should deserve innovative preventive means.

References

1. Bryan AC (1974) Conference on the scientific basis of respiratory therapy. Pulmonary physiotherapy in the pediatric age group. Comments of a devil's advocate. Am Rev Respir Dis 110:143–144
2. Slutsky AS, Ranieri VM (2013) Ventilator-induced lung injury. N Engl J Med 369:2126–2136
3. Gattinoni L, Taccone P, Carlesso E, Marini JJ (2013) Prone position in acute respiratory distress syndrome. Rationale, indications, and limits. Am J Respir Crit Care Med 188:1286–1293
4. Mure M, Martling CR, Lindahl SG (1997) Dramatic effect on oxygenation in patients with severe acute lung insufficiency treated in the prone position. Crit Care Med 25:1539–1544
5. Langer M, Mascheroni D, Marcolin R, Gattinoni L (1988) The prone position in ARDS patients. A clinical study. Chest 94:103–107
6. Blanch L, Mancebo J, Perez M, Martinez M, Mas A, Betbese AJ, Joseph D, Ballus J, Lucangelo U, Bak E (1997) Short-term effects of prone position in critically ill patients with acute respiratory distress syndrome. Intensive Care Med 23:1033–1039
7. Jolliet P, Bulpa P, Chevrolet JC (1998) Effects of the prone position on gas exchange and hemodynamics in severe acute respiratory distress syndrome. Crit Care Med 26:1977–1985
8. Guerin C, Badet M, Rosselli S, Heyer L, Sab JM, Langevin B, Philit F, Fournier G, Robert D (1999) Effects of prone position on alveolar recruitment and oxygenation in acute lung injury. Intensive Care Med 25:1222–1230
9. Sud S, Friedrich JO, Taccone P, Polli F, Adhikari NK, Latini R, Pesenti A, Guerin C, Mancebo J, Curley MA, Fernandez R, Chan MC, Beuret P, Voggenreiter G, Sud M, Tognoni G, Gattinoni L (2010) Prone ventilation reduces mortality in patients with acute respiratory failure and severe hypoxemia: systematic review and meta-analysis. Intensive Care Med 36:585–599
10. ARDSnet (2000) Ventilation with lower tidal volumes as compared with traditional tidal volumes for acute lung injury and the acute respiratory distress syndrome. The Acute Respiratory Distress Syndrome Network. N Engl J Med 342:1301–1308
11. Slutsky AS, Tremblay LN (1998) Multiple system organ failure. Is mechanical ventilation a contributing factor? Am J Respir Crit Care Med 157:1721–1725
12. Pappert D, Rossaint R, Slama K, Gruning T, Falke KJ (1994) Influence of positioning on ventilation-perfusion relationships in severe adult respiratory distress syndrome. Chest 106:1511–1516
13. Richter T, Bellani G, Scott Harris R, Vidal Melo MF, Winkler T, Venegas JG, Musch G (2005) Effect of prone position on regional shunt, aeration, and perfusion in experimental acute lung injury. Am J Respir Crit Care Med 172:480–487
14. Gattinoni L, Pelosi P, Vitale G, Pesenti A, D'Andrea L, Mascheroni D (1991) Body position changes redistribute lung computed-tomographic density in patients with acute respiratory failure. Anesthesiology 74:15–23
15. Papazian L, Paladini MH, Bregeon F, Thirion X, Durieux O, Gainnier M, Huiart L, Agostini S, Auffray JP (2002) Can the tomographic aspect characteristics of patients presenting with acute respiratory distress syndrome predict improvement in oxygenation-related response to the prone position? Anesthesiology 97:599–607
16. Protti A, Chiumello D, Cressoni M, Carlesso E, Mietto C, Berto V, Lazzerini M, Quintel M, Gattinoni L (2009) Relationship between gas exchange response to prone position and lung recruitability during acute respiratory failure. Intensive Care Med 35:1011–1017

17. Pelosi P, Tubiolo D, Mascheroni D, Vicardi P, Crotti S, Valenza F, Gattinoni L (1998) Effects of the prone position on respiratory mechanics and gas exchange during acute lung injury. Am J Respir Crit Care Med 157:387–393
18. Mentzelopoulos SD, Roussos C, Zakynthinos SG (2005) Prone position reduces lung stress and strain in severe acute respiratory distress syndrome. Eur Respir J 25:534–544
19. Chiumello D, Cressoni M, Racagni M, Landi L, Li Bassi G, Polli F, Carlesso E, Gattinoni L (2006) Effects of thoraco-pelvic supports during prone position in patients with acute lung injury/acute respiratory distress syndrome: a physiological study. Crit Care 10:R87
20. Mancebo J, Fernandez R, Blanch L, Rialp G, Gordo F, Ferrer M, Rodriguez F, Garro P, Ricart P, Vallverdu I, Gich I, Castano J, Saura P, Dominguez G, Bonet A, Albert RK (2006) A multicenter trial of prolonged prone ventilation in severe acute respiratory distress syndrome. Am J Respir Crit Care Med 173:1233–1239
21. Guérin C, Reignier J, Richard J-C, Beuret P, Gacouin A, Boulain T, Mercier E, Badet M, Mercat A, Baudin O, Clavel M, Chatellier D, Jaber S, Rosselli S, Mancebo J, Sirodot M, Hilbert G, Bengler C, Richecoeur J, Gainnier M, Bayle F, Bourdin G, Leray V, Girard R, Baboi L, Ayzac L (2013) Prone positioning in severe acute respiratory distress syndrome. N Engl J Med 368:2159–2168
22. Galiatsou E, Kostanti E, Svarna E, Kitsakos A, Koulouras V, Efremidis SC, Nakos G (2006) Prone position augments recruitment and prevents alveolar overinflation in acute lung injury. Am J Respir Crit Care Med 174:187–197
23. Cornejo RA, Diaz JC, Tobar EA, Bruhn AR, Ramos CA, Gonzalez RA, Repetto CA, Romero CM, Galvez LR, Llanos O, Arellano DH, Neira WR, Diaz GA, Zamorano AJ, Pereira GL (2013) Effects of prone positioning on lung protection in patients with acute respiratory distress syndrome. Am J Respir Crit Care Med 188:440–448
24. Beitler JR, Guerin C, Ayzac L, Mancebo J, Bates DM, Malhotra A, Talmor D (2015) PEEP titration during prone positioning for acute respiratory distress syndrome. Crit Care 19:436
25. Cakar N, der Kloot TV, Youngblood M, Adams A, Nahum A (2000) Oxygenation response to a recruitment maneuver during supine and prone positions in an oleic acid-induced lung injury model. Am J Respir Crit Care Med 161:1949–1956
26. Amato MB, Meade MO, Slutsky AS, Brochard L, Costa EL, Schoenfeld DA, Stewart TE, Briel M, Talmor D, Mercat A, Richard JC, Carvalho CR, Brower RG (2015) Driving pressure and survival in the acute respiratory distress syndrome. N Engl J Med 372:747–755
27. Talmor D, Sarge T, Malhotra A, O'Donnell CR, Ritz R, Lisbon A, Novack V, Loring SH (2008) Mechanical ventilation guided by esophageal pressure in acute lung injury. N Engl J Med 359:2095–2104
28. Papazian L, Gainnier M, Marin V, Donati S, Arnal JM, Demory D, Roch A, Forel JM, Bongrand P, Bregeon F, Sainty JM (2005) Comparison of prone positioning and high-frequency oscillatory ventilation in patients with acute respiratory distress syndrome. Crit Care Med 33:2162–2171
29. Broccard A, Shapiro RS, Schmitz LL, Adams AB, Nahum A, Marini JJ (2000) Prone positioning attenuates and redistributes ventilator-induced lung injury in dogs. Crit Care Med 28:295–303
30. Valenza F, Guglielmi M, Maffioletti M, Tedesco C, Maccagni P, Fossali T, Aletti G, Porro GA, Irace M, Carlesso E, Carboni N, Lazzerini M, Gattinoni L (2005) Prone position delays the progression of ventilator-induced lung injury in rats: does lung strain distribution play a role? Crit Care Med 33:361–367
31. Park MS, He Q, Edwards MG, Sergew A, Riches DW, Albert RK, Douglas IS (2012) Mitogen-activated protein kinase phosphatase-1 modulates regional effects of injurious mechanical ventilation in rodent lungs. Am J Respir Crit Care Med 186:72–81
32. Gattinoni L, Tognoni G, Pesenti A, Taccone P, Mascheroni D, Labarta V, Malacrida R, Di Giulio P, Fumagalli R, Pelosi P, Brazzi L, Latini R (2001) Effect of prone positioning on the survival of patients with acute respiratory failure. N Engl J Med 345:568–573
33. Guerin C, Gaillard S, Lemasson S, Ayzac L, Girard R, Beuret P, Palmier B, Le QV, Sirodot M, Rosselli S, Cadiergue V, Sainty JM, Barbe P, Combourieu E, Debatty D, Rouffineau J,

Ezingeard E, Millet O, Guelon D, Rodriguez L, Martin O, Renault A, Sibille JP, Kaidomar M (2004) Effects of systematic prone positioning in hypoxemic acute respiratory failure: a randomized controlled trial. JAMA 292:2379–2387
34. Taccone P, Pesenti A, Latini R, Polli F, Vagginelli F, Mietto C, Caspani L, Raimondi F, Bordone G, Iapichino G, Mancebo J, Guerin C, Ayzac L, Blanch L, Fumagalli R, Tognoni G, Gattinoni L (2009) Prone positioning in patients with moderate and severe acute respiratory distress syndrome: a randomized controlled trial. JAMA 302:1977–1984
35. Sud S, Friedrich JO, Adhikari NK, Taccone P, Mancebo J, Polli F, Latini R, Pesenti A, Curley MA, Fernandez R, Chan MC, Beuret P, Voggenreiter G, Sud M, Tognoni G, Gattinoni L, Guerin C (2014) Effect of prone positioning during mechanical ventilation on mortality among patients with acute respiratory distress syndrome: a systematic review and meta-analysis. CMAJ 186:E381–E390
36. Albert RK, Keniston A, Baboi L, Ayzac L, Guérin C (2014) Prone position-induced improvement in gas exchange does not predict improved survival in the acute respiratory distress syndrome. Am J Respir Crit Care Med 189:494–496
37. Gattinoni L, Vagginelli F, Carlesso E, Taccone P, Conte V, Chiumello D, Valenza F, Caironi P, Pesenti A (2003) Decrease in PaCO2 with prone position is predictive of improved outcome in acute respiratory distress syndrome. Crit Care Med 31:2727–2733
38. Lemasson S, Ayzac L, Girard R, Gaillard S, Pavaday K, Guerin C (2006) Does gas exchange response to prone position predict mortality in hypoxemic acute respiratory failure? Intensive Care Med 32:1987–1993
39. Jozwiak M, Teboul JL, Anguel N, Persichini R, Silva S, Chemla D, Richard C, Monnet X (2013) Beneficial hemodynamic effects of prone positioning in patients with acute respiratory distress syndrome. Am J Respir Crit Care Med 188:1428–1433
40. Danek SJ, Lynch JP, Weg JG, Dantzker DR (1980) The dependence of oxygen uptake on oxygen delivery in the adult respiratory distress syndrome. Am Rev Respir Dis 122:387–395
41. Repesse X, Charron C, Vieillard-Baron A (2016) Acute respiratory distress syndrome: the heart side of the moon. Curr Opin Crit Care 22:38–44
42. Guérin C, Matthay MA (2016) Acute cor pulmonale in ARDS. Intensive Care Med 42(5):934–936.
43. Boissier F, Katsahian S, Razazi K, Thille AW, Roche-Campo F, Leon R, Vivier E, Brochard L, Vieillard-Baron A, Brun-Buisson C, Mekontso Dessap A (2013) Prevalence and prognosis of cor pulmonale during protective ventilation for acute respiratory distress syndrome. Intensive Care Med 39:1725–1733
44. Vieillard-Baron A, Charron C, Caille V, Belliard G, Page B, Jardin F (2007) Prone positioning unloads the right ventricle in severe ARDS. Chest 132:1440–1446
45. Mekontso Dessap A, Boissier F, Charron C, Bégot E, Repessé X, Legras A, Brun-Buisson C, Vignon P, Vieillard-Baron A (2016) Acute cor pulmonale during protective ventilation for acute respiratory distress syndrome: prevalence, predictors, and clinical impact. Intensive Care Med 42:862–870
46. Melsen WG, Rovers MM, Bonten MJ (2013) Attributable mortality of ventilator-associated pneumonia – Authors' reply. Lancet Infect Dis 13:1015
47. Ayzac L, Girard R, Baboi L, Beuret P, Rabilloud M, Richard J, Guerin C (2016) Ventilator associated pneumonia in ARDS patients: the impact of prone positioning. A secondary analysis of the PROSEVA trial. Intensive Care Med 42:871–878
48. Meade MO, Cook DJ, Guyatt GH, Slutsky AS, Arabi YM, Cooper DJ, Davies AR, Hand LE, Zhou Q, Thabane L, Austin P, Lapinsky S, Baxter A, Russell J, Skrobik Y, Ronco JJ, Stewart TE (2008) Ventilation strategy using low tidal volumes, recruitment maneuvers, and high positive end-expiratory pressure for acute lung injury and acute respiratory distress syndrome: a randomized controlled trial. JAMA 299:637–645
49. Mercat A, Richard JC, Vielle B, Jaber S, Osman D, Diehl JL, Lefrant JY, Prat G, Richecoeur J, Nieszkowska A, Gervais C, Baudot J, Bouadma L, Brochard L (2008) Positive end-expiratory pressure setting in adults with acute lung injury and acute respiratory distress syndrome: a randomized controlled trial. JAMA 299:646–655

50. Peek GJ, Mugford M, Tiruvoipati R, Wilson A, Allen E, Thalanany MM, Hibbert CL, Truesdale A, Clemens F, Cooper N, Firmin RK, Elbourne D (2009) Efficacy and economic assessment of conventional ventilatory support versus extracorporeal membrane oxygenation for severe adult respiratory failure (CESAR): a multicentre randomised controlled trial. Lancet 374:1351–1363
51. Papazian L, Forel JM, Gacouin A, Penot-Ragon C, Perrin G, Loundou A, Jaber S, Arnal JM, Perez D, Seghboyan JM, Constantin JM, Courant P, Lefrant JY, Guerin C, Prat G, Morange S, Roch A (2010) Neuromuscular blockers in early acute respiratory distress syndrome. N Engl J Med 363:1107–1116
52. Ferguson ND, Cook DJ, Guyatt GH, Mehta S, Hand L, Austin P, Zhou Q, Matte A, Walter SD, Lamontagne F, Granton JT, Arabi YM, Arroliga AC, Stewart TE, Slutsky AS, Meade MO, Investigators OT, Canadian Critical Care Trials G (2013) High-frequency oscillation in early acute respiratory distress syndrome. N Engl J Med 368:795–805
53. Young D, Lamb SE, Shah S, MacKenzie I, Tunnicliffe W, Lall R, Rowan K, Cuthbertson BH, Group OS (2013) High-frequency oscillation for acute respiratory distress syndrome. N Engl J Med 368:806–813
54. Esteban A, Anzueto A, Frutos F, Alia I, Brochard L, Stewart TE, Benito S, Epstein SK, Apezteguia C, Nightingale P, Arroliga AC, Tobin MJ (2002) Characteristics and outcomes in adult patients receiving mechanical ventilation: a 28-day international study. JAMA 287:345–355
55. Esteban A, Ferguson ND, Meade MO, Frutos-Vivar F, Apezteguia C, Brochard L, Raymondos K, Nin N, Hurtado J, Tomicic V, Gonzalez M, Elizalde J, Nightingale P, Abroug F, Pelosi P, Arabi Y, Moreno R, Jibaja M, D'Empaire G, Sandi F, Matamis D, Montanez AM, Anzueto A (2008) Evolution of mechanical ventilation in response to clinical research. Am J Respir Crit Care Med 177:170–177
56. Esteban A, Frutos-Vivar F, Muriel A, Ferguson ND, Penuelas O, Abraira V, Raymondos K, Rios F, Nin N, Apezteguia C, Violi DA, Thille AW, Brochard L, Gonzalez M, Villagomez AJ, Hurtado J, Davies AR, Du B, Maggiore SM, Pelosi P, Soto L, Tomicic V, D'Empaire G, Matamis D, Abroug F, Moreno RP, Soares MA, Arabi Y, Sandi F, Jibaja M, Amin P, Koh Y, Kuiper MA, Bulow HH, Zeggwagh AA, Anzueto A (2013) Evolution of mortality over time in patients receiving mechanical ventilation. Am J Respir Crit Care Med 188:220–230
57. Girard R, Baboi L, Ayzac L, Richard JC, Guerin C, Proseva Trial Group (2014) The impact of patient positioning on pressure ulcers in patients with severe ARDS: results from a multicentre randomised controlled trial on prone positioning. Intensive Care Med 40:397–403

Partial or Total Extracorporeal Support 7

Nicolò Patroniti, Stefano Isgrò, and Michela Bombino

7.1 Introduction

Extracorporeal membrane oxygenation (ECMO) is one of the terms used to describe a number of different techniques used for prolonged cardiac and/or respiratory support. During ECMO a fraction of the patient venous return is diverted through an artificial lung for gas exchange (oxygenation and CO_2 removal) and then returned to the patient. Depending on the returning vessel (venous or arterial), ECMO can be used for cardiac (veno-arterial bypass (VA-ECMO)) or respiratory support. For respiratory support blood can be drained either from a venous vessel (veno-venous ECMO (VV-ECMO)) or from an arterial vessel (arteriovenous bypass (AV-ECMO)). During VV and VA-ECMO, the blood is withdrawn from the patient through the action of a pump, whereas during AV-ECMO, the blood flow is driven by the patient's arterial pressure. For respiratory support in ARDS patients, VV-ECMO represents the simplest and more rational choice [1]. Depending on the extracorporeal blood flow (ECBF), VV-ECMO can be used to support both oxygenation and CO_2 removal (ECBF 3–7 l/min, total extracorporeal support) or to provide mainly CO_2 removal (ECBF 0.5–2.5 l/min, partial extracorporeal support). This chapter will focus mainly on the application of VV-ECMO in ARDS patient.

N. Patroniti (✉)
School of Medicine and Surgery, University of Milan-Bicocca,
Via Cadore 48, Monza 20900 (MB), Italy

Department of Emergency and Intensive Care, San Gerardo Hospital,
Via Pergolesi 33, Monza 20900 (MB), Italy
e-mail: nicolo.patroniti@unimib.it

S. Isgrò • M. Bombino
Department of Emergency and Intensive Care, San Gerardo Hospital,
Via Pergolesi 33, Monza 20900 (MB), Italy
e-mail: stefano.isgro@gmail.com; michela.bombino@gmail.com

D. Chiumello (ed.), *Acute Respiratory Distress Syndrome (ARDS)*,
DOI 10.1007/978-3-319-41852-0_7

7.2 Principles of VV-ECMO

7.2.1 Components of ECMO Circuit

Basic components necessary for VV-ECMO are the cannulas for vascular access, a pump to propel the blood and an artificial lung to provide gas exchange.

The oxygenator or membrane lung (ML) is the fundamental unit of the ECMO circuit. Modern MLs consist of microporous hollow fibre membranes, made of hydrophobic polymers. MLs of polymethylpentene have become the standard for long-term applications [2–6]. The sweep gas flows through the inner part of the fibres while blood flows on their outside. The membrane avoids any direct contact between gases and blood while allowing transfer of both oxygen and carbon dioxide. A third compartment for heat exchange is commonly present. For each compartment, there is an input and an output port.

The blood flows through the ECMO circuit under the driving force of a pump. Centrifugal pumps have become the standard for long-term applications completely replacing roller pumps. In order to eliminate the stagnation, thrombosis and heat production associated with earlier centrifugal pump models, modern centrifugal pumps are built with a hole in the centre of the rotor (Mendler design) [7] and use both a magnetically suspended and a magnetically driven pump. The pump unit always incorporate a sensor for flow measurements and alarm settings.

Blood is drained from, and returned to, the patient throughout special vascular cannulas [8]. ECMO cannulas have a thin wall, commonly made of polyurethane, and are wire reinforced to prevent kinking or collapse. Cannulas of different design, size and length are available for different cannula configurations and different ECMO indications. All components of the ECMO circuit are available also with *heparin-coated* surfaces to increase biocompatibility and reduce activation of the clotting cascade [8].

7.2.2 Physiology of VV-ECMO

The effect of VV-ECMO on oxygenation and CO_2 removal is a function of a complex interplay between several factors. During VV-ECMO the ML and the native lung (NL) are in series (Fig. 7.1). We can understand the physiology of VV-ECMO by following the changes in blood gas content from the blood leaving the organs to the arterial blood. Delivery of oxygen and removal of CO_2 during VV-ECMO involve different mechanisms and different efficiencies that ultimately result in different ECMO indication possibilities. For this reason, it is useful to discuss separately the effects of VV-ECMO on oxygenation and on CO_2 removal.

7.2.2.1 Oxygen Delivery During VV-ECMO

During VV-ECMO, the arterial oxygen content (CaO_2) will depend on the O_2 delivering contributions of both the ML and the NL (Fig. 7.1).

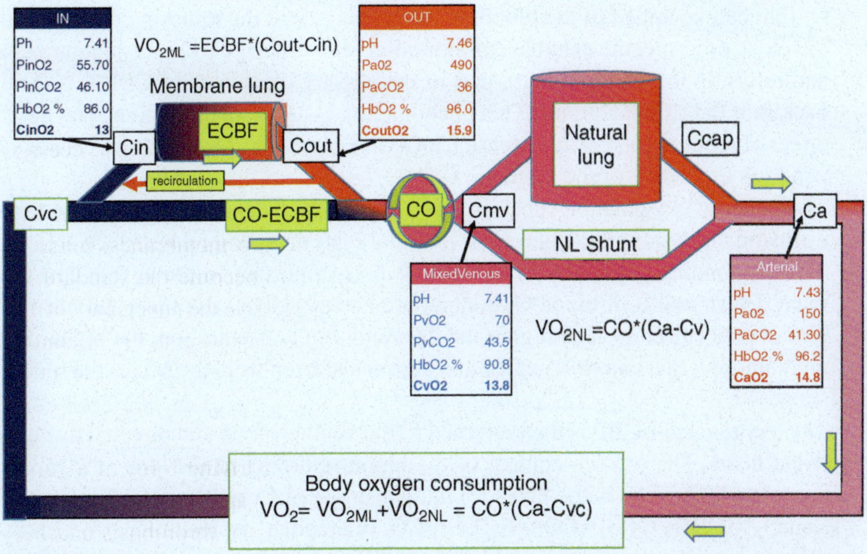

Fig. 7.1 A schematic of a model of O_2 delivery and consumption during VV-ECMO. Part of the blood returning from the body with a low oxygen content (Cv) is diverted to the membrane lung (ML). In the ML lung the blood is fully saturated (Cout) and returned to the rest of the venous return. Cin and Cout are the oxygen content of the blood entering and exiting the ML, respectively. In the presence of recirculation, Cin is higher than Cv. The blood entering the lung (mixed venous blood (Cmv)) is determined by ECMO blood flow (ECBF) relative to patients' cardiac output (CO). The arterial blood (Ca) is determined by the intrapulmonary shunt (NL shunt) relative to CO. An example is reported with relevant gas analytic values and oxygen content computation. The total oxygen delivery corresponds to total patient's oxygen consumption (VO_2) and is the sum of the oxygen contribution of the NL (VO_{2NL}) and of ML (VO_{2NL}). A more detailed description is provided in the text

Venous blood returns from the peripheral tissues with low oxygen content (CvO_2). The blood pump generates the extracorporeal blood flow (ECBF) diverting part of the venous return, i.e. cardiac output (CO), towards the ML. The ML loads the ECBF with oxygen, raising the oxygen content from the inlet ($CinO_2$) to the outlet ($CoutO_2$) of an amount corresponding to the oxygen delivery of the ML ($VO_{2ML} = ECBF * (CoutO_2 - CinO_2)$).

The VO_{2ML} and then the contribution of ML to total oxygen delivery depend on three main factors:

1. The ECBF is the most important factor: VO_{2ML} will increase directly with the increase in ECBF. However, depending on intrinsic characteristics of the membrane lung, there is a limit to the oxygenator flow ("rated flow") above which no more O_2 can be added to the blood.
2. The O_2 pressure gradient between the extracorporeal sweep gas flow (ECGF) and the inlet blood: on the gas side, the O_2 partial pressure depends on the FiO_2 of the ECGF. On the blood side, the higher the $CinO_2$, the lower the quantity of

O_2 that can be added to the blood. If the drainage and the returning cannula are too close or in specific cannula configuration (e.g. drainage from the jugular vein and return in the femoral vein), part of the already oxygenated ECBF is sucked back into the ECMO circuit. This phenomenon is called recirculation. The main effect of recirculation is to increase $CinO_2$ and decrease VO_{2ML} and then the oxygenation efficiency of the system.

3. The intrinsic oxygenation capability of the ML which depends on the membrane diffusion characteristics (thickness, material) and the membrane surface area.
4. The O_2-bonding capability of the blood: It is important to remember that the main determinants of blood O_2 content are haemoglobin saturation and haemoglobin concentration. The higher the haemoglobin concentration, the higher the amount of O_2 that can be bounded and then transferred from the ML to the blood.

The oxygenated ECBF is then returned to the venous blood and directed towards the right heart. The oxygen content of the blood returning to the lung (the mixed venous blood, $CmvO_2$) is the flow-weighted average of $CoutO_2$ and CvO_2: $CmvO_2 = [CoutO_2*ECBF+ CvO_2*(CO - ECBF)]/CO$. In practice, the resulting effect of the membrane lung is to increase the O_2 content of the blood returning to the lung from CvO_2 to $CmvO_2$. With the given CvO_2, $CmvO_2$ and then the mixed O_2 saturation are directly proportional to ratio between ECBF and CO.

The oxygen contribution of the native lung ($VO_{2NL} = (CaO_2 - CmvO_2)*CO$) depends on its residual gas exchange capability which depends on both the severity of the lung disease (i.e. the intrapulmonary shunt fraction) and the ventilator management.

The sum of VO_{2NL} and VO_{2ML}, i.e. the total oxygen delivered, corresponds to the total oxygen consumption of the patient ($VO_2Tot = VO_{2NL} + VO_{2ML}$). Consequently, the lower the NL contribution, the higher must be the contribution of the ML and then the oxygen delivery efficiency of the ECMO system. A highly efficient VV-ECMO system, able to deliver a high VO_{2ML}, requires high ECBF, minimal recirculation and low $CinO_2$.

7.2.2.2 Effect of VV-ECMO on CO_2 Removal

While the efficiency in delivering O_2 has several limitations, removal of CO_2 during VV-ECMO is much easier to achieve. While the amount of O_2 delivery is limited by full saturation of arterialized blood and by haemoglobin concentration, a substantial amount of CO_2 can be removed from venous blood. In fact, normal venous blood carries around 50 mL of CO_2/100 mL of blood, most of which in the form of bicarbonate ion. When the ECBF flows through the ML, dissolved CO_2 is transferred from the blood to the gas side, while new dissolved CO_2 is released from carbonic ion assuring a continuous availability of dissolved transferable CO_2. In this process, the main limiting factor to the amount of removable CO_2 is the partial pressure of CO_2 on the gas side, which depends on the ECGF. High ECGF will maintain the partial pressure of CO_2 on the gas side close to zero, thus maintaining a high CO_2 partial pressure gradient. Indeed, contrary to oxygen delivery, efficient CO_2 removal can be obtained with relatively lower ECBF.

7.2.3 Cannulation and Cannula Configurations for VV-ECMO

Achieving proper vascular access is a fundamental step in implementing an ECMO treatment [9–15]. An important historical step in cannulation for ECMO has been the availability of thin-walled cannulas, in the early 1990s, that allowed to move from surgical to percutaneous cannulation techniques. The percutaneous approach has several advantages: reduced risk of bleeding, shorter operative time and easier mobilization and nursing of the patient. This reason has become the standard technique for VV-ECMO [9–15].

Choice of vessels, cannulas type and size and configuration are mainly dictated by the maximum ECBF needed for the support of the patient, the maximum recirculation tolerable, the patient comfort, the patient anatomical features, the presence of some obstructed vein and local preferences.

The size and position of the drainage cannula are the main determinants of ECBF. For ECBF higher than 3–4 l/min, drainage cannula size to up 23–28 Fr is necessary. The best position is the intrahepatic portion of the inferior vena cava or in the right atrium. Cannulas with multiple holes distributed along the cannulas are available to enhance blood drainage (multiple-stage drainage cannulas). The reimmission cannulas normally have holes only in a short portion near to their extremity.

For VV-ECMO four different cannula configurations are available (Fig. 7.2):

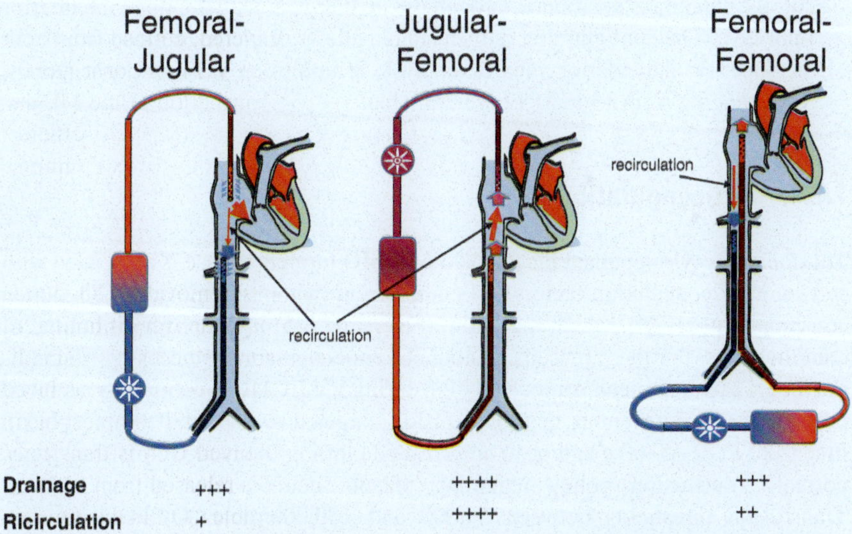

Fig. 7.2 A schematic of cannula configuration using single-lumen cannulas. Independently from the reimmission cannula, the drainage cannula should be placed with the tip above renal veins. Drainage performance and recirculation rate are reported on the bottom. Though drainage is considered easier with the jugular-femoral approach, recirculation is higher and the effective extracorporeal blood flow is lower than with the other configurations

1. Femoral-jugular configuration: The drainage cannula (21–28 Fr, 38–55 cm long) is inserted through the femoral vein and positioned with the tip in the inferior vena cava, while the reimmission cannula (19–21 Fr, 15–38 cm long) is inserted through the jugular vein with the tip in the right atrium. This represents the most used and also the easiest configuration. ECBF rates up to 6–7 L/min are easily obtained with minimal recirculation [16].
2. Femoro-femoral configuration: The drainage cannula (21–28 Fr, 38–55 cm long) is inserted through the femoral vein and positioned with the tip in the inferior vena cava, while the reimmission cannula (21–23 Fr, 50–55 cm long) is inserted through the contralateral femoral vein with the tip positioned in the inferior vena cava (but higher than the drainage cannula) or in the right atrium. The femoro-femoral approach offers safer access and less possibility of accidental cannula dislocation. Mobilization of the patient's head is facilitated, but at the expense of lower limb mobilization. With this approach, minimization of recirculation requires careful positioning of the cannula tips.
3. Jugular-femoral configuration: The drainage cannula (21–25 Fr, 15–38 cm long) is inserted through the jugular vein and positioned with the tip in the right atrium, while the reimmission cannula (19–23 Fr, 15–55 cm long) is inserted through the femoral vein. Though popular in some centre, this approach is not much diffused given the high recirculation.
4. Single-vessel double-lumen cannula: A single double-lumen cannula is inserted through the jugular vein. Different types of double-lumen cannulas are available. The most popular is the AVALON ELITE® Bi-Caval Dual Lumen Catheter [17–20]: the cannula is positioned through the jugular vein with the tip in the inferior vena cava. The configuration of the cannula allows drainage of blood from both the superior and inferior vena cava, while reimmission is in the right atrium. Sizes ranging from 13 to 31 Fr are available.

7.2.4 Anticoagulation

The contact between patient blood and the ECMO foreign surface is associated with activation of coagulation factors and complement factors, platelets and fibrinogen consumption [21–24], which may lead to bleeding [25] and thromboembolic [26] complications. For these reasons, continuous anticoagulation is necessary throughout the ECMO treatment. Anticoagulation during VV-ECMO is commonly achieved by continuous intravenous heparin infusion, targeted to a partial thromboplastin time (aPTT) of 45–60 s and/or to an activated clotting time (ACT) of 1.5–2 times normal. Transfusion policy regarding platelet count varies among centres. Transfusion thresholds between 50,000 and 100,000/μL have been reported. Activation of the coagulation cascade and clot formation in the circuit are accompanied by a progressive decrease in platelet count and fibrinogen level and consumption of coagulation factors that may lead to a syndrome similar to disseminated intravascular coagulation. For this reason, activation of the coagulation and circuit thrombosis, along with oxygenator performance and/or increase of transmembrane pressure, must be monitored to understand the need for a prompt replacement of ECMO circuit. D-dimer levels have been shown to be a reliable variable to detect circuit thrombosis.

7.3 ECMO for ARDS: A Historical Perspective

Long-term applications of ECMO support are an evolution of heart-lung machine use in cardiac surgery. The first successful use of prolonged ECMO in an adult ARDS patient was reported by Hill et al. in 1972 [27]. After only 2 years from first successful cases, the National Institute of Health commissioned a multicentre randomized clinical trial on prolonged ECMO for adults with ARDS [28]. At the time, the main indication for ECMO in ARDS patients was to correct the hypoxaemia while buying time for the lungs to heal [29]. As such, high ECMO blood flow rates were necessary to improve oxygenation, and the veno-arterial configuration was the standard. Following the negative results of the study, which failed to show any survival benefit from ECMO, only few investigators continued studying and improving the technique. Contrary to adult applications, applications in newborn showed encouraging results [30–35]. This contributed to maintain some interest on ECMO.

A landmark contribution to the evolution of adult ECMO came from the pioneering work done in the laboratory of T. Kolobow at the NIH. In a series of study, Kolobow and Gattinoni showed that [36–40] (1) nearly all the metabolic CO_2 production could be removed through an artificial lung using much lower extracorporeal blood flows than those required to oxygenate the blood and (2) removal of CO_2 through the membrane lung allows to reduce, virtually to zero, ventilation of the native lung. Based on these observations, they developed the concept of extracorporeal CO_2 removal ($ECCO_2R$) and proposed the use of a VV bypass configuration instead of the classical VA mode and the use of low-frequency ventilation to allow lung rest [40]. Unfortunately, a single-centre, randomized controlled trial conducted by Morris et al. in 40 ARDS patients failed to show a benefit from this technique [41]. Nevertheless, few centres around the world continued to apply ECMO in adult patients, contributing to improve the ECMO technique for long-term applications [42–45].

Following the concept of lung rest developed by Kolobow et al., several animal and human studies have demonstrated that, though necessary to preserve life, mechanical ventilation (MV) can exacerbate lung damage eventually contributing to mortality [46–54]. This has led to the concept of *ventilator-induced lung injury* (VILI) [54] and of "protective ventilatory strategy", mainly consisting of low Vt (6–8 mL/Kg PBW) and limitation of plateau airway pressures (Pplat <28–30 cmH_2O). ECMO is a unique technique to master protective ventilation and lung rest since, as Kolobow foresaw, it allows to minimize the need for mechanical ventilation allowing for using extremely low tidal volumes and to apply safe plateau pressures even in the most severe patients. Finally, in 2009, Peek et al. published the results of the Conventional Ventilation or ECMO for Severe Adult Respiratory Failure (CESAR) trial [55]. The study enrolled 180 adult patients

(18–65 years) with severe but potentially reversible acute respiratory failure, defined as a Murray score ≥3 or uncompensated hypercapnia with a pH < 7.20. Patients randomized to receive ECMO were transferred to the Leicester ECMO centre, while controls remained in designated treatment centres. The trial showed a survival advantage (47% vs 63% at 6 months) associated with the use of ECMO in adults. Unfortunately, the enthusiasm for the positive results has been mitigated by important limitations of the study. First, not all patients allocated to the ECMO group received ECMO, because they died before or during transportation (five patients) or they improved with conventional treatment after transportation to the ECMO centre (17 patients). Second, as there was no standardized protocol for mechanical ventilation in the control group, significantly fewer patients in the control group received a protective ventilatory strategy. However, despite these limitations, the results of the study have led to an increase in interest in ECMO worldwide. Incidentally, publication of the study almost coincided with the outbreak of H1N1 influenza in 2009. Following the successful use of ECMO in patients with H1N1-induced severe ARDS reported from the Australian and New Zealand experience [50], several countries recurred to the use of ECMO, even organizing national network able to centralize the most severe patients. The published case series from these experiences report survival rates ranging from 68 to 83% [56–63].

Since 2009, the use of respiratory ECMO in adults has continued to grow. The relative simplification of the technique together with the acquisition of experience has push more and more centres to institute specialized ECMO teams able to employ different ECMO techniques for different indications.

7.4 Indications to VV-ECMO

There are two main indications to VV-ECMO in ARDS (Fig. 7.3):

1. Refractory hypoxia: This is the classical indication. The aim is to deliver oxygen and improve oxygenation in patients with hypoxaemia unresponsive to other treatments. For this indication, VV-ECMO is employed with high ECBF that provide both oxygen delivery with improvement of oxygenation and CO_2 removal to decrease tidal volume and plateau pressure reducing the burden of injurious mechanical ventilation. This VV-ECMO application is generally identified as total extracorporeal support.
2. Injurious ventilation: In some patient nearly acceptable blood gas values can be obtained but at the expense of high minute ventilation with high tidal volumes/respiratory rates and high inspiratory plateau pressures. Given the higher efficiency of VV-ECMO in removing CO_2, decrease of minute ventilation, tidal volume, respiratory rate and consequently airway pressures can be obtained with relatively low ECBF (<2 l/min). When CO_2 removal is the main indication and VV-ECMO is employed at relatively low ECBF, we talk of partial extracorporeal support.

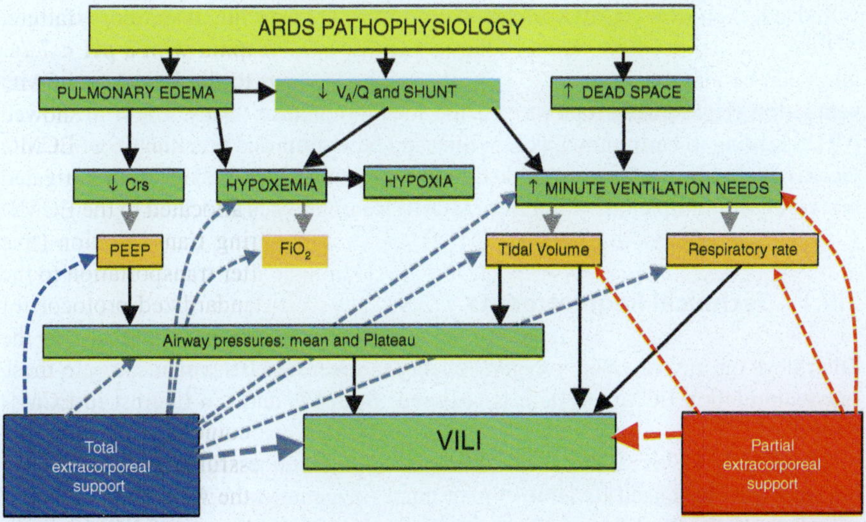

Fig. 7.3 A schematic of different pathophysiological effects of total and partial extracorporeal support. Main pathophysiological alteration of ARDS (*green boxes*) and therapeutic implications (*orange boxes*) are reported. Total extracorporeal support allows to relieve hypoxia (and consequently decrease FiO_2 and PEEP requirements) and to minimize ventilator-induced lung injury (VILI) (allowing to decrease tidal volume, respiratory rate and consequently airway pressures). Partial extracorporeal support is indicated only to minimize VILI as it does not have any positive effect on patient oxygenation. *VA/Q* ventilation perfusion ratio, *SHUNT* intrapulmonary shunt, *Crs* respiratory system compliance

7.5 Total Respiratory Extracorporeal Support

Total respiratory extracorporeal support refers to ECMO application in the most severe acute respiratory failure patients with hypoxaemia refractory to lung-protective ventilation and adjunctive therapies like inhaled nitric oxide, prone positioning and recruitment manoeuvres. The aim is to provide viable oxygenation when the natural lung becomes unable to provide it and prevent the mechanical ventilation-associated lung damage. Therefore, total extracorporeal respiratory support is viewed as a rescue therapy for severely hypoxaemic ARDS patients.

The reason to institute ECMO in severe ARDS is to break the "vicious cycle" of tissue hypoxia (Fig. 7.3) [64]. Refractory hypoxaemia leads in the most severe cases to tissue hypoxia; in this setting the weapons that conventional mechanical ventilation uses to relieve hypoxaemia are the increase of FiO_2 up to 1 and the increase of mean airway pressure (PEEP, I:E ratio manipulation, plateau, recruitment manoeuvres). The increase in intrathoracic pressures leads in turn to haemodynamic compromise defacing, in the most severe cases, the effects of the relief of hypoxaemia on tissue hypoxia. In this setting, institution of high-flow total ECMO support can provide viable delivery of oxygen to the tissues also when gas exchange through the natural lung is completely abolished.

Indeed, high-flow ECMO provides also total CO_2 removal, abolishing the need of tidal ventilation of the natural lung to remove CO_2. During ECMO the natural lungs can be maintained "at rest" avoiding high plateau pressures and high minute ventilation requirements that stretch the low-compliance "baby lungs" of severe ARDS leading to barotrauma, volutrauma and biotrauma and breaking therefore the vicious cycle of ventilator-associated lung injury (VALI or VILI) and the final dismal result of multiple organ failures (MOFs) leading to death [65].

7.5.1 Technical Requirements

To achieve the aim of viable oxygen delivery in severe ARDS patients, a high-flow, low-recirculation ECMO system is required. Both VA and VV-ECMO configurations can be used.

In the early 1970s, at the dawn of ECMO application in severe ARDS [28], the VA approach was used to achieve maximum oxygenation. VA-ECMO is characterized by high blood flow and null recirculation and therefore is an efficient system to oxygenate the blood, but in the setting of severe lung injury, its use has been abandoned due to the high rate of complications related to the arterial cannulation (bleeding, compartment syndrome, embolization) and the development of differential hypoxia (Harlequin syndrome) if the arterial cannula is not positioned centrally at the level of the aortic arch. Nowadays, the percutaneous VV configuration is used in more than 70% of severe refractory hypoxaemic patients, as reported by data from the Extracorporeal Life Support Organization (ELSO) registry [66, 67].

ECBF as stated before is the main determinant of oxygenation during total respiratory ECMO support. Reported ECBF in the refractory hypoxaemic patients ranges from greater than 3–6 l/min. The amount of cardiac output (CO) oxygenated by the artificial lung, i.e. the ECBF indexed to CO (ECBF/CO), must be greater than 60% to obtain an arterial O_2 saturation >90% or a PaO_2 >60 mmHg [68].

Large-bore drainage cannulas are a prerequisite for achieving the goal of a high ECBF in the setting of refractory ARDS. The other important factor is their location in relation to the position of the return cannula (Fig. 7.2). If the drainage and return cannula are in the inferior vena cava, through a femoro-femoral approach, the distance between the tip of the two cannulas is critical to minimize recirculation. The best VV configuration in terms of effective ECBF (total ECBF-recirculated ECBF) is the femoro-jugular approach. In contrast, the jugulo-femoral approach is the least efficient in terms of recirculation, followed by the femoro-femoral one. In the recent years the use of a single-vessel approach gathered the favours of the ECMO community; a double-lumen large-bore cannula (AVALON ELITE® Bi-Caval Dual Lumen Catheter) is inserted percutaneously in the internal jugular vein and drains blood from both inferior and superior vena cava if correctly positioned. The inner return cannula has a hole that is directed towards the tricuspid valves, minimizing recirculation of oxygenated blood [69].

7.5.2 What Is Refractory Hypoxaemia? Who Are the Candidates for Rescue ECMO Support?

Refractory hypoxaemia is reported as a cause of death in only 10–15% of ARDS patients, being multiple organ failure and sepsis the leading causes in the majority of the cases [70].

Esan et al. [71] defined refractory hypoxaemia as PaO_2/FiO_2 ratio <100 mmHg or inability to maintain Pplat <30 cmH_2O despite a tidal volume of 4 mL/kg IBW or the development of barotrauma or an oxygenation index >30. According to the Berlin definition of ARDS [72], the candidates for ECMO as a rescue therapy are in the most severe category group characterized by PaO_2/FiO_2 <100 mmHg with PEEP ≥5 cmH_2O. In the recently published LUNG SAFE study [73], ECMO was used as a rescue therapy in 48 out of 729 patients with severe ARDS (6.6%) in the 4 weeks enrolment period; assuming that the main reason for ECMO in this group was refractory hypoxaemia, the figure is slightly lower than the 10–15% incidence reported previously and can be explained by the more widespread use in the last 10 years of adjunctive manoeuvres and the adherence to lung-protective mechanical ventilation.

For the ELSO guidelines [74] ECMO "*should be considered* in hypoxic respiratory failure due to any cause (primary or secondary) when the risk of mortality is 50% or greater (PaO_2/FiO_2 <150 mmHg on FiO_2 >90% and/or Murray score 2-3), and *is indicated* when the risk of mortality is 80% or greater (PaO_2/FiO_2 <100 mmHg on FiO_2 >90% and/or Murray score 3-4 despite optimal care for 6 h or more)".

In Table 7.1 we report the main criteria of selection reported in some clinical series and in published and ongoing ECMO trials [28, 41, 55, 56, 60–63, 75–78, 80], whereas in Table 7.2 the real pre-ECMO baseline data are reported from the largest published series in the last 10 years [55, 56, 60–63, 66, 68, 76–79, 81–86].

The idea to insert total ECMO support as a rescue therapy in severe ARDS with persistent hypoxaemia despite "optimal" conventional mechanical ventilation and other less invasive adjunctive treatments (iNO, proning) dates back to the late 1990s from the German and Austrian groups [87, 88]. Interestingly, "optimal" conventional ventilation was already defined to use a protective tidal volume 5–7 mL/kg and a peak pressure limit <35 cmH_2O [88], and early referral to specialized centres was already claimed to be important in the overall clinical management of the most severely ill ARDS patients [87].

7.5.3 The Natural Lung Maintenance During Total Respiratory ECMO

As stated above, the provision of total gas exchange with ECMO could make mechanical ventilation worthless. Nevertheless, some airway pressure to maintain the lung not completely collapsed is used by all the ECMO providers. Two different

Table 7.1 Reported indications/contraindications for total extracorporeal respiratory support in ARDS

References	ECMO indications	ECMO contraindications
Zapol [28] Morris [41]	Fast entry: PaO_2 <50 mmHg with FiO_2 1.0 and PEEP ≥ 5 cmH_2O Slow entry: PaO_2 <50 mmHg for >12 h with FiO_2 0.6 and PEEP ≥ 5 cmH_2O with shunt fraction >30%	
Linden [75]	Fast entry: PaO_2/FiO_2 <60 and shunt fraction >30% on FiO_2 >0.9 for 2 h and diffuse infiltrates in four quadrants Slow entry: unresponsive to prone positioning, iNO and HFO; persistent hypercapnia	Age >60 Advanced MOFs Underlying severe disease Severe immunosuppression
Hemmila [76]	PaO_2/FiO_2 <100 on FiO_2 of 1.0, alveolar-arterial gradient ($AaDO_2$) >600 mmHg, or shunt fraction >30% despite and after optimal treatment	Age >70
Peek [55]	Severe, potentially reversible ARF, Murray Lung Injury score (LIS) ≥ 3·0, or uncompensated hypercapnia with pH < 7·20 despite optimum conventional treatment	High pressure (peak inspiratory pressure >30 cmH_2O) or high FiO_2 (>0.8) ventilation >7 days Signs of intracranial bleeding Any other contraindication to limited heparinization Any contraindication to continuation of active treatment
ANZ ECMO [56]	Refractory hypoxaemia (PaO_2/FiO_2 <60 mmHg), or hypercarbia ($PaCO_2$ >100 mmHg, with PaO_2/FiO_2 <100)	Significant pre-existing comorbidities Weight >120 kg Pulmonary hypertension Cardiac arrest
Roch [62]	PaO_2/FiO_2 <70 mmHg for at least 2 h at FiO_2 1 and PEEP level adjusted to obtain Pplat 30 cmH_2O, or PaO_2/FiO_2 <100 mmHg with Pplat >35 cmH_2O, or respiratory acidosis with pH ≤7.15 despite RR ≥35/min	
Patroniti [61]	At least one of the following criteria: OI >30 PaO_2/FiO_2 <70 with PEEP ≥ 15 cmH_2O (patient already admitted to an ECMOnet centre); PaO_2/FiO_2 <100 with PEEP ≥10 cmH_2O (patients still to be transferred) pH <7.25 for at least 2 h Haemodynamic instability	Absolute: Intracranial bleeding or other major contraindication to anticoagulation Previous severe disability Poor prognosis because of the underlying disease Relative: 1. MV >7 days
Noah [60]	CESAR criteria for transfer ECMO instituted if adequate gas exchange could not be achieved with conventional lung-protective ventilation	

Table 7.1 (continued)

References	ECMO indications	ECMO contraindications
Schmid [77]	$PaO_2/FiO_2 \leq 80$ mmHg with FiO_2 of 1.0, PEEP 18 cmH_2O and refractory respiratory acidosis (pH ≤7.25), despite optimization of conservative therapy	
Lindskov [78]	Before 2010: acute potentially reversible and potentially fatal respiratory failure Fast entry and slow entry criteria as reported by Zapol After 2010: PaO_2/FiO_2 <100 mmHg on FiO_2 >0.9 and LIS 3–4 $PaCO_2$ >100 mmHg because of asthma or permissive hypercapnia (plateau ≤ 30 cmH_2O) Severe air leak syndromes	Before 2010: Mechanical ventilation >5 days and FiO_2 1.0 >3 days Cancer Nonreversible CNS injury Chronic disease with short life expectancy Profound uncontrollable sepsis After 2010: There are no absolute contraindications to ECLS. Each patient is considered individually with respect to risks and benefits
Pham [63]	Severe ARDS defined as: LIS >3 Arterial pH less than 7.21 PaO_2/FiO_2 <100 mmHg Arterial oxygen saturation <90%	
Lehle [79]	Severe ARDS with LIS 3–4 and PaO_2/FiO_2 <80 mmHg on high PEEP (generally >15 cmH_2O) despite optimization Relative indication for vvECMO: LIS 2–3 and a PaO_2/FiO_2 <150 mmHg Severe respiratory acidosis (pH < 7.25) Inspiratory pressure over 30 cmH_2O Severe air leaks	
EOLIA trial [80]	PaO_2/FiO_2 <50 mmHg with FiO_2 >0.8 for >3 h, despite optimization of mechanical ventilation (Vt 6 mL/kg and PEEP >10 cmH_2O) and despite adjunctive therapies (NO, recruitment manoeuvres, prone position, HFO ventilation, almitrine infusion)	Intubation and mechanical ventilation >7 days Pregnancy Weight >1 kg/cm or BMI >45 kg/m^2

philosophies to manage the natural lungs emerge from the international surveys [89, 90] and reviews [91, 92] recently published on this topic.

The first one aims to the achievement of "resting" ventilatory setting with low FiO_2 around 0.4 and PEEP of 10 cmH_2O, low respiratory rate (5–10) and low tidal volume to maintain plateau pressure <25–30 cmH_2O. This strategy exploits the ECMO support treatment to its limits. If the lung collapses completely, the "baby ARDS lung" accomplishes no gas exchange, and hypoxaemia, despite total ECMO, could become an issue. Another drawback of this ventilatory rest approach is the possible ensuing of right heart failure due to the development of high pulmonary

Table 7.2 Baseline characteristics and outcome of severe ARDS reported in large VV-ECMO series published in the last 10 years

References	n. pts	Age years	PaO_2/FiO_2 mmHg	$PaCO_2$	pH	PEEP cmH_2O	PIP cmH_2O	Plateau cmH_2O	Pre-ECMO MV (days)	LIS	SOFA	ECMO days	Survival %
Schmidt [68]	2355	41 (28–54)	59 (48–75)	56 (44–73)	7.3 (7.2–7.4)	13 (10–16)	36 (31–43)	–	2.4 (0.8–6.3)	–	–	7 (4–13)	57
Brogan [66]	1473	35 (22–53)	57 (45–71)	–	7.3 (7.2–7.4)	13 (10–16)	40 (35–48)	–	2.2 (0.8–6.7)	–	–	23 ± 20	50
Lehle [79]	317	50 (37–62)	64 (51–79)		7.2 (7.1–7.3)					3.3 (3.3–3.7)		9 (6–15)	62
Enger [81]	304	46 (43–48)	69 (65–74)	–	7.2 (7.2–7.3)	16 (16–17)	35 (34–36)	–	5 (4–7)	3.5 (3.4–3.5)	11 (11–12)	10 (9–11)	59
Hemmila [76]	280	38 ± 13	55 ± 16	–	7.3 ± 0.1	13 ± 5	44 ± 11	–	4 ± 3	–	–	9 ± 8	52
Schmid [77]	176	48.0 ± 16.7	77 ± 47	70 ± 30	7.2 ± 0.2	18 ± 6	35 ± 6	–	6.1 ± 10.2	3.4 ± 0.5	12.3 ± 3.8	12 ± 9 (1–67)	56
Schmidt [82]	140	44 (30–56)	53 (43–60)	63 (51–77)	7.2 (7.2–7.3)	10 (8–12)	–	32 (30–35)	5 (1–11)	–	12 (10–15)	15 (8–30)	60
Lindskov [78]	124	42 (16–67)	48 (37–60)	57	7.26 ± 0.15	–	–	37 (35–41)	–	3.7	13	9 (1–23)	71
Noah [60]	123	34 (28–46)	54.9 ± 14.3	–	–	–	–	–	–	–	9.1 ± 2.9	–	73
Roch [62]	85	47 ± 15	60 (50–70)	59 (50–73)	7.1 ± 0.2	–	–	32 (29–35)	2 (1–8)	3.5 (3.3–3.7)	9 (7–11)	9 (7–13)	44
Rega [83]	70	43 ± 18	56 ± 18	–	7.22 ± 0.18	13 ± 3	44 ± 11	–	4.5 ± 7.4	–	–	7 ± 5	43
Pham [63]	69	42 (32–53)	63 ± 21	57 ± 18	7.26 ± 0.12	13 ± 4	–	32 ± 5	2 (1–5)	3.4 ± 0.6	9.5 ± 4	–	64
Peek [55]	68	40 ± 13	76 ± 30	–	7.1 ± 0.1	14 ± 9	–	–	1,5 (0.7–4.3)	3.5 ± 0.6	–	10 (5–23)	63
Davies [56]	68	36 (27–45)	56 (48–63)	69 (54–83)	7.2 (7.1–7.3)	18 (15–20)	36 (33–38)	–	2 (1–5)	3.8 (3.5–4.0)		10 (7–15)	75
Chiu [84]	65	48.0 ± 17.3	60.7 ± 30.6	56.8 ± 20.7	7.25 ± 0.14	13.2 ± 2.2	35.7 ± 7.2	–	3.8 ± 3.6	3.62± 0.32	11.3 ± 2.7		48
Weber-Carstens [85]	61	42 (39–45)	87 (74–101)	–	–	20 (18–21)	–	34 (32–36)	–	–	12 (12–13)	–	46
Klinzing [86]	51	48 (33–58)	57 (49–74)	57 (47–76)	7.3 (7.1–7.4)	12 (10–15)	34 (31–37)	---	2 (1–8)	–	12 (9–13)		55
Patroniti [61]	49	39 (32–46)	63 (56–79)	57 (48–72)	7.3 (7.2–7.4)	16 (14–19)	33 (30–39)	33 (30–35)	2 (1–5)	3.8 (3.3–3.8)	7 (6–9)	10 (7–17)	71

vascular resistance due to parenchymal collapse. ECMO centres that use this ventilatory strategy report a high rate of switches to VA-ECMO or necessity to add a second drainage cannula to achieve the ECMO blood flow necessary to match the metabolic requirements of the entire body of these severely compromised patients [56, 93].

The second approach utilized higher PEEP levels trying to maintain the natural lung expanded at a minimal functional residual capacity. The rational is that the lungs kept open with higher PEEP associated with very low tidal ventilation (< than 4 mL/kg PBW) are less prone to superinfection and have better surfactant function [94].

Recent surveys highlighted the variability of ventilatory approach during total ECMO [89–92]. Some general rules can be depicted:

ECMO initiation phase:

1. Patients are mainly kept sedated and paralyzed in a controlled mode of ventilation. Pressure control was the most commonly used mechanical ventilation mode (64.4%) in a recent survey [90].
2. When ECMO starts, a reduction of TV and RR is gradually instituted increasing the sweep gas flow of the artificial lung. The reduction in minute ventilation must be gradual not allowing huge swings of $PaCO_2$ and pH.
3. The main goal is to achieve a "safe and protective" plateau pressure (Pplat), at least <30 cmH_2O. In some ECMO centres, this goal is achieved only with the reduction of TV in an ultraprotective range (<4 mL/Kg IBW) maintaining the PEEP level unchanged or even increased to avoid brisk changes in mean airway pressure that can lead to alveolar flooding due to capillary leak. In other ECMO centres the Pplat goal is achieved through a reduction in TV combined with a decrease of PEEP to 10 cmH_2O; mean airway pressure is roughly maintained with an increase in inspiratory time. If the respiratory rate is reduced to 8–12 breaths/min and an I/E ratio of 1:1 is maintained, the inspiratory time would result to 2.5–3.5 s.
4. The second goal is to minimize O_2 toxicity reducing the FiO_2 of the natural lung to 0.3–0.4, thus avoiding resorption atelectasis.

ECMO maintenance phase:

1. In the most recent survey on mechanical ventilation during VV-ECMO, the median PEEP during ECMO was 10 cmH_2O, but 22.6% centres set PEEP <10 cmH_2O and 15.5% used 15–20 cmH_2O. PEEP was maintained fixed in the majority (63%) of the cases. A "lung rest" strategy was reported by 45.7% while an "open lung" strategy in 44.2% of the centres.
2. Recruitment manoeuvres were seldom used.
3. Turning the patient prone during ECMO is feasible and has been reported as safe in the most experienced ECMO centres, but it is a demanding task and utilized only as a rescue manoeuvre in case of refractory hypoxaemia during ECMO [95–97].

4. Tracheostomy is performed on ECMO in 71.3% of the centres despite large variability in its timing.
5. Some centres favour restoring spontaneous breathing early despite severe hypoxaemia (SpO_2 <80%) claiming that this approach is the most "protective" and allow the patient to be fully awake. The most will prefer to move to assisted spontaneous breathing when the natural lung function starts to improve.

ECMO weaning phase:

1. The contribution of VV-ECMO to the whole oxygen requirement of the body is reduced mainly by means of step ward decreases in FiO_2 of sweep gas. Only in cases in which ECMO blood flow was greatly increased (5–6 l/min), due to refractory hypoxaemia, its reduction to a lower target is preferred as the first weaning step.
2. Pressure support assisted spontaneous breathing (pressure support ventilation, PSV) remains the most common mode of ventilatory assistance during the weaning phase from VV-ECMO. Downward titration of the sweep gas flow through the artificial lung allows to restore spontaneous breathing efforts and some clearance of CO_2 through the natural lung. If asynchrony became an issue, mainly in those patients with still very low lung compliance, the neurally adjusted ventilatory assist (NAVA) mode can allow a better patient-ventilator interaction and a more "protective" ventilation [98, 99].
3. Finally ECMO sweep gases are turned off for some hours to test the endurance of the patient in maintaining acid-base balance through the natural lung CO_2 clearance without falling back to a non-protective dangerous ventilation. If the test is successful, the ECMO circuit can be removed.

7.5.4 Management of Persistent Severe Hypoxaemia During VV-ECMO

Severe hypoxaemia can persist despite total ECMO support or ensue during the ECMO run due to complete loss of gas exchange capabilities of the natural lung (i.e. intrapulmonary shunt around 100%) or important increase of total O_2 requirements.

To overcome this event, different strategies are proposed [100–102]:

1. Optimize the ECMO blood flow, eventually inserting a second drainage cannula if necessary, or move to hybrid configurations like veno-venous-arterial ECMO.
2. Identify and correct recirculation through repositioning of the cannulas.
3. Optimize residual native lung function with recruitment manoeuvres and prone position.
4. Identify oxygenator failure and replace it.
5. Optimize the effective ECMO blood flow (i.e. the ratio ECBF/CO) through a reduction of cardiac output (avoid fever, active cooling, beta-blockers).

6. Liberal blood transfusions to increase the arterial oxygen content and therefore O_2 delivery.

7.5.5 Complications and Limits of Total Extracorporeal Support

The major limit of extracorporeal support still lies in the need of anticoagulation to prevent thrombus formation and the related risk of bleeding.

Murphy and coworkers recently reviewed the haemostatic complications related to ECMO [103]. The contact of blood with the non-endothelial surfaces of the circuit leads to activation of the coagulation and fibrinolytic pathways and excites a complement-mediated inflammatory response. Anticoagulants, mainly unfractionated heparin, are used trying to inhibit this prothrombotic state. "Bleeding is the Achilles heel of ECMO support" [103] and adversely affects the outcome of the patients. Many factors play a role in the increased risk of bleeding during ECMO; some are related to the necessary anticoagulation, some are patient related and some are related to the ECMO circuit per se. Common alterations that can lead to bleeding complications are thrombocytopenia, hyperfibrinolysis, disseminated intravascular coagulation and acquired von Willebrand syndrome. Surgical site bleeding is the most common complication reported; therefore any invasive procedure undertaken during ECMO must be weighted against the potential for its subsequent bleeding.

The costs of ECMO support, not only the equipment-related ones but also the manpower associated with the overall care of these severe patients, are another reported limitation of the technique. Despite cost-effectiveness in terms of quality of life has been proved by the Cesar trial [55] and despite high survival rates with no long-term sequelae reported in the major patients' series, the widespread and increasing use of the technique [104] arises questions about patient selection and ECMO centres' capabilities. Some outcome prediction scores [68, 81, 82, 84, 86, 105–107] have recently been proposed to help answering the question "which ARDS patient deserves ECMO support?". Major factors contributing to outcome are patient age, comorbidities, other organ failures (SOFA score), immunosuppression and days of mechanical ventilation before ECMO institution. A score will never give the final answer about the single patient we are caring of. As Parhar and Vuylsteke conclude, "There is at present no definite tool to tell the clinician when ECMO should or should not be used. We can only, at best, list a few reasons why it should not" [107].

Another important point that showed an impact on outcome of ECMO-supported ARDS patients is the early retrieval to a high-volume referral centre [108], not only able to conduit "good ECMO" but also with full knowledge of the best care of ARDS per se and with the multidisciplinary skills to face all the possible complications ensuing during the ECMO run. This idea was proposed already in the late 1990s [87] and has recently stated by the position paper of the International ECMO Network (ECMOnet) [109, 110] and the Consensus Conference on ECMO held by the Société de Réanimation de Langue Française (SRLF) [111]. In both documents the requirements of an ECMO referral centre are clearly stated: "possess all human and material means essential to the care of ARDS patients and to setting up and use of extracorporeal life support techniques"; an ECMO support mobile team should be available 24 h a day, 7 days a week; the centre must perform continuing medical education and training in ECMO and manage at least 20 ECMO cases/year with 12 being respiratory ones.

ECMO is used in ARDS as a bridge to recovery. Sometimes the time required to reach the respiratory autonomy of the patient from ECMO can be very long. A lot of ECMO centres report long (>1 month) ECMO runs with a good outcome, rarely the ECMO-supported ARDS patients can be considered candidates for lung transplantation [112–115]. Therefore, in the longest runs, ethical issues regarding the continuation or withdrawal of this life-sustaining procedure can arise [116].

7.6 Partial Extracorporeal Support

We have previously seen that the efficiency of VV-ECMO in providing CO_2 removal is much higher than the efficiency in delivering oxygen and that a high amount of CO_2 can be removed from the ML with lower ECBF requiring smaller cannulas and simpler systems. The key advantage of removing CO_2 through these devices is that it is possible to reduce the minute ventilation required through the native lung. Potential indications include:

1. Decrease of ventilatory needs in patients with exacerbations of chronic obstructive pulmonary disease (COPD) or severe asthma, to reduce dynamic hyperinflation and avoid endotracheal intubation or facilitate weaning from mechanical ventilation [117–122].
2. Immunocompromised patients, with the goal of facilitating extubation or even avoiding intubation.
3. Bridge to lung transplantation [123–128].
4. Decrease of tidal volume, respiratory rate and plateau airway pressure in ARDS patients for "ultraprotective ventilation". In this chapter we will focus on the use of partial VV-ECMO for ultraprotective ventilation in ARDS patients.

7.6.1 Techniques for Partial Extracorporeal Support

Depending on the range of operative blood flows and cannula configurations, techniques may be classified as follows:

1. VV-ECCO$_2$R. This is the classical ECCO$_2$R techniques as proposed by Gattinoni [39]. A standard adult ECMO system runs with ECBF ranging from 1.5 to 2.5 L/min. With modern technology, it is possible to use low-medium surface oxygenators with small-size tubes and cannulas that provide ECBF ranges from 500 mL/min up to 2–2.5 L/min.

2. Low flow $ECCO_2R$ ($LF\text{-}ECCO_2R$). Various devices have been recently implemented to specifically provide CO_2 removal operating with very low extracorporeal blood flow, ranging from 250 to 500 mL/min [121, 129–132]. Depending on the level of CO_2 content in the venous blood, these systems allow removal of up to about 80–120 mL of CO_2/min. Most of these systems can be employed with double-lumen catheters similar to those used for continuous renal replacement techniques (size 14–17 Fr).
3. Arteriovenous CO_2 removal ($AVCO_2R$). Femoral vein and artery are both cannulated with percutaneous approach. The oxygenators (Novalung®) offer extremely low resistance to blood flow (surface area 1.3 m^2), which is driven by patient's arteriovenous pressure gradient. Effective blood flow is conditioned by the size of arterial cannula (13–15–17Fr) and by mean systemic pressure, ranging from 0.6 to 1.8 L/min [133]. No heat exchanger is provided. This technique can be associated with bleeding and limb ischaemia due to cannulation of the femoral artery [134, 135].

7.6.2 Partial Extracorporeal Support for Protective Ventilatory Strategies in ARDS

The idea of ultraprotective ventilation follows from the observation of Terragni et al. [52] and Bellani et al. [53] that, despite the use of a "protective" tidal volume, a substantial amount of hyperinflated lung can still be present and that further reduction of tidal volume may be beneficial. However, especially in most severe patients, the possibility of further reduced tidal volume is limited by the level of respiratory acidosis we can accept. Extracorporeal CO_2 removal allows to extend the degree of protective ventilation and prevent VILI while maintaining adequate gas exchange. Using $AVCO_2R$ in 90 ARDS patients, Bein et al. were able to reduce minute ventilation to less injurious settings [136]. However, in 22% of the cases, major complications were observed, the most serious being ischaemia of the leg.

Terragni and coworkers in 2009 [131] applied a $LF\text{-}ECCO_2R$ technique in a group of ARDS patients at risk of VILI (Pplat higher than 28 cmH_2O). They were able to lower tidal volume from 6 to 4 mL/Kg while keeping constant CO_2 and pH levels. They found a reduction in inflammatory and morphologic biomarkers of lung inflammation. Of note, to avoid potential atelectasis associated with low tidal volume, PEEP was increased by 2–4 cmH_2O while oxygenation significantly improved.

Bein and coworkers in 2013 published a randomized controlled trial, the "Xtravent-study" [134]: the study compared two groups ventilated with a tidal volume of 3 and 6 mL/Kg/PBW; PEEP was managed according to ARDSnet high PEEP/FiO_2 table in both groups. Though there was no difference in ventilator-free days between groups in the overall population, a post hoc analysis demonstrated a reduction in ventilator-free days in the group of patients with PaO_2/FiO_2 lower than 150 mmHg. As in the study by Terragni et al., the group with 3 mL/kg/PBW received a higher PEEP level [137].

In summary, the available literature demonstrates that ultraprotective ventilation combined with some form of extracorporeal CO_2 removal is feasible without major side effects. The rational is strong, but further studies are required to demonstrate potential survival benefits from the use of ultraprotective ventilatory strategies in ARDS patients.

References

1. Fan E, Gattinoni L, Combes A, Schmidt M, Peek G, Brodie D, Muller T, Morelli A, Ranieri VM, Pesenti A, Brochard L, Hodgson C, Van Kiersbilck C, Roch A, Quintel M, Papazian L (2016) Venovenous extracorporeal membrane oxygenation for acute respiratory failure: a clinical review from an international group of experts. Intensive Care Med 42(5):712–724
2. Horton S, Thuys C, Bennett M, Augustin S, Rosenberg M, Brizard C (2004) Experience with the Jostra Rotaflow and QuadroxD oxygenator for ECMO. Perfusion 19:17–23
3. Eash HJ, Jones HM, Hattler BG, Federspiel WJ (2004) Evaluation of plasma resistant hollow fiber membranes for artificial lungs. ASAIO J 50:491–497
4. Thiara APS, Hoel TN, Kristiansen F, Karlsen HM, Fiane AE, Svennevig JL (2007) Evaluation of oxygenators and centrifugal pumps for long-term pediatric extracorporeal membrane oxygenation. Perfusion 22:323–326
5. Haworth WS (2003) The development of the modern oxygenator. Ann Thorac Surg 76:2216–2219
6. Montoya JP, Shanley CJ, Merz SI, Bartlett RH (1992) Plasma leakage through microporous membranes. Role of phospholipids. ASAIO J 38:M399–M405
7. Mendler N, Podechtl F, Feil G, Hiltmann P, Sebening F (1995) Seal-less centrifugal blood pump with magnetically suspended rotor: rot-a-flot. Artif Organs 19(7):620–624
8. Kohler K, Valchanov K, Nias G, Vuylsteke A (2012) ECMO cannula review. Perfusion 28:114–124
9. Kohler K, Valchanov K, Nias G, Vuylsteke A (2013) ECMO cannula review. Perfusion 28:114–124
10. Paulsen MJ, Orizondo R, Le D et al (2012) A simple, standard method to characterize pressure/flow performance of vascular access cannulas. ASAIO J 59:24–29
11. Ngatchou W, Ramadan ASE, Van Nooten G, Antoine M (2012) Left tilt position for easy extracorporeal membrane oxygenation cannula insertion in late pregnancy patients. Interact Cardiovasc Thorac Surg 15:285–287
12. Weiner MM, Geldard P, Mittnacht AJ (2013) Ultrasound-guided vascular access: a comprehensive review. J Cardiothorac Vasc Anesth 27:345–360
13. Troianos CA, Hartman GS, Glas KE et al (2011) Guidelines for performing ultrasound guided vascular cannulation: recommendations of the American Society of Echocardiography and the Society of Cardiovascular Anesthesiologists. J Am Soc Echocardiogr 24:1291–1318
14. Pranikoff T, Hirschl RB, Remenapp R, Swaniker F, Bartlett RH (1999) Venovenous extracorporeal life support via percutaneous cannulation in 94 patients. Chest 115:818–822
15. Grasselli G, Pesenti A, Marcolin R, Patroniti N, Isgró S, Tagliabue P, Lucchini A, Fumagalli R (2010) Percutaneous vascular cannulation for extracorporeal life support (ECLS): a modified technique. Int J Artif Organs 33:553–557
16. Rich PB, Awad SS, Crotti S et al (1988) A prospective comparison of atrio-femoral and femoro-atrial flow in adult venovenous extracorporeal life support. J Thorac Cardiovasc Surg 116:628–632
17. Wang D, Zhou X, Liu X et al (2008) Wang-Zwische double lumen cannula-toward a percutaneous and ambulatory paracorporeal artificial lung. ASAIO J 54:606–661
18. Javidfar J, Brodie D, Wang D et al (2011) Use of bicaval dual-lumen catheter for adult venovenous extracorporeal membrane oxygenation. Ann Thorac Surg 91:1763–1769

19. Bermudez CA, Rocha RV, Sappington PL et al (2010) Initial experience with single cannulation for venovenous extracorporeal oxygenation in adults. Ann Thorac Surg 90:991–995
20. Camboni D, Philipp A, Lubnow M et al (2012) Extracorporeal membrane oxygenation by single-vessel access in adults: advantages and limitations. ASAIO J 58:616–621
21. Heiden D, Mielke CH, Rodvien R et al (1975) Platelets, hemostasis, and thromboembolism during treatment of acute respiratory insufficiency with extracorporeal membrane oxygenation. J Thorac Cardiovasc Surg 70(4):644–655
22. Rodvien R (1978) Hematologic observations made in patients with acute respiratory distress syndrome in the cooperative ECMO project. Artif Organs 2(1):12–18
23. Gardinali M, Cicardi M, Frangi D et al (1985) Studies of complement activation in ARDS patients treated by long-term extracorporeal CO2 removal. Int J Artif Organs 8(3):135–140
24. Uziel L, Cugno M, Fabrizi I, Pesenti A, Gattinoni L, Agostoni A (1990) Physiopathology and management of coagulation during long-term extracorporeal respiratory assistance. Int J Artif Organs 13(5):280–287
25. Frenckner B, Ehrén H, Palmér K (1991) Patient complications during extracorporeal membrane oxygenation (ECMO). Eur J Pediatr Surg 1(6):339–342
26. Kasirajan V, Smedira NG, McCarthy JF et al (1999) Risk factors for intracranial hemorrhage in adults on extracorporeal membrane oxygenation. Eur J Cardiothorac Surg 15(5):508–514
27. Hill JD, O'Brien TG, Murray JJ, Dontigny L, Bramson ML, Osborn JJ, Gerbode F (1972) Prolonged extracorporeal oxygenation for acute post-traumatic respiratory failure (shock-lung syndrome). Use of the Bramson membrane lung. N Engl J Med 286(12):629–634
28. Zapol WM, Snider MT, Hill JD, Fallat RJ, Bartlett RH, Edmunds LH, Morris AH, Peirce EC 2nd, Thomas AN, Proctor HJ, Drinker PA, Pratt PC, Bagniewski A, Miller RG Jr (1979) Extracorporeal membrane oxygenation in severe acute respiratory failure: a randomized prospective study. JAMA 242:2193–2196
29. Zapol WM, Kitz RJ (1972) Buying time for the lungs to heal. N Engl J Med 286(12):657–658
30. Bartlett RH, Gazzaniga AB, Jefferies MR, Huxtable RF, Haiduc NJ, Fong SW (1976) Extracorporeal membrane oxygenation (ECMO) cardiopulmonary support in infancy. Trans Am Soc Artif Intern Organs 22:80–93
31. Bartlett RH, Andrews AF, Toomasian JM, Haiduc NJ, Gazzaniga AB (1982) Extracorporeal membrane oxygenation for newborn respiratory failure: forty-five cases. Surgery 92(2):425–433
32. Kirkpatrick BV, Krummel TM, Mueller DG, Ormazabal MA, Greenfield LJ, Salzberg AM (1983) Use of extracorporeal membrane oxygenation for respiratory failure in term infants. Pediatrics 72(6):872–876
33. Trento A, Griffith BP, Hardesty RL (1986) Extracorporeal membrane oxygenation experience at the University of Pittsburgh. Ann Thorac Surg 42(1):56–59
34. Bartlett RH, Roloff DW, Cornell RG, Andrews AF, Dillon PW, Zwischenberger JB (1985) Extracorporeal circulation in neonatal respiratory failure: a prospective randomized study. Pediatrics 76(4):479–487
35. O'Rourke PP, Crone RK, Vacanti JP, Ware JH, Lillehei CW, Parad RB, Epstein MF (1989) Extracorporeal membrane oxygenation and conventional medical therapy in neonates with persistent pulmonary hypertension of the newborn: a prospective randomized study. Pediatrics 84(6):957–963
36. Kolobow T, Solca M, Gattinoni L, Pesenti A (1981) Adult respiratory distress syndrome (ARDS): why did ECMO fail? Int J Artif Organs 4(2):58–59
37. Kolobow T, Gattinoni L, Tomlinson TA, Pierce JE (1977) Control of breathing using an extracorporeal membrane lung. Anesthesiology 46(2):138–141
38. Kolobow T, Gattinoni L, Tomlinson T, Pierce JE (1978) An alternative to breathing. J Thorac Cardiovasc Surg 75(2):261–266
39. Gattinoni L, Agostoni A, Pesenti A, Fumagalli R, Rossi F, Iapichino G, Romagnoli G, Uziel L, Agostoni A (1980) Treatment of acute respiratory failure with low-frequency positive-pressure ventilation and extracorporeal removal of CO_2. Lancet 2:292–294

40. Gattinoni G, Pesenti A, Mascheroni D, Marcolin R, Fumagalli R, Rossi F, Iapichino G, Romagnoli G, Uziel L, Agostoni A, Kolobow T, Damia G (1986) Low-frequency positive pressure ventilation with extracorporeal CO_2 removal in severe acute respiratory failure. JAMA 256:881–896
41. Morris AH, Wallace CJ, Menlove RL, Clemmer TP, Orme JF Jr, Weaver LK, Dean NC, Thomas F, East TD, Pace NL, Suchyta MR, Beck E, Bombino M, Sittig DF, Böhm S, Hoffmann B, Becks H, Butler S, Pearl J, Rasmusson B (1994) Randomized clinical trial of pressure—controlled inverse ratio ventilation and extracorporeal CO_2 removal for adult respiratory distress syndrome. Am J Respir Crit Care Med 149(2 Pt 1):295–305
42. Kolla S, Awad SS, Rich PB, Schreiner RJ, Hirschl RB, Bartlett RH (1997) Extracorporeal life support for 100 adult patients with severe respiratory failure. Ann Surg 226(4):544–564
43. Bartlett RH, Roloff DW, Custer JR, Younger JG, Hirschl RB (2000) Extracorporeal life support: the University of Michigan experience. JAMA 283:904–908
44. Mols G, Loop T, Geiger K, Farthmann E, Benzing A (2000) Extracorporeal membrane oxygenation: a ten-year experience. Am J Surg 180:144–154
45. Lewandowski K (2000) Extracorporeal membrane oxygenation for severe acute respiratory failure. Crit Care 4:156–168
46. Tremblay LN, Slutsky AS (2006) Ventilator-induced lung injury: from the bench to the bedside. Intensive Care Med 32:24–33
47. Webb HH, Tierney DF (1974) Experimental pulmonary edema due to intermittent positive pressure ventilation with high inflation pressures: protection by positive pressures end-expiratory pressure. Am Rev Respir Dis 110:556–565
48. Dreyfuss D, Soler P, Basset G, Saumon G (1988) High inflation pressure pulmonary edema: respective effects of high airway pressure, high tidal volume and positive end-expiratory pressure. Am Rev Respir Dis 137:1159–1164
49. Muscedere JG, Mullen JBM, Gari K, Slutsky AS (1994) Tidal ventilation at low airway pressures can augment lung injury. Am J Respir Crit Care Med 149:1327–1334
50. Tremblay L, Valenza F, Ribeiro SP, Li J, Slutsky AS (1997) Injurious ventilatory strategies increase cytokines and c-fos m-RNA expression in an isolated rat lung model. J Clin Invest 99:944–952
51. The acute respiratory distress syndrome network (2000) Ventilation with lower tidal volumes as compared with traditional tidal volumes for acute lung injury and the acute respiratory distress syndrome. N Engl J Med 342:1301–1308
52. Terragni PP, Rosboch G, Tealdi A, Corno E, Menaldo E, Davini O, Gandini G, Herrmann P, Mascia L, Quintel M, Slutsky AS, Gattinoni L, Ranieri VM (2009) Tidal hyperinflation during low tidal volume ventilation in acute respiratory distress syndrome. Am J Respir Crit Care Med 175:160–166
53. Bellani G, Messa C, Guerra L, Spagnolli E, Foti G, Patroniti N, Fumagalli R, Musch G, Fazio F, Pesenti A (2009) Lungs of patients with acute respiratory distress syndrome show diffuse inflammation in normally aerated regions: a [18F]-fluoro-2-deoxy-D-glucose PET/CT study. Crit Care Med 37(7):2216–2222
54. Slutsky AS, Ranieri VM (2013) Ventilator-induced lung injury. N Engl J Med 369: 2126–2136
55. Peek G, Mugford M, Tiruvoipati R, Wilson A, Allen E, Thalanany MM, Hibbert CL, Truesdale A, Clemens F, Cooper N, Firmin RK, Elbourne D, CESAR trial collaboration (2009) Efficacy and economic assessment of conventional ventilatory support versus extracorporeal membrane oxygenation for severe adult respiratory failure (CESAR): a multicentre randomised controlled trial. Lancet 374(9698):1351–1136
56. Davies A, Jones D, Bailey M, Beca J, Bellomo R, Blackwell N et al (2009) Extracorporeal membrane oxygenation for 2009 influenza A(H1N1) acute respiratory distress syndrome. JAMA 302(17):1888–1895
57. Freed DH, Henzler D, White CW, Fowler R, Zarychanski R, Hutchison J, Arora RC, Manji RA, Legare JF, Drews T, Veroukis S, Kesselman M, Guerguerian AM, Kumar A, Canadian Critical Care Trials Group (2010) Extracorporeal lung support for patients who had severe

respiratory failure secondary to influenza A (H1N1) 2009 infection in Canada. Can J Anaesth 57(3):240–247
58. Nair P, Davies AR, Beca J, Bellomo R, Ellwood D, Forrest P, Jackson A, Pye R, Seppelt I, Sullivan E, Webb S (2011) Extracorporeal membrane oxygenation for severe ARDS in pregnant and postpartum women during the 2009 H1N1 pandemic. Intensive Care Med 37(4):648–654
59. Turner DA, Rehder KJ, Peterson-Carmichael SL, Ozment CP, Al-Hegelan MS, Williford WL, Peters MA, Noble PW, Cheifetz IM (2011) Extracorporeal membrane oxygenation for severe refractory respiratory failure secondary to 2009 H1N1 influenza A. Respir Care 56(7):941–946
60. Noah MA, Peek GJ, Finney SJ, Griffiths MJ, Harrison DA, Grieve R, Sadique MZ, Sekhon JS, McAuley DF, Firmin RK, Harvey C, Cordingley JJ, Price S, Vuylsteke A, Jenkins DP, Noble DW, Bloomfield R, Walsh TS, Perkins GD, Menon D, Taylor BL, Rowan KM (2011) Referral to an extracorporeal membrane oxygenation center and mortality among patients with severe 2009 influenza A(H1N1). JAMA 306(15):1659–1668
61. Patroniti N, Zangrillo A, Pappalardo F, Peris A, Cianchi G, Braschi A, Iotti GA, Arcadipane A, Panarello G, Ranieri VM, Terragni P, Antonelli M, Gattinoni L, Oleari F, Pesenti A (2011) The Italian ECMO network experience during the 2009 influenza A (H1N1) pandemic: preparation for severe respiratory emergency outbreaks. Intensive Care Med 37(9):1447–1457
62. Roch A, Lepaul-Ercole R, Grisoli D, Bessereau J, Brissy O, Castanier M, Dizier S, Forel JM, Guervilly C, Gariboldi V, Collart F, Michelet P, Perrin G, Charrel R, Papazian L (2010) Extracorporeal membrane oxygenation for severe influenza A (H1N1) acute respiratory distress syndrome: a prospective observational comparative study. Intensive Care Med 36(11): 1899–1905
63. Pham T, Combes A, Rozé H, Chevret S, Mercat A, Roch A, Mourvillier B, Ara-Somohano C, Bastien O, Zogheib E, Clavel M, Constan A, Marie Richard JC, Brun-Buisson C, Brochard L, REVA Research Network (2013) Extracorporeal membrane oxygenation for pandemic influenza A(H1N1)-induced acute respiratory distress syndrome: a cohort study and propensity-matched analysis. Am J Respir Crit Care Med 187(3):276–285
64. Tiruvoipati R, Botha J, Peek G (2012) Effectiveness of extracorporeal membrane oxygenation when conventional ventilation fails: valuable option or vague remedy? J Crit Care 27: 192–198
65. Bigatello LM, Pesenti A (2009) Ventilator-induced lung injury: less ventilation, less injury. Anesthesiology 111(4):699–700
66. Brogan TV, Thiagarajan RR, Rycus PT et al (2009) Extracorporeal membrane oxygenation in adults with severe respiratory failure: a multi-center database. Intensive Care Med 35(12): 2105–2114
67. Schmidt M, Bailey M, Sheldrake J et al (2014) Predicting survival after extracorporeal membrane oxygenation for severe acute respiratory failure. The Respiratory Extracorporeal Membrane Oxygenation Survival Prediction (RESP) Score. Am J Respir Crit Care Med 189(11):1374–1382
68. Schmid C, Tachon G, Devilliers C et al (2013) Blood oxygenation and decarboxylation determinants during venovenous ECMO for respiratory failure in adults. Intensive Care Med 39:838–846
69. Abrams D, Brodie D; Extracorporeal Life Support Organization (ELSO) (2015) Identification and management of recirculation in venovenous ECMO. http://www.elsoorg/resources/Guidelines.aspx. Accessed 13 Mar 3016
70. Stapleton RD, Wang BM, Hudson LD et al (2005) Causes and timing of death in patients with ARDS. Chest 128(2):525–532
71. Esan A, Hess DR, Raoof S et al (2010) Severe hypoxemic respiratory failure: part 1 – ventilatory strategies. Chest 137(5):1203–1216
72. The ARDS Definition Task Force (2012) Acute respiratory distress syndrome-The Berlin Definition. JAMA 307(23):2526–2533

73. Bellani G, Laffey JG, Pham T et al (2016) Epidemiology, patterns of care, and mortality for patients with acute respiratory distress syndrome in Intensive Care Units in 50 countries. JAMA 315(8):788–800
74. Extracorporeal Life Support Organization (ELSO) (2013) Guidelines for adult respiratory failure. Supplement to the ELSO general guidelines version 13. http://www.elsoorg/resources/Guidelines.aspx. Accessed 13 Mar 2016
75. Lindén V, Palmér K, Reinhard J et al (2000) High survival in adult patients with acute respiratory distress syndrome treated by extracorporeal membrane oxygenation, minimal sedation, and pressure supported ventilation. Intensive Care Med 26(11):1630–1637
76. Hemmila MR, Rowe SA, Boules TN et al (2004) Extracorporeal life support for severe acute respiratory distress syndrome in adults. Ann Surg 240(4):595–605
77. Schmid C, Philipp A, Hilker M et al (2012) Venovenous extracorporeal membrane oxygenation for acute lung failure in adults. J Heart Lung Transplant 31(1):9–15
78. Lindskov C, Jensen RH, Sprogoe P et al (2013) Extracorporeal membrane oxygenation in adult patients with severe acute respiratory failure. Acta Anaesthesiol Scand 57(3):303–311
79. Lehle K, Philipp A, Hiller K-A et al (2014) Efficiency of gas transfer in venovenous extracorporeal membrane oxygenation: analysis of 317 cases with four different ECMO systems. Intensive Care Med 40:1870–1877
80. Extracorporeal Membrane Oxygenation for Severe Acute Respiratory Distress Syndrome (EOLIA trial). https://clinicaltrials.gov/show/NCT01470703. Accessed 17 March 2016
81. Enger T, Philipp A, Videm V et al (2014) Prediction of mortality in adult patients with severe acute lung failure receiving veno-venous extracorporeal membrane oxygenation: a prospective observational study. Crit Care 18(2):R67. doi:10.1186/cc13824
82. Schmidt M, Zogheib E, Rozé H et al (2013) The PRESERVE mortality risk score and analysis of long-term outcomes after extracorporeal membrane oxygenation for severe acute respiratory distress syndrome. Intensive Care Med 39:1704–1713
83. Rega FR, Evrard V, Bollen H et al (2007) pH 48 h after onset of extracorporeal membrane oxygenation is an independent predictor of survival in patients with respiratory failure. Artif Organs 31(5):384–389
84. Chiu LC, Tsai FC, Hu HC et al (2015) Survival predictors in acute respiratory distress syndrome with extracorporeal membrane oxygenation. Ann Thorac Surg 99(1):243–250
85. Weber-Carstens S, Goldmann A, Quintel M et al (2013) Extracorporeal lung support in H1N1 provoked acute respiratory failure—the experience of the German ARDS network. Dtsch Arztebl Int 110(33–34):543–549
86. Klinzing S, Wenger U, Steiger P et al (2015) External validation of scores proposed for estimation of survival probability of patients with severe adult respiratory distress syndrome undergoing extracorporeal membrane oxygenation therapy: a retrospective study. Crit Care 19:142. doi:10.1186/s13054-015-0875-z
87. Lewandowski K, Rossaint R, Pappert D et al (1997) High survival rate in 122 ARDS patients managed according to a clinical algorithm including extracorporeal membrane oxygenation. Intensive Care Med 23(8):819–835
88. Ullrich R, Lorber C, Röder G et al (1999) Controlled airway pressure therapy, nitric oxide inhalation, prone position, and extracorporeal membrane oxygenation (ECMO) as components of an integrated approach to ARDS. Anesthesiology 91(6):1577–1586
89. Marhong JD, Telesnicki T, Munshi L et al (2014) Mechanical ventilation during extracorporeal membrane oxygenation. An International Survey. Ann Am Thorac Soc 11(6):956–961
90. Camporota L, Nicoletti E, Malafronte M et al (2015) International survey on the management of mechanical ventilation during ECMO in adults with severe respiratory failure. Minerva Anestesiol 81(11):1170–1183
91. Schmidt M, Pellegrino V, Combes A et al (2014) Mechanical ventilation during extracorporeal membrane oxygenation. Crit Care 18:203

92. Marhong JD, Munshi L, Detsky M et al (2015) Mechanical ventilation during extracorporeal life support (ECLS): a systematic review. Intensive Care Med 41(6):994–1003
93. Holzgraefe B, Broomé M, Kalzén H et al (2010) Extracorporeal membrane oxygenation for pandemic H1N1 2009 respiratory failure. Minerva Anestesiol 76:1043–1051
94. Haitsma JJ, Lachmann B (2006) Lung protective ventilation in ARDS: the open lung maneuver. Minerva Anestesiol 72:117–132
95. Goettler CE, Pryor JP, Hoey BA et al (2002) Prone positioning does not affect cannula function during extracorporeal membrane oxygenation or continuous renal replacement therapy. Crit Care 6:452–455
96. Culbreth RE, Goodfellow LT (2016) Complications of prone positioning during extracorporeal membrane oxygenation for respiratory failure: a systematic review. Respir Care 61(2):249–254
97. Litmathe J, Sucker C, Easo J et al (2012) Prone and ECMO – a contradiction per se? Perfusion 27:78–82
98. Karagiannidis C, Lubnow M, Philipp A et al (2010) Autoregulation of ventilation with neutrally adjusted ventilatory assist on extracorporeal lung support. Intensive Care Med 36: 2038–2044
99. Mauri T, Bellani G, Grasselli G et al (2013) Patient-ventilator interaction in ARDS patients with extremely low compliance undergoing ECMO: a novel approach based on diaphragm electrical activity. Intensive Care Med 39(2):282–291
100. Nunes LB, Mendes PV, Hirota AS et al (2014) Severe hypoxemia during veno-venous extracorporeal membrane oxygenation: exploring the limits of extracorporeal respiratory support. Clinics 69(3):173–178
101. Montisci A, Maj G, Zangrillo A et al (2015) Management of refractory hypoxemia during venovenous extracorporeal membrane oxygenation for ARDS. ASAIO J 61:227–236
102. Levy B, Taccone FS, Guarracino F (2015) Recent developments in the management of persistent hypoxemia under veno-venous ECMO. Intensive Care Med 41:508–510
103. Murphy DA, Hockings LE, Andrews RK et al (2015) Extracorporeal membrane oxygenation-hemostatic complications. Transfus Med Rev 29(2):90–101
104. Sauer CM, Yuh DD, Bonde P (2015) Extracorporeal membrane oxygenation use has increased by 433% in adults in the United States from 2006 to 2011. ASAIO J 61(1):31–36
105. Pappalardo F, Pieri M, Greco T et al (2013) Predicting mortality risk in patients undergoing venovenous ECMO for ARDS due to influenza A (H1N1) pneumonia: the ECMOnet score. Intensive Care Med 39(2):275–281
106. Scmidt M, Combes A, Pilcher D (2014) What's new with survival prediction models in acute respiratory failure patients requiring extracorporeal membrane oxygenation. Intensive Care Med 40(8):1555–1558
107. Parhar K, Vuylsteke A (2014) What's new in ECMO: scoring the bad indications. Intensive Care Med 40(11):1734–1737
108. Barbaro RP, Odetola FO, Kidwell KM et al (2015) Association of hospital-level volume of extracorporeal membrane oxygenation cases and mortality. Analysis of the extracorporeal life support organization registry. Am J Respir Crit Care Med 191(8):894–901
109. Fan E, Brodie D (2015) Higher volumes, better outcomes: the end or just the beginning of the story for extracorporeal membrane oxygenation? Am J Respir Crit Care Med 191(8): 864–866
110. Combes A, Brodie D, Bartlett R et al (2014) Position paper for the organization of extracorporeal membrane oxygenation programs for acute respiratory failure in adult patients. Am J Respir Crit Care Med 190(5):488–496
111. Richard C, Argaud L, Blet A et al (2014) Extracorporeal life support for patients with acute respiratory distress syndrome: report of a consensus conference. Ann Intensive Care 4:15. doi:10.1186/2110-5820-4-15
112. Camboni D, Philipp A, Lubnow M, et al (2011) Support time dependent outcome analysis for veno-venous extracorporeal membrane oxygenation. Eur J Cardiothorac Surg 40:1341–6; discussion 1346–1347.

113. Kon ZN, Dahi S, Evans CF et al (2015) Long-term venovenous extracorporeal membrane oxygenation support for acute respiratory distress syndrome. Ann Thorac Surg 100(6):2059–2063
114. Posluszny J, Rycus PT, Bartlett RH et al (2016) Outcome of adult respiratory failure patients receiving prolonged (≥14 Days) ECMO. Ann Surg 263(3):573–581
115. Rosenberg AA, Haft JW, Bartlett R et al (2013) Prolonged duration ECMO for ARDS: futility, native lung recovery, or transplantation? ASAIO J 59(6):642–650
116. Abrams DC, Prager K, Blinderman CD et al (2014) Ethical dilemmas encountered with the use of extracorporeal membrane oxygenation in adults. Chest 145(4):876–882
117. Cardenas VJ Jr, Lynch JE, Ates R, Miller L, Zwischenberger JB (2009) Venovenous carbon dioxide removal in chronic obstructive pulmonary disease: experience in one patient. ASAIO J 55(4):420–422
118. Garcia JP, Kon ZN, Evans C, Wu Z, Iacono AT, McCormick B, Griffith BP (2011) Ambulatory veno-venous extracorporeal membrane oxygenation: innovation and pitfalls. J Thorac Cardiovasc Surg 142(4):755–761
119. Burki NK, Mani RK, Herth FJ, Schmidt W, Teschler H, Bonin F, Becker H, Randerath WJ, Stieglitz S, Hagmeyer L, Priegnitz C, Pfeifer M, Blaas SH, Putensen C, Theuerkauf N, Quintel M, Moerer O (2013) A novel extracorporeal CO(2) removal system: results of a pilot study of hypercapnic respiratory failure in patients with COPD. Chest 143(3):678–686
120. Kluge S, Braune SA, Engel M, Nierhaus A, Frings D, Ebelt H et al (2012) Avoiding invasive mechanical ventilation by extracorporeal carbon dioxide removal in patients failing noninvasive ventilation. Intensive Care Med 38(10):1632–1639
121. Del Sorbo L, Pisani L, Filippini C, Fanelli V, Fasano L, Terragni P et al (2015) Extracorporeal Co2 removal in hypercapnic patients at risk of noninvasive ventilation failure. Crit Care Med 43(1):120–127
122. Sklar MC, Beloncle F, Katsios CM, Brochard L, Friedrich JO (2015) Extracorporeal carbon dioxide removal in patients with chronic obstructive pulmonary disease: a systematic review. Intensive Care Med 41(10):1752–1762
123. Lang G, Taghavi S, Aigner C, Rényi-Vámos F, Jaksch P, Augustin V, Nagayama K, Ghanim B, Klepetko W (2012) Primary lung transplantation after bridge with extracorporeal membrane oxygenation: a plea for a shift in our paradigms for indications. Transplantation 93:729–736
124. Fischer S, Simon AR, Welte T, Hoeper MM, Meyer A, Tessmann R, Gohrbandt B, Gottlieb J, Haverich A, Strueber M (2011) Bridge to lung transplantation with the novel pumpless interventional assist device Novalung. J Thorac Cardiovasc Surg 131:719–723
125. Hammainen P, Schersten H, Lemstrom K et al (2011) Usefulness of extracorporeal membrane oxygenation as a bridge to lung transplantation: a descriptive study. J Heart Lung Transplant 30:103–107
126. Bermudez CA, Rocha RV, Zaldonis D et al (2011) Extracorporeal membrane oxygenation as a bridge to lung transplant: midterm outcomes. Ann Thorac Surg 92:1226–1232
127. Ricci D, Boffini M, Del Sorbo L, El Qarra S, Comoglio C, Ribezzo M, Bonato R, Ranieri VM, Rinaldi M (2010) The use of CO2 removal devices in patients awaiting lung transplantation: an initial experience. Transplant Proc 42(4):1255–1258
128. Fuehner T, Kuehn C, Hadem J, Wiesner O, Gottlieb J, Tudorache I, Olsson KM, Greer M, Sommer W, Welte T, Haverich A, Hoeper MM, Warnecke G (2012) Extracorporeal membrane oxygenation in awake patients as bridge to lung transplantation. Am J Respir Crit Care Med 185(7):763–768
129. Livigni S, Maio M, Ferretti E, Longobardo A, Potenza R, Rivalta L, Selvaggi P, Vergano M, Bertolini G (2006) Efficacy and safety of a low-flow veno-venous carbon dioxide removal device: results of an experimental study in adult sheep. Crit Care 10(5):R151
130. Fanelli V, Ranieri MV, Mancebo J, Moerer O, Quintel M, Morley S et al (2016) Feasibility and safety of low-flow extracorporeal carbon dioxide removal to facilitate ultra-protective ventilation in patients with moderate acute respiratory distress syndrome. Critical Care (London, England) 20(1):36
131. Terragni PP, Del Sorbo L, Mascia L, Urbino R, Martin EL, Birocco A et al (2009) Tidal volume lower than 6 mL/kg enhances lung protection. Anesthesiology 111(4):826–835

132. Turani F, Martini S, Marinelli A, Falco M, Barchetta R, Candidi F, Gargano F (2013) ECCO2 removal with a phosphorylcholine-coated membrane oxygenator in difficult respiratory weaning patients. Crit Care 17(2):1
133. Lund LW, Federspiel WJ (2013) Removing extra CO2 in COPD patients. Curr Respir Care Rep 2:131–138
134. Bein T, Weber-Carstens S, Goldmann A, Müller T, Staudinger T, Brederlau J et al (2013) Lower tidal volume strategy (≈3 mL/kg) combined with extracorporeal CO2 removal versus "conventional" protective ventilation (6 mL/kg) in severe ARDS: the prospective randomized Xtravent-study. Intensive Care Med 39(5):847–856
135. Zimmermann M, Bein T, Arlt M, Philipp A, Rupprecht L, Mueller T et al (2009) Pumpless extracorporeal interventional lung assist in patients with acute respiratory distress syndrome: a prospective pilot study. Critical Care (London, England) 13(1):R10
136. Bein T, Weber F, Philipp A, Prasser C, Pfeifer M, Schmid FX, Butz B, Birnbaum D, Taeger K, Schlitt HJ (2006) A new pumpless extracorporeal interventional lung assist in critical hypoxemia/hypercapnia. Crit Care Med 34(5):1372–1377
137. Terragni P, Ranieri VM, Brazzi L (2015) Novel approaches to minimize ventilator-induced lung injury. Curr Opin Crit Care 21(1):20–25

Hemodynamic Monitoring and Fluid Management in ARDS

8

Dusan Hanidziar and Edward A. Bittner

8.1 Introduction

Acute respiratory distress syndrome (ARDS) is a major cause of morbidity and mortality in the ICU affecting as many as 10% of critically ill patients and almost a quarter of mechanically ventilated patients [1, 2]. ARDS is characterized by increased permeability of the alveolar-capillary membrane due to dysregulated, tissue-destructive inflammation. Pulmonary edema, the result of fluid maldistribution, has an adverse impact on respiratory function at several levels including decreased lung compliance, impaired gas exchange, reduction of surfactant levels, and pulmonary hypertension [3]. In the early phase of ARDS, a systemic inflammatory state is usually responsible for hypovolemia. In this phase, early and adequate fluid resuscitation is essential to prevent the development of multiorgan dysfunction, which can impact mortality in patients with ARDS [4]. As the inflammatory state resolves, the excessive fluid can have a detrimental impact on patient outcome. Transition from one phase to another is complex and can often be difficult to distinguish. However, identifying the transition between these two phases is likely to be important for optimization of fluid balance and improving patient outcomes.

Hemodynamic monitoring and modulation of fluid status in patients with ARDS have been the focus of a number of studies – some promising and others disappointing in their physiological effects and impact on patient outcomes. While such investigations may ultimately improve patient-centered outcomes, fluid management in ARDS continues to be a source of great controversy. Fluid management is a complex issue and one of the most challenging aspects of critical care. The focus of this chapter is to review the current literature on hemodynamic monitoring and fluid management of patients with ARDS with a goal toward improving patient outcomes and identifying opportunities for further investigation.

D. Hanidziar, MD, PhD (✉) • E.A. Bittner, MD, PhD
Anesthesia, Critical Care and Pain Medicine,
Massachusetts General Hospital/Harvard Medical School, Boston, MA, USA
e-mail: dhanidziar@partners.org; ebittner@mgh.harvard.edu

D. Chiumello (ed.), *Acute Respiratory Distress Syndrome (ARDS)*,
DOI 10.1007/978-3-319-41852-0_8

8.2 Pathophysiology

An understanding of the pathophysiology of ARDS with its associated fluid maldistribution and accumulation is essential for developing an approach to management. While ARDS can be triggered by a wide range of pulmonary and extrapulmonary processes, the syndrome shares a common pattern of an acutely developed alveolar-capillary injury. The early phase of ARDS is characterized by diffuse alveolar damage, with disruption of the alveolar epithelial and endothelial cell layers. As a result of increased alveolar-capillary permeability, protein-rich pulmonary edema fluid accumulates in the alveolar spaces, along with neutrophils, macrophages, and erythrocytes. Fibrin-rich hyaline membranes form along the denuded basement membrane [5]. Airspace filling is likely exacerbated by epithelial injury and a decrease in the capacity of the injured alveolar epithelium to reabsorb edema fluid [6]. Edema reabsorption requires that the fluid leak be reduced not only by reduction of endothelial permeability but also by restoration of the functional, more impermeable epithelial layer.

Increased interstitial hydrostatic pressure and pulmonary edema weight have been suggested to be among the key mechanisms of atelectasis formation according to the "sponge theory of ARDS," postulating a fall in lung compliance combined with compression and collapse of dependent small airways [7]. In ARDS, the greater the degree of pulmonary microvascular permeability, the more outward fluid filtration from microvessels will occur, at any given level of pulmonary vascular hydrostatic pressure [8]. Also, if the pulmonary vascular hydrostatic pressure increases as frequently occurs during fluid resuscitation, the increase in pulmonary edema is even more pronounced. With severe ARDS, pulmonary hypertension may develop with increased pulmonary capillary pressure and/or cardiac failure adding a hydrostatic component to the edema formation. Although alveolar-capillary barrier dysfunction primarily causes the pulmonary edema seen in this disease, reduced colloid osmotic pressure may contribute to the generation and persistence of pulmonary edema as well [9]. In fact, hypoproteinemia is one of the strongest predictors of the development of ARDS among patients with sepsis [10].

In noninjured lungs, pulmonary edema is strictly controlled by the lymphatic drainage system, which constantly removes extravascular lung water (EVLW) from the interstitial tissue and drains it into the superior vena cava via the thoracic duct. In the early stages of ARDS, the increase in interstitial edema is regulated by a compensatory increase of lymphatic drainage. However, as the amount of interstitial edema increases, lymphatic drainage is overwhelmed, and interstitial edema enters the alveoli [11, 12]. The first accumulation site for this pulmonary edema is the loose peri-bronchovascular connective tissue of the lung hila, since this area has both low resistance to fluid flux and major compliance. While interstitial pressure in this area remains low, there is little resorption of interstitial edema, and the pressure gradient remains in favor of further transudation from pulmonary vasculature toward the interstitium thereby worsening fluid maldistribution. Lung weight increases from the accumulation of pulmonary edema producing compression atelectasis with impairment of pulmonary mechanics and gas exchange. Furthermore, increased intrathoracic pressure resulting from positive-pressure mechanical ventilation leads to the activation of feedback systems designed to maintain intravascular volume and arterial pressures [13]. In particular, the renal aldosterone-angiotensin system is activated leading to water and salt retention. Therefore, in ARDS, in addition to the original inflammatory protein-rich edema accumulation, there is a superimposed tendency to retain the infused fluids with further water accumulation.

8.3 Adverse Effects of Fluid Overload

The accumulation of interstitial and alveolar fluid in the lungs plays a central role in the pathogenesis of ARDS. The detrimental impact of pulmonary edema may not be immediately apparent clinically because the quantity of pulmonary edema fluid, which is reflected by extravascular lung water, can increase two- to threefold prior to a significant decrease in arterial oxygenation [14]. However, clinical data suggest that the quantity of edema fluid in patients appears to be an important determinant of hospital morbidity and mortality in patients with ARDS. Almost 30 years ago, Simmons et al. observed that an increase in body weight and fluid balance in ARDS patients was correlated with survival [15]. Humphrey et al. subsequently demonstrated that patients with ARDS who achieved goal-directed fluid removal had a statistically greater hospital survival compared to those not attaining this therapeutic end point [16]. In a later study, Sakr et al. showed that even after controlling for degree of organ dysfunction and size of tidal volumes, patients with ARDS who survived their ICU stay had a net negative fluid balance compared to nonsurvivors [17]. The association between positive fluid balance and adverse outcome has also been reported in the pediatric population [18]. Other studies have focused on quantification of the amount of pulmonary edema using measures of extravascular lung water (EVLW) obtained by thermodilution techniques and evaluated the influence on outcome in patients at risk for ARDS. Sakka et al. retrospectively analyzed 373 intensive care unit (ICU) patients and found that the maximum quantity of EVLW was significantly higher in nonsurvivors than in survivors [19]. However, the prognostic effect of the quantity of edema fluid, measured by thermodilution, was not found in patients presenting with ARDS in this study. However, studies where EVLW was indexed to ideal body weight (extravascular lung water index, EVLWI) have found EVLW to be a significant predictor of mortality. Phillips et al. found that the EVLWI measured on day 1 of ARDS was found to be predictive of mortality [20]. In another study, Cordemans et al. reported that the maximum difference between EVLWI measurements during the patient's stay in the ICU was related to poor prognosis [21]. More recently, Jozwiak et al. reported that in patients with ARDS, both the EVLWI and pulmonary vascular permeability index, a measure of the integrity of the alveolar-capillary barrier obtained by thermodilution, were independent risk factors for mortality [22].

8.4 Benefits of Fluid Restriction

Given the evidence that excessive lung water is associated with worsened outcomes in patients with ARDS, a fundamental question is whether an aggressive approach to reducing the amount of lung water when guided by EVLW measurement or other clinical parameters can improve outcomes. The landmark Fluid and Catheter Treatment Trial (FACTT) evaluated the benefits of fluid restriction in patients with ARDS [23]. In this study, the fluid management was based on measuring central venous pressure (CVP) or pulmonary capillary wedge pressure. Patients without evidence of shock with a central venous catheter were randomized to maintain a target central venous pressure of less than 4 mmHg in the conservative group compared with 10–14 mmHg in the liberal treatment group. Patients with a pulmonary artery catheter had a target pulmonary capillary wedge pressure of less than 8 mmHg in the conservative group compared with 14–18 mmHg in the liberal strategy. Patients assigned to the conservative fluid management group had a significantly improved mean oxygenation index, the lung injury score, an increased number of ventilator-free days, and decreased length of stay in the ICU, although they demonstrated no difference in hospital mortality compared with the liberal fluid management group. Despite the importance of these findings, the exclusion of hemodynamically unstable patients or patients with renal failure makes it impossible to generalize these results or to create a simple protocol for management of the fluid status in all ARDS patients. In most patients, ARDS occurs within the context of a generalized process of systemic inflammation resulting from conditions such as severe sepsis, burn injury, hemorrhagic shock, and necrotizing pancreatitis that are responsible for hemodynamic dysfunction. A number of guidelines for these conditions recommend an aggressive and early fluid resuscitation, based on the body of evidence showing that rapid repletion of fluid deficit in shock prevents the critical decrease of oxygen delivery, attenuates the severity of multiple organ dysfunction, and reduces mortality [24–26]. However, when these conditions are complicated by coinciding ARDS, the optimal fluid management remains unknown. A study of septic patients with acute lung injury showed that mortality was increased in patients who did not receive adequate early fluid management [27]. However, excessive early fluid administration can be accompanied by intense fluid accumulation in the tissues, particularly in the lungs, leading to increase in pulmonary edema. This fluid administration dilemma forces the clinician to modify the early goal-directed resuscitation approach and consider "permissive hypovolemia" [28]. Whether this approach is optimal for ARDS patients is unclear; however, if undertaken, it is probably best implemented in the settings of advanced volumetric and metabolic monitoring.

8.5 Fluid Measurement and Monitoring

8.5.1 Measurement of Pulmonary Edema

8.5.1.1 Clinical

Accurate measurement and quantification of pulmonary edema are important for diagnostic and therapeutic interventions. Clinically pulmonary edema can be detected on physical examination by the presence of rales and may be confirmed by chest radiography. However, it has been shown to be difficult to quantify the amount of pulmonary edema based on chest radiography alone [29]. Other indirect radiological estimates of lung water, such as CT scanning and MRI, while more accurate, are impractical for real-time measurement in critically ill patients.

8.5.1.2 Extravascular Lung Water

Limitations of indirect measures of lung water led to the development of thermal dye techniques to allow estimation of lung water at the bedside. Currently, the single transpulmonary thermodilution technique is considered the clinical gold standard of lung water estimation [30]. Using this technique, the extravascular lung water (EVLW), which is the amount of fluid that is accumulated in the interstitial and alveolar spaces, can be calculated. EVLW obtained via the single transpulmonary thermodilution technique has been shown to compare favorably with other methods of lung water assessment including the double-indicator dilution technique and the ex vivo gravimetric method [31]. Compared to non-indexed EVLW, EVLW adjusted for body weight (EVLWI, mL/kg) is better correlated with the severity of lung injury and the oxygenation in patients with ARDS [32]. An increased value of EVLWI is a pathophysiological hallmark of hydrostatic as well as inflammatory lung edema, and this technique can detect small (10–20%) increases in lung water [33]. The normal value for EVLWI is reported to be approximately 7 mL/kg and results from the equilibrium between fluid leakage and lymphatic drainage [34]. Values of the EVLWI exceeding 30 mL/kg have been reported during severe pulmonary edema [22].

8.5.1.3 Pulmonary Vascular Permeability Index

Transpulmonary thermodilution also provides a method for estimation of the integrity of the alveolar-capillary barrier of the lung referred to as the pulmonary vascular permeability index (PVPI) [35]. The PVPI is the ratio between the volume of fluid that has leaked into the extravascular space (EVLWI) and the volume of fluid that has remained in the intravascular compartment (pulmonary blood volume). The value of PVPI has been validated in both animal and human studies showing that it was significantly higher in patients with ARDS than in patients with hydrostatic pulmonary edema [12]. A PVPI value of 3 is considered to be the maximal normal value [36]. As with EVLWI, elevated PVPI values have also been shown to predict mortality in patients with ARDS [22]. Clinically, both the EVLWI and PVPI may be complementarily useful to guide fluid management of patients at risk of fluid overload, as in patients with ARDS. For a given value of EVLWI, the higher the PVPI, the greater the risk of increase in extravascular lung water during fluid administration.

8.5.1.4 Ultrasound

An accumulating body of evidence suggests that lung ultrasound is useful for management of patients with ARDS. Lung ultrasound can provide a semiquantitative estimate of the presence and dynamic changes in lung water and assist in confirming the diagnosis of ARDS [37]. In the presence of interstitial-alveolar fluid, vertical artifacts arising from the pleura ("B lines") are detectable, and evidence suggests real-time matching of B-line quantity with changes in EVLW and total body water [38]. Scores based on number and thickness of B lines have been developed which permit a semiquantitative evaluation of the amount of extravascular lung water and lung density [39, 40]. Recently, a quantitative lung ultrasound method has been proposed [41]. A small study of pulmonary edema patients suggests that bedside lung ultrasound may be useful in distinguishing between inflammatory and hydrostatic edema [42]. Inflammatory edema is suggested by spared areas, pleural abnormalities, and consolidation, whereas large effusions, a smooth thin pleural line, and diffuse homogenous alveolar-interstitial syndrome (or white lung) suggest hydrostatic edema. Given its diagnostic ability, ready availability, and ease of use, ultrasound is a useful point of care tool for this estimation.

8.5.2 Hemodynamic Monitoring

8.5.2.1 General Principles/Strategies

In most patients, ARDS is part of an early and generalized systemic inflammation that is responsible for hemodynamic dysfunction. While conservative fluid management in later ARDS is associated with improved outcomes, optimal fluid management in this early period remains unclear. Methods of hemodynamic optimization and fluid management which account for dynamic changes over time are most likely to have a positive impact on patient outcomes. The risks associated with excessive fluid administration have led to development of strategies to assess "fluid responsiveness" before performing volume expansion. In principle, the only reason to administer fluid is to increase stroke volume (SV); if SV does not increase, fluid administration serves no rational purpose and is likely to be harmful [43]. Studies in heterogeneous groups of critically ill and injured patients have consistently demonstrated that only about 50% of hemodynamically unstable patients are fluid responsive, that is, their SV will increase by greater than 10–15% following a fluid bolus [44, 45]. These considerations suggest that determining whether a patient is fluid responsive as well as determining the patient's "position" on his or her Frank-Starling curve should occur prior to each fluid bolus. According to the Frank-Starling principle, as the preload increases, left ventricular SV increases until the optimal preload is achieved at which point the SV remains relatively constant [46]. A necessary requirement for this model is that both ventricles are operating on similar points of their Frank-Starling curve. In patients with RV dysfunction, SV may not increase with fluid loading (it may actually decrease) even though the LV is preload responsive. The adverse effects of fluid loading occur as the patient reaches the plateau of his or her Frank-Starling curve, when atrial pressures increase sharply, increasing venous and pulmonary hydrostatic pressures, which causes a shift of fluid into the interstitial space with an increase in pulmonary and peripheral tissue edema. Furthermore, increased cardiac filling pressures increase the release of natriuretic peptides which cleave membrane-bound proteoglycans and glycoproteins off the endothelial glycocalyx, thereby further increasing endothelial permeability [47, 48].

8.5.2.2 Static Parameters

Static markers of cardiac preload, such as the central venous pressure or pulmonary artery occlusion pressure, have been used for decades for testing fluid responsiveness; however, recent literature has questioned their reliability [44, 49]. The major reason for this unreliability is that the slope of the cardiac function curve depends on the cardiac systolic function that varies among patients. Therefore, an absolute value of any "static" measure of preload could correspond to either preload dependence or preload independence. An additional element of unreliability in the use of static markers of preload comes from errors that can occur in their measurement and interpretation [50]. Although static markers of preload cannot reliably be used to predict fluid responsiveness, they may have utility in confirming that the fluid administered has actually filled the cardiac chambers. In addition, cardiac filling pressures may have a role as safety parameters during fluid administration, i.e., a large increase in filling pressures can help to decide to stop fluid administration [51]. To address the shortcomings of the static indices for prediction of fluid responsiveness, a variety of dynamic indices have been developed. These dynamic indices are based on observing the changes in cardiac output or stroke volume resulting from heart-lung interactions during mechanical ventilation, by postural maneuvers, or fluid challenges [52]. This section will briefly review several "dynamic" indices of fluid responsiveness and their role in hemodynamic management of patients with ARDS.

8.5.2.3 Dynamic Parameters

Pulse Pressure Variation

During positive-pressure mechanical ventilation, intrathoracic pressure increases with lung insufflation, which reduces venous return to the right heart. If the right ventricle is preload-dependent, this will inevitably reduce the right ventricular outflow and ultimately result in a reduced left ventricular preload. Hence, positive-pressure mechanical ventilation induces cyclic changes in intrathoracic pressure that transiently affect ventricular preload, resulting in greater cyclic changes in stroke volume (SV) when the ventricle operates on the steep (responder) rather than on the flat (nonresponder) portion of the Frank-Starling curve. These cyclic changes in SV can be evaluated by changes in pulse pressure over the respiratory cycle because the pulse pressure is proportional to SV [53].

A number of studies have demonstrated that pulse pressure variation (PPV) is a reliable indicator of fluid responsiveness in critically ill patients including those with ARDS, provided that the conditions of its validity are fulfilled. Pulse pressure variation (ΔPP) has been proposed to predict fluid responsiveness in patients with ARDS [54, 55]. However, the respiratory variation in pulse pressure as a marker of fluid responsiveness is not valid under some conditions that commonly affect patients with ARDS. First, in the setting of spontaneous breathing activity, stroke volume variations are related more to the respiratory irregularity rather than to preload dependence [56]. Second, in the setting of cardiac arrhythmias, the variation of stroke volume is related more to arrhythmia itself than to heart-lung interactions

[57]. A third important limitation occurs in the setting of low tidal volume ventilation and/or with low lung compliance which are common in patients with ARDS. In this setting the low tidal volumes and lung compliance can reduce the transmission of changes in alveolar pressure to the intrathoracic structures, thereby diminishing the magnitude of the ventilation-induced changes of intravascular pressure [55]. This may result in false-negative predictions of fluid responsiveness by PPV. To improve the performance of ΔPP for assessment of fluid responsiveness in patients managed with low tidal volume, a recent study reported correction of ΔPP by pleural pressure changes. ΔPpl values facilitate discrimination between responders and nonresponders. In their analysis, a ΔPP/ΔPpl greater than 2 predicted fluid responsiveness with a sensitivity of 92.3% and a specificity of 93.2% [58]. While this work shows promise, further validation is needed.

Respiratory Variation of the Inferior Vena Cava

The increase in intrathoracic pressure with positive-pressure mechanical ventilation can induce changes in the diameter of the inferior vena cava (IVC). Due to the IVC's high compliance, the changes are more likely to be observed in the case of hypovolemia than in normo- or hypervolemia. In patients receiving positive-pressure ventilation, respiratory variation of the diameter of the IVC has been demonstrated to be a reliable predictor of fluid responsiveness [59]. As with other dynamic measures based on heart-lung interactions, IVC variation has only limited predictive value in the case of spontaneous breathing activity [60]. Additionally, low lung compliance and mechanical ventilation with a low tidal volume should theoretically minimize the effect of ventilation on the vena cava diameter and may thus invalidate the method. By contrast, IVC collapsibility to assess fluid responsiveness can be used in the setting of cardiac arrhythmias. The respiratory variation of the inferior vena cava is simple to measure by transthoracic echocardiography, which represents an important advantage. In fact, the subcostal ultrasonic window may prove to be the only window providing an acceptable image in patients with ARDS due to the increased echogenicity of the lungs. Ultrasonic assessment of the IVC may be particularly useful for assessing volume responsiveness in the early phase of care, before arterial cannulation has been performed.

Fluid Challenge

The most intuitive way to test fluid responsiveness is to administer a fluid challenge and observe its effects on cardiac output. The disadvantage of the "common" fluid challenge is that it consists of administering 250–500 mL of fluid. This volume of fluid may seem negligible at first; however, performing fluid challenges repeatedly, as can occur in the early phase of shock, may contribute to significant fluid overload. A "mini fluid challenge" has been described as an alternative [61, 62]. Nevertheless, small amounts of fluid can only induce small changes in stroke volume and cardiac output. Thus, this test requires a very precise technique for measuring cardiac output. Whether the "mini fluid challenge" is effective for clinical decision-making requires further investigation.

The Passive Leg-Raising Maneuver

An alternative to the fluid bolus for assessing fluid responsiveness is the passive leg-raising (PLR) maneuver. The PLR maneuver is performed by lifting the patient's legs passively from the horizontal position, and it is associated with the gravitational transfer of blood from the lower extremities to the intrathoracic compartment [63]. Beyond its ease of use, this method has the advantage of reversing its effects once the legs are returned to the horizontal position. Therefore, the PLR maneuver may be considered a reversible "self-volume challenge" [64]. Since the maximal hemodynamic effects of PLR occur within the first minute of leg elevation, it is important to assess these effects with a method able to track real-time changes in SV. The change in blood pressure following a PLR or fluid challenge is a poor guide to fluid responsiveness; SV may increase without a significant change in blood pressure. The reliability of PLR as a test of preload responsiveness has been confirmed in multiple studies performed in critically ill patients [65].

EVLW as a Therapeutic Target

EVLW is a sensitive marker of the development of pulmonary edema correlating with markers of lung injury, including the PaO_2/FiO_2 oxygenation ratio, lung compliance, chest radiograph, and lung injury score. Patients with ARDS may therefore benefit from management guided by EVLW. An early diagnosis of the pathological accumulation of EVLW during resuscitation may allow for earlier interventions and changes in the therapeutic plan [12]. In addition, monitoring of EVLW may identify the point when de-resuscitation should be started, namely, the institution of an aggressive negative fluid balance once the hemodynamic status stabilizes. While this approach seems promising, further clinical studies are required to demonstrate the benefit of such a strategy.

8.6 Fluid Restriction and Edema Clearance

8.6.1 Practical Considerations

Recovery from ARDS requires that the pulmonary edema resolves [66, 67]. The primary methods to decrease pulmonary edema are the use of loop diuretics, such as furosemide and/or hemofiltration. The inherent risk of these methods is the induction of organ hypoperfusion. Monitoring strategies to guide the edema clearance by furosemide or hemofiltration before inducing organ hypoperfusion should be beneficial for outcomes, although data to support this assertion is limited. Recently the E/Ea ratio, an ultrasound-derived marker of left ventricular filling pressure, has been reported to be a discriminating factor for identifying ARDS patients who will not tolerate negative fluid balance [68]. The FACTT trial demonstrated that for patients with ARDS that are not in shock, adopting a conservative fluid management strategy improves pulmonary-related outcome. However, despite the benefit, the FACTT protocol was complex and practically difficult to implement in routine clinical practice. The protocol contained a total of 18 different cells with

Table 8.1 Simplified fluid and catheter treatment trial "FACTT Lite" protocol[a]

Central venous pressure	Urine output <0.5 mL/kg/h	Urine output ≥0.5 mL/kg/h
>8	Furosemide[b]	Furosemide[c]
4–8	Fluid bolus[b]	Furosemide[c]
<4	Fluid bolus[b]	No intervention[c]

Adapted from Grissom et al. [69]
[a]Recommended for patients with mean arterial pressure ≥60 mmHg and off vasopressors for ≥12 h
[b]Reassess in 1 h
[c]Reassess in 4 h

instructions that include dobutamine infusion, fluid bolus, or furosemide administration. To more easily operationalize a fluid restrictive strategy in subsequent trials, the ARDS Network investigators developed a simplified conservative fluid protocol, "FACTT Lite" (Table 8.1) [69]. The FACTT Lite provided three possible instructions determined by the CVP and urine output: furosemide administration, fluid bolus, or no intervention. As with the original FACTT Conservative protocol, FACTT Lite contained instructions to withhold furosemide until the patient achieved a mean arterial pressure greater than 60 mmHg off of vasopressors for at least 12 h.

A retrospective comparison of the performance of FACTT Lite with FACTT Conservative and FACTT Liberal was recently reported. Fluid management with FACTT Lite resulted in a significantly greater average cumulative fluid balance (+2.05 L) over 7 days than FACTT Conservative but a significantly lower average cumulative fluid balance compared to FACTT Liberal (+5.07 L mL) over the same time period. In subjects without baseline shock, in whom the fluid protocol was applied throughout the duration of the study, management with FACTT Lite resulted in an equivalent cumulative fluid balance to FACTT Conservative and had similar clinical outcomes of ventilator-free days, ICU-free days, and mortality as FACTT Conservative and significantly greater ventilator-free days and ICU-free days than FACTT Liberal. Interestingly, development of new-onset shock during the study was lower in the FACTT Lite group than in the FACTT Conservative group. This might be explained by a less aggressive diuresis in the first 2 days in the FACTT Lite group compared with the FACTT Conservative group.

8.6.2 Enhancing Edema Clearance

8.6.2.1 Modulation of Oncotic Pressure

Endogenous albumin is an important regulator of endothelial integrity [70, 71]. From a hemodynamic point of view, hypoalbuminemia results in a decrease in plasma oncotic pressure; therefore, pulmonary edema forms at a lower hydrostatic pressure because the oncotic pressure gradient between plasma and the interstitium decreases [72]. Administration of albumin to raise oncotic pressure and promote the water movement from the interstitial to the intravascular space has been suggested as a method to reduce pulmonary edema. This approach can be combined with the use of furosemide to facilitate the removal of the excess fluid from the plasma. The efficacy of this approach was initially evaluated by Martin et al. in a trial of 37 hypoproteinemic patients with acute lung injury randomized to receive protocolized albumin replacement and continuous infusion of furosemide versus double placebo [73]. The patients treated with albumin and furosemide showed improvement of oxygenation with better hemodynamics and fluid balance compared with controls. Based on the results of this study, it was estimated that the albumin/furosemide protocol accelerated the edema clearance, by 3–4 days compared with its natural evolution [74]. The beneficial effect of albumin administration was subsequently evaluated in a small trial which compared the efficacy of furosemide and albumin compared to furosemide alone [75]. This trial suggested that albumin is a critical component of this regimen, for both maintenance of hemodynamic stability and improved oxygenation. While these studies suggest promise, it is important to stress, however, that both studies excluded patients with hemodynamic instability and/or receiving vasopressor support suggesting that the full-blown phase of ARDS was already overcome in the enrolled patients. Larger trials are needed to confirm the findings and define the optimal timing of colloid/diuretic administration.

8.6.2.2 Pharmacologic Therapies

The resolution of alveolar edema does not occur by normalization of vascular pressures alone but is driven by active transport of sodium and chloride ions from the alveolar luminal space across the epithelial cells, thereby creating an osmotic gradient for the reabsorption of water. The use of pharmacologic agents to promote sodium (and water) transport out of the alveoli is an appealing and complementary way to enhance the edema clearance. Even with severe epithelial injury, alveolar clearance may be pharmacologically stimulatable [76]. Several experimental studies have shown that the exogenous administration of cAMP agonists, in particular $\beta_2$agonists, accelerates the resolution of edema [77]. The action of $\beta_2$agonists principally occurs through an increase in the quantity and activity of Na/K pumps in the basal membrane and sodium channels in the pneumocyte apical membrane. The net effect of these actions is to increase the sodium gradient between the alveoli and the interstitium and thereby increase the absorption of water.

A randomized trial in 40 ARDS patients by Perkins et al. suggested that the infusion of salbutamol compared with placebo for 7 days was able to significantly diminish the quantity of pulmonary water measured by transpulmonary thermodilution without affecting oxygenation and duration of mechanical ventilation [78]. Unfortunately, the suggested benefit was not demonstrated in successive trials. In fact, a multicenter trial by the same investigators that randomly assigned ARDS patients to intravenous salbutamol or placebo was terminated early because of excess mortality in the treatment group [79]. In the related trial which compared aerosolized albuterol or saline treatment in acute lung injury, there was also no benefit in either ventilator-free days or mortality [80]. A number of possible explanations have been proposed for failure of $\beta_2$agonist therapy to improve outcomes in these clinical trials including inadequate aerosol drug delivery, downregulation of beta-2 receptors, and inability of injured alveolar epithelium to respond to a

$\beta_2$agonist. Finally, it is possible that with lung-protective ventilation and a fluid-conservative hemodynamic strategy, there was little opportunity to further enhance alveolar fluid clearance with the $\beta_2$agonist. While some questions remain, such as whether or not there may be a benefit with a different cAMP agonist or benefit in specific subpopulations, the available data do not support the use of $\beta_2$agonist to facilitate edema clearance.

8.7 General Paradigm for Resuscitation in ARDS

In addition to the amount of fluid administered, it is increasingly being recognized that timing of fluid administration during the course of critical illness is crucial: both immediate commencements of resuscitation with target end points in the early phase of critical illness followed by fluid restriction and mobilization when shock resolves are of utmost importance in achieving best outcomes. This process has recently been more formally divided into four phases that are distinguishable based on the time course of critical illness denoted by the acronym "ROSE": rescue, optimization, stabilization, and evacuation (Table 8.2) [81]. In each of these four stages of treatment modalities, goals and monitoring tools can substantially differ. Adaptation of this paradigm to the hemodynamic management of patients with ARDS may be beneficial for patient management and is described in the following section and summarized in Table 8.2.

The *rescue* phase encompasses the period of initial stabilization of the patient with severe systemic hypotension and evidence of tissue hypoperfusion. In this phase, the immediate goal is to correct the shock, and intravenous fluids are typically first line therapy. Fluid administration is expected to increase cardiac preload and, in the case of preload dependence, to increase cardiac output and eventually improve tissue oxygenation. Evidence is lacking to support the use of specific resuscitation protocols for patients with ARDS during this period. The volume of fluid required during this phase must be individualized and will necessarily vary between patients. However, patients with coincident conditions such as sepsis may benefit from a protocolized approach developed for that condition. Since the need for intervention is immediate, only those readily available tools and targets should be considered. Multiple fluid boluses may need to be administered to achieve a predefined blood pressure target, often with limited hemodynamic monitoring such as routine bedside vital signs. During the resuscitative phase, fluids must be administered in a timely and targeted manner with appropriate limits to fluid administration.

Maintaining the mean arterial pressure above the lower autoregulatory threshold for perfusion of the most vulnerable organs (heart, brain, kidneys) is essential. Invasive blood pressure monitoring should be initiated to allow continuous blood pressure display. Consideration of the patients' individual premorbid conditions (e.g., hypertension, CHF) may be more beneficial in establishing resuscitation goals rather than what is recommended as a universal target in the guidelines. Maintaining adequate mean arterial pressure in mechanically ventilated patients with permissive hypercapnia is critical given that impaired cerebral autoregulation can predispose

Table 8.2 Paradigm for fluid resuscitation/hemodynamic management in patients with ARDS

Stage	Patient characteristics	Hemodynamic goals	Strategy	Targets and monitoring tools
Rescue	Severe hypotension Evidence of tissue hypoperfusion	Rapid correction of shock Maintain lower autoregulatory limits for organ perfusion	Rapid fluid bolusing to increase cardiac preload and CO	Clinical signs/symptoms Macrohemodynamics (MAP, CO) Lactate Dynamic parameters (PPV, IVC variation, fluid bolus, PLR)
Optimization	Evidence of tissue hypoperfusion	Improve cardiac output and oxygen delivery Maintain tissue perfusion	Titrate fluids Continue fluid boluses in responders and avoid in nonresponders Initiate vasoactive agents early in fluid nonresponders Inotropic support if poor cardiac performance coupled with signs of organ hypoperfusion	Organ perfusion (MAP, CO, $ScvO_2$) Fluid responsiveness EVLW and PVPI as safety parameters
Stabilization	No evidence of tissue hypoperfusion Stable or decreasing doses of vasopressors	Maintain even to negative fluid balance	Restrict fluids	Daily and cumulative fluid balance, body weight
Evacuation	No evidence of tissue hypoperfusion No requirement for vasopressors	Mobilize accumulated fluid while avoiding organ hypoperfusion	Administer diuretics +/− albumin Extracorporeal removal if poor response to diuretics	Negative daily and cumulative fluid balance, body weight Ultrasound (E/Ea ratio)

Adapted from Malbrain et al. [81]

patients with decreased cerebrovascular reserve to cerebral ischemia [82]. Besides, standard hemodynamic monitors, ultrasonography, and echocardiography may offer valuable advanced information on heart function, including preload, contractility, and ventricular performance.

In the *optimization* phase, the therapeutic goal is to maintain tissue perfusion. This phase should be monitored using clinical judgment as well as physiologic and biochemical parameters individualized to the patient. Conventional indicators of the adequacy of resuscitation, such as the resolution of oliguria, a decrease in lactate levels, and improving $ScvO_2$, can be helpful but may not occur in every patient. However, it is important to acknowledge that none of these indices have a high enough sensitivity on their own to be used as a target in every patient; therefore, a "multimodal" approach to optimization may be necessary. Monitoring of EVLW and PVPI may be valuable to prevent fluid overload. Vasoactive agents should be initiated early in fluid nonresponders in order to minimize the pathological pooling of blood and help mobilizing the unstressed volume. Providing inotropic support should be reserved for those patients who after optimizing both pre- and afterload still show unsatisfactory cardiac performance coupled with signs of organ hypoperfusion.

Fluid administration is often a necessary component of optimization, but unmonitored volume resuscitation in patients with persistent hypoperfusion increases the likelihood of fluid overload. The absence of fluid responsiveness or evidence of fluid overload should be used to determine when to stop giving fluid challenges in patients who fail to achieve their resuscitation goals. The importance of this approach in patients with ARDS is demonstrated by a recently published retrospective analysis of the FACTT trial which examined the effect of fluid bolus administration in the patients randomized to the pulmonary artery catheter arm of the study [83]. Importantly, less than a quarter of the patients were fluid responders (increase in CI >15%). Furthermore, fluid boluses were unlikely to result in an increase in urine output, and only small changes in heart rate or mean arterial pressure after a fluid bolus were noted. Therefore, routine administration of fluids to patients with shock or oliguria who were previously resuscitated may not improve organ function.

In the *stabilization* phase, there is adequate tissue perfusion, and although patients may still require vasopressor support, the doses of these medications are stable or decreasing. In the absence of evidence suggesting hypoperfusion, fluid administration should be restricted. Fluid challenges should not be routinely given, even in those who are fluid responsive. Maintenance fluids are usually not required and should be discontinued when possible as critically ill patients frequently receive sufficient fluids with medications and nutrition to account for insensible losses.

In the *evacuation* phase, interventions are targeted at fluid removal. There is no consensus about the optimal timing of fluid removal, and there are limited data to guide a specific recommendation. In the FACTT and FACTT Lite trials, patients were required to have been off vasopressor therapy for at least 12 h before diuretics were administered. A reasonable approach is to begin with restricting fluids when patients achieve hemodynamic stability and/or normal tissue perfusion and then to consider initiating diuresis in patients with clinical evidence of fluid overload that are unable to achieve a negative fluid balance spontaneously. Negative fluid balance may be achieved by the combined administration of furosemide alone or together with albumin. However, in some patients the response to diuretics remains poor. In these cases an active de-resuscitation by extracorporeal means may be considered. There are concerns about the risk of organ hypoperfusion associated with active fluid removal, and the data providing guidance for this phase of management are still limited. Consequently, fluid removal should be performed cautiously with clear limits and appropriate safety monitoring to avoid inducing hypovolemia. The use of hemodynamic indices such as the E/Ea ratio, EVLWI, and PVPI may aid in facilitating edema clearance without compromising end-organ function.

Conclusion

Fluid overload in patients with ARDS is a preventable complication that is associated with increased morbidity and mortality. Two aspects of fluid management appear to be helpful in preventing fluid overload in patients with ARDS. First, during resuscitation, excessive fluid administration should be avoided. Second, removal of excess fluid should be promoted in patients whose shock has been resolved. A stage-targeted approach to hemodynamic management for patients with ARDS which combines clinical judgment along with sophisticated monitoring tools may be beneficial to guide management. Rational fluid management strategies should be implemented during each phase of resuscitation to help mitigate the effects of fluid overload and, thereby, improve outcomes. Initial fluid resuscitation should be guided by an assessment of fluid responsiveness until stabilization occurs, while later management requires a conservative fluid approach or even active fluid removal. Whether specific protocol-directed resuscitation for ARDS-associated shock improves outcome remains to be determined, while in established ARDS, a fluid-conservative approach is the minimum requirement. Further research on how to best personalize fluid therapy for the critically ill patients with ARDS is needed.

References

1. Bellani G, Laffey JG, Pham T et al (2016) Epidemiology, patterns of care, and mortality for patients with acute respiratory distress syndrome in intensive care units in 50 countries. JAMA 315:788–800
2. Phua J, Badia JR, Adhikari NK et al (2009) Has mortality from acute respiratory distress syndrome decreased over time?: a systematic review. Am J Respir Crit Care Med 179:220–227
3. Roch A, Guervilly C, Papazian L (2011) Fluid management in acute lung injury and ards. Ann Intensive Care 1:16
4. Stapleton RD, Wang BM, Hudson LD et al (2005) Causes and timing of death in patients with ARDS. Chest 128:525–532
5. Matthay MA, Ware LB, Zimmerman GA (2012) The acute respiratory distress syndrome. J Clin Invest 122:2731–2740
6. Matthay MA, Zimmerman GA (2005) Acute lung injury and the acute respiratory distress syndrome: four decades of inquiry into pathogenesis and rational management. Am J Respir Cell Mol Biol 33:319–327
7. Gattinoni L, Caironi P, Pelosi P, Goodman LR (2001) What has computed tomography taught us about the acute respiratory distress syndrome? Am J Respir Crit Care Med 164:1701–1711
8. Staub NC (1978) Pulmonary edema: physiologic approaches to management. Chest 74:559–564
9. Arif SK, Verheij J, Groeneveld AB, Raijmakers PG (2002) Hypoproteinemia as a marker of acute respiratory distress syndrome in critically ill patients with pulmonary edema. Intensive Care Med 28:310–317

10. Mangialardi RJ, Martin GS, Bernard GR et al (2000) Hypoproteinemia predicts acute respiratory distress syndrome development, weight gain, and death in patients with sepsis. Ibuprofen in Sepsis Study Group. Crit Care Med 28:3137–3145
11. Ware LB, Matthay MA (2005) Clinical practice. Acute pulmonary edema. N Engl J Med 353:2788–2796
12. Jozwiak M, Teboul J-L, Monnet X (2015) Extravascular lung water in critical care: recent advances and clinical applications. Ann Intensive Care 5:38
13. Koyner JL, Murray PT (2008) Mechanical ventilation and lung-kidney interactions. Clin J Am Soc Nephrol 3:562–570
14. Maharaj R (2012) Extravascular lung water and acute lung injury. Cardiol Res Pract 2012:Article ID 407035 6 pages
15. Simmons RS, Berdine GG, Seidenfeld JJ et al (1987) Fluid balance and the adult respiratory distress syndrome. Am Rev Respir Dis 135:924–929
16. Humphrey H, Hall J, Sznajder I et al (1990) Improved survival in ARDS patients associated with a reduction in pulmonary capillary wedge pressure. Chest 97:1176–1180
17. Sakr Y, Vincent JL, Reinhart K et al (2005) High tidal volume and positive fluid balance are associated with worse outcome in acute lung injury. Chest 128:3098–3108
18. Flori HR, Church G, Liu KD et al (2011) Positive fluid balance is associated with higher mortality and prolonged mechanical ventilation in pediatric patients with acute lung injury. Crit Care Res Pract 2011:854142
19. Sakka SG, Klein M, Reinhart K et al (2002) Prognostic value of extravascular lung water in critically ill patients. Chest 122:2080–2086
20. Phillips CR, Chesnutt MS, Smith SM (2008) Extravascular lung water in sepsis-associated acute respiratory distress syndrome: indexing with predicted body weight improves correlation with severity of illness and survival. Crit Care Med 36:69–73
21. Cordemans C, De Laet I, Van Regenmortel N, Schoonheydt K, Dits H, Huber W, Malbrain ML (2012) Fluid management in critically ill patients: the role of extravascular lung water, abdominal hypertension, capillary leak, and fluid balance. Ann Intensive Care 2(Suppl 1):S1
22. Jozwiak M, Silva S, Persichini R et al (2013) Extravascular lung water is an independent prognostic factor in patients with acute respiratory distress syndrome. Crit Care Med 41:472–480
23. National Heart, Lung, and Blood Institute Acute Respiratory Distress Syndrome (ARDS) Clinical Trials Network, Wiedemann HP, Wheeler AP, Bernard GR et al (2006) Comparison of two fluid-management strategies in acute lung injury. N Engl J Med 354:2564–2575
24. Dellinger RP, Levy MM, Rhodes A et al (2013) Surviving Sepsis Campaign: international guidelines for management of severe sepsis and septic shock, 2012. Intensive Care Med 39:165–228
25. Tenner S, Baillie J, DeWitt J, Vege SS (2013) American College of Gastroenterology guideline: management of acute pancreatitis. Am J Gastroenterol 108:1400–1415 ; 1416
26. Pham TN, Cancio LC, Gibran NS, American Burn Association (2008) American Burn Association practice guidelines burn shock resuscitation. J Burn Care Res 29:257–266
27. Murphy CV, Schramm GE, Doherty JA et al (2009) The importance of fluid management in acute lung injury secondary to septic shock. Chest 136:102–109
28. Kirov MY (2012) Pulmonary edema in hypovolemic patients: how can we predict it in clinical practice? Crit Care Med 40:994–995
29. Halperin BD, Feeley TW, Mihm FG, Chiles C, Guthaner DF, Blank NE (1985) Evaluation of the portable chest roentgenogram for quantitating extravascular lung water in critically ill adults. Chest 88:649–652
30. Shyamsundar M, Attwood B, Keating L, Walden AP (2013) Clinical review: the role of ultrasound in estimating extra-vascular lung water. Crit Care 17:237
31. Michard F (2007) Bedside assessment of extravascular lung water by dilution methods: temptations and pitfalls. Crit Care Med 35:1186–1192
32. Kushimoto S, Endo T, Yamanouchi S et al (2013) Relationship between extravascular lung water and severity categories of acute respiratory distress syndrome by the Berlin definition. Crit Care 17:R132

33. Fernández-Mondéjar E, Rivera-Fernández R, García-Delgado M, Touma A, Machado J, Chavero J (2005) Small increases in extravascular lung water are accurately detected by transpulmonary thermodilution. J Trauma 59:1420–1423
34. Tagami T, Kushimoto S, Yamamoto Y et al (2010) Validation of extravascular lung water measurement by single transpulmonary thermodilution: human autopsy study. Crit Care 14:R162
35. Monnet X, Anguel N, Osman D, Hamzaoui O, Richard C, Teboul JL (2007) Assessing pulmonary permeability by transpulmonary thermodilution allows differentiation of hydrostatic pulmonary edema from ALI/ARDS. Intensive Care Med 33:448–453
36. Kushimoto S, Taira Y, Kitazawa Y et al (2012) The clinical usefulness of extravascular lung water and pulmonary vascular permeability index to diagnose and characterize pulmonary edema: a prospective multicenter study on the quantitative differential diagnostic definition for acute lung injury/acute respiratory distress syndrome. Crit Care 16:R232
37. Corradi F, Brusasco C, Pelosi P (2014) Chest ultrasound in acute respiratory distress syndrome. Curr Opin Crit Care 20:98–103
38. Bataille B, Rao G, Cocquet P et al (2015) Accuracy of ultrasound B-lines score and E/Ea ratio to estimate extravascular lung water and its variations in patients with acute respiratory distress syndrome. J Clin Monit Comput 29:169–176
39. Baldi G, Gargani L, Abramo A, D'Errico L et al (2013) Lung water assessment by lung ultrasonography in intensive care: a pilot study. Intensive Care Med 39:74–84
40. Enghard P, Rademacher S, Nee J et al (2015) Simplified lung ultrasound protocol shows excellent prediction of extravascular lung water in ventilated intensive care patients. Crit Care 19:36
41. Corradi F, Ball L, Brusasco C et al (2013) Assessment of extravascular lung water by quantitative ultrasound and CT in isolated bovine lung. Respir Physiol Neurobiol 187:244–249
42. Copetti R, Soldati G, Copetti P (2008) Chest sonography: a useful tool to differentiate acute cardiogenic pulmonary edema from acute respiratory distress syndrome. Cardiovasc Ultrasound 6:16
43. Marik PE, Lemson J (2014) Fluid responsiveness: an evolution of our understanding. Br J Anaesth 112:617–620
44. Marik PE, Cavallazzi R (2013) Does the Central Venous Pressure (CVP) predict fluid responsiveness: an update meta-analysis and a plea for some common sense. Crit Care Med 41:1774–1781
45. Cecconi M, Parsons AK, Rhodes A (2011) What is a fluid challenge? Curr Opin Crit Care 17:290–295
46. Starling EH (1918) The Linacre lecture on the law of the heart, given at Cambridge, 1915, vol 27. Longmans, London
47. Bruegger D, Jacob M, Rehm M et al (2005) Atrial natriuretic peptide induces shedding of endothelial glycocalyx in coronary vascular bed of guinea pig hearts. Am J Physiol Heart Circ Physiol 289:H1993–H1999
48. Bruegger D, Schwartz L, Chappell D et al (2011) Release of atrial natriuretic peptide precedes shedding of the endothelial glycocalyx equally in patients undergoing on- and off-pump coronary artery bypass surgery. Basic Res Cardiol 106:1111–1121
49. Osman D, Ridel C, Ray P, Monnet X, Anguel N, Richard C et al (2007) Cardiac filling pressures are not appropriate to predict hemodynamic response to volume challenge. Crit Care Med 35:64–68
50. Rizvi K, Deboisblanc BP, Truwit JD et al (2005) Effect of airway pressure display on interobserver agreement in the assessment of vascular pressures in patients with acute lung injury and acute respiratory distress syndrome. Crit Care Med 33:98–103
51. Guerin L, Monnet X, Teboul JL (2013) Monitoring volume and fluid responsiveness from static to dynamic indicators. Best Pract Res Clin Anaesthesiol 2:177–185
52. Monnet X, Teboul JL (2013) Assessment of volume responsiveness during mechanical ventilation: recent advances. Crit Care 17:217
53. Marik PE, Cavallazzi R, Vasu T, Hirani A (2009) Dynamic changes in arterial waveform derived variables and fluid responsiveness in mechanically ventilated patients: a systematic review of the literature. Crit Care Med 37:2642–2647

54. Michard F, Descorps-Declere A, Lopes MR (2008) Using pulse pressure variation in patients with acute respiratory distress syndrome. Crit Care Med 36:2946–2948
55. Teboul JL, Monnet X (2013) Pulse pressure variation and ARDS. Minerva Anestesiol 79:398–407
56. Teboul JL, Monnet X (2008) Prediction of volume responsiveness in critically ill patients with spontaneous breathing activity. Curr Opin Crit Care 14:334–339
57. Muller L, Louart G, Bousquet PJ et al (2010) The influence of the airway driving pressure on pulsed pressure variation as a predictor of fluid responsiveness. Intensive Care Med 36:496–503
58. Liu Y, Wei LQ, Li GQ, Yu X, Li GF, Li YM (2016) Pulse pressure variation adjusted by respiratory changes in pleural pressure, rather than by tidal volume, reliably predicts fluid responsiveness in patients with acute respiratory distress syndrome. Crit Care Med 44:342–351
59. Feissel M, Michard F, Faller JP, Teboul JL (2004) The respiratory variation in inferior vena cava diameter as a guide to fluid therapy. Intensive Care Med 30:1834–1837
60. Zhang Z, Xu X, Ye S, Xu L (2014) Ultrasonographic measurement of the respiratory variation in the inferior vena cava diameter is predictive of fluid responsiveness in critically ill patients: systematic review and meta-analysis. Ultrasound Med Biol 40:845–853
61. Muller L, Toumi M, Bousquet PJ et al (2011) An increase in aortic blood flow after an infusion of 100 ml colloid over 1 minute can predict fluid responsiveness: the mini-fluid challenge study. Anesthesiology 115:541–547
62. Mallat J, Meddour M, Durville E et al (2015) Decrease in pulse pressure and stroke volume variations after mini-fluid challenge accurately predicts fluid responsiveness†. Br J Anaesth 115:449–456
63. Monnet X, Rienzo M, Osman D et al (2006) Passive leg raising predicts fluid responsiveness in the critically ill. Crit Care Med 34:1402–1407
64. Monnet X, Teboul JL (2015) Passive leg raising: five rules, not a drop of fluid! Crit Care 19:18
65. Cavallaro F, Sandroni C, Marano C et al (2010) Diagnostic accuracy of passive leg raising for prediction of fluid responsiveness in adults: systematic review and meta-analysis of clinical studies. Intensive Care Med 36:1475–1483
66. Ware LB, Matthay MA (2001) Alveolar fluid clearance is impaired in the majority of patients with acute lung injury and the acute respiratory distress syndrome. Am J Respir Crit Care Med 163:1376–1383
67. Berthiaume Y, Matthay MA (2007) Alveolar edema fluid clearance and acute lung injury. Respir Physiol Neurobiol 159:350–359
68. Allyn J, Allou N, Dib M et al (2013) Echocardiography to predict tolerance to negative fluid balance in acute respiratory distress syndrome/acute lung injury. J Crit Care 28:1006–1010
69. Grissom CK, Hirshberg EL, Dickerson JB, National Heart Lung and Blood Institute Acute Respiratory Distress Syndrome Clinical Trials Network et al (2015) Fluid management with a simplified conservative protocol for the acute respiratory distress syndrome*. Crit Care Med 43:288–295
70. Lum H, Siflinger-Birnboim A, Blumenstock F, Malik AB (1991) Serum albumin decreases trans-endothelial permeability to macromolecules. Microvasc Res 42:91–102
71. Dull RO, Jo H, Sill H, Hollis TM, Tarbell JM (1991) The effect of varying albumin concentration and hydrostatic pressure on hydraulic conductivity and albumin permeability of cultured endothelial monolayers. Microvasc Res 41:390–407
72. Guyton AC (1965) Interstitial fluid pressure. II. Pressure-volume curves of interstitial space. Circ Res 16:452–460
73. Martin GS, Mangialardi RJ, Wheeler AP et al (2002) Albumin and furosemide therapy in hypoproteinemic patients with acute lung injury. Crit Care Med 30:2175–2182
74. Gattinoni L, Caspani ML (2002) Albumin and furosemide in acute lung injury: a little step forward? Crit Care Med 30:2376–2377
75. Martin GS, Moss M, Wheeler AP et al (2005) A randomized, controlled trial of furosemide with or without albumin in hypoproteinemic patients with acute lung injury. Crit Care Med 33:1681–1687

76. Roch A, Hraiech S, Dizier S, Papazian L (2013) Pharmacological interventions in acute respiratory distress syndrome. Ann Intensive Care 3:20
77. Mehta D, Bhattacharya J, Matthay MA, Malik AB (2004) Integrated control of lung fluid balance. Am J Phys Lung Cell Mol Phys 287:L1081–L1090
78. Perkins GD, McAuley DF, Thickett DR, Gao F (2006) The beta-agonist lung injury trial (BALTI): a randomized placebo-controlled clinical trial. Am J Respir Crit Care Med 173:281–287
79. Gates S, Perkins GD, Lamb SE, Kelly C, Thickett DR, Young JD et al (2013) Beta-Agonist Lung injury TrIal-2 (BALTI-2): a multicentre, randomised, double-blind, placebo-controlled trial and economic evaluation of intravenous infusion of salbutamol versus placebo in patients with acute respiratory distress syndrome. Health Technol Assess 17:1–87
80. Matthay MA, Brower RG, Carson S et al (2011) Randomized, placebo-controlled clinical trial of an aerosolized β_2-agonist for treatment of acute lung injury. Am J Respir Crit Care Med 184:561–568
81. Malbrain ML, Marik PE, Witters I et al (2014) Fluid overload, de-resuscitation, and outcomes in critically ill or injured patients: a systematic review with suggestions for clinical practice. Anaesthesiol Intensive Ther 46:361–380
82. Taccone FS, Castanares-Zapatero D, Peres-Bota D et al (2010) Cerebral autoregulation is influenced by carbon dioxide levels in patients with septic shock. Neurocrit Care 12:35–42
83. Lammi MR, Aiello B, Burg GT et al (2015) Response to fluid boluses in the fluid and catheter treatment trial. Chest 148:919–926

Weaning in ARDS

9

Ross Freebairn

9.1 Introduction

Depending upon case mix, about one in four ventilated in an ICU has ARDS-induced respiratory failure [1]. Mechanical ventilation (MV), the mainstay of support for ARDS and also a driver of intensive care costs, is associated with complications that pose risks to patients [2, 3]. Increasing the duration of MV increases that risk [4]. As respiratory function improves, MV needs to be withdrawn at the earliest possible juncture. Very few randomized trials of MV weaning have had a primary focus on patients suffering from ARDS. For reasons outlined below, substituting results acquired from general populations or applying techniques developed in non-ARDS patient groups may have limitations.

In patients with ARDS, reversal or control of the precipitant of the respiratory failure is essential before the "weaning" can begin. This entails correction or attenuation of the precipitating cause of the ARDS as well as restoring the respiratory systems to a stable, functional state. ARDS impact is not confined to the respiratory system, and thus weaning is not solely ventilator focused. Restoration of cardiovascular, neuromuscular, neurological, and psychiatric homeostasis is required for successful weaning [5, 6].

9.1.1 Definitions

Weaning is the successful separation (or liberation) of the patient from the ventilator. Weaning definitions range from being totally free of MV support to just being free of invasive ventilation [7]. The lack of standard definitions and the varied end

R. Freebairn, FANZCA, FRCPE, FCICM
Intensive Care Services, Hawke's Bay Hospital, Hastings, New Zealand

Chinese University of Hong Kong, Hong Kong, China
e-mail: ross.freebairn@xtra.co.nz

D. Chiumello (ed.), *Acute Respiratory Distress Syndrome (ARDS)*,
DOI 10.1007/978-3-319-41852-0_9

points for weaning complicate analysis [7, 8]. Prolonged MV also has a myriad of definitions including MV periods for as brief as 2 days to as long as 29 days [9–11]. A 2004 consensus defined prolonged MV as greater than or equal to 21 consecutive days of MV, for greater than or equal to 6 h/d [10].

The end of the weaning process also lacks agreed definitions and is variously defined as first extubation, successful extubation, unassisted breathing for 24 or 72 h, the first spontaneous breathing trial (SBT) or successful SBT, or an ill-defined "successful weaning" [7, 12–17]. The spectrum of transitioning supportive therapy such as high-flow nasal cannula (HFNC) as adjuncts to weaning adds further complexity [18–21].

9.1.2 Routine Weaning

Standard weaning should be employed early in the ICU stay. Once the need for muscle paralysis, deep sedation, prone positioning, and other complex respiratory interventions is no longer needed, active weaning should commence.

Generally, once the underlying condition is reversed, the majority of patients can be weaned by simple sequential cessation of neuromuscular blocking agents, sedation, and respiratory support, with wakefulness, spontaneous breathing, and extubation following without significant delay. However, a smaller number, dependent on case mix but usually about one third of patient number, require a more complex process. The truly "difficult-to-wean patient" represents one in six of all MV patients in the ICU [3, 22, 23].

Respiratory failure is due to ARDS that may be solely due to community-, hospital-, or ICU-acquired ARDS, or it can be contributed to by coexisting respiratory conditions, such as chronic lung disease (CLD) [23]. These coexisting conditions all carry different morbidities and associated mortalities, and influence the duration of support required, difficulty of weaning, and outcomes achieved [23]. Unfortunately, ARDS, particularly severe ARDS, while not exclusively confined to one group, makes up a significant portion of "difficult-to-wean" patients. Of this difficult-to-wean group, about one third of patients require more than 3 weeks of weaning makeup representing about one a patient in 20 of all ICU MV patients [10, 24, 25]

9.2 Progress Toward Weaning

Weaning has been extensively studied, but existing data does not include any large trial where patients with ARDS were the sole or majority of subjects. In the absence of ARDS-specific trials, the consensus view appears to be that the principles applied to weaning with other causes of respiratory failure are valid and that unnecessary prolongation of MV should be avoided by timely recognition of readiness to wean and readiness to extubate [26, 27].

The first step is the reversal of the underlying condition. ARDS is not a disease but is precipitated by a pathological condition; both its severity and duration are dependent upon that condition [23]. As the underlying condition may influence the ability to wean, management of the underlying and comorbid pathologies is crucial but beyond the scope of this review. While it is prudent to consider weaning during early recovery, if the precipitating cause is an ongoing process, such as unresolved sepsis or recurrent pancreatitis, attempts at early weaning may be interrupted by recurrence or by nosocomial complication and may represent backward steps in any weaning program [5]. However, the alternative of waiting until complete resolution of the underlying condition will unduly delay recovery and precipitate increased debilitation. The earliest return to spontaneous respiratory effort is important as even short intervals of complete diaphragmatic inactivity during MV may increase diaphragmatic proteolysis and atrophy of diaphragm muscle [28, 29].

9.2.1 Weaning Criteria Assessment

The patient's capacity to breathe spontaneously is often underestimated. With severe ARDS, early weaning must be balanced against the risks of spontaneous breathing [30, 31]. Neither clinical assessment nor objective assessments are reliable or accurate in assessing readiness to wean. While some patients fail weaning trials having satisfied weaning criteria, up to one third of patients judged by criteria "not to be ready to wean" can wean successfully. Under half of patients in the defining weaning studies were ventilated because of ARDS, and many studies were limited to those ventilated for less than 2 weeks. Patients with ARDS are typically ventilated for 8 days with a quarter receiving ventilated for double that period [1].

Weaning predictors are often incorporated in protocols to predict weaning outcome for patients on MV. The traditional weaning algorithm was based upon moving from controlled to other modes over a relatively short period. The addition of complex modes to the ventilator armamentarium that support weaning means that the historic criteria are not necessarily relevant and has blurred the line between "ventilation" and "weaning" [32–34]. One of the most common tools, the frequency–TV ratio (or rapid shallow breathing index), has been shown not to convey a survival benefit and did not assist in avoiding tracheostomy or extubation failure [35]. Routine application of weaning predictors is not recommended, but a bedside assessment checklist for clinicians may be a prompt weaning [4, 36, 37].

The performance of most weaning indices remains below expectation, and there is a need for a robust predictive tool [38, 39]. Only five assessment tools were associated with weaning success or failure [37, 40]:

1. Negative inspiratory force (maximal inspiratory pressure)
2. Minute ventilation
3. Respiratory frequency
4. Tidal volume
5. Frequency–TV ratio (f/VT)

9.2.2 Spontaneous Breathing Trials

Once it is determined that weaning is possible, and desirable, the next step is usually a "spontaneous breathing trial" (SBT). A SBT comprises an assessment of a patient's capacity to breathe and is advocated as the best method to ascertain extubation readiness [4, 41].

A SBT generally comprises 30–60 min on low levels of pressure support ventilation (PSV) ranging from 0–8 cmH_20 and continuous positive airway pressure (CPAP) delivered by the ventilator or other CPAP devices or using a T-piece attached to the endotracheal tube. A recent Cochrane systematic review confirms earlier reports that no difference in overall weaning success is based on the SBT method, although PSV was more effective than T-tube for successful SBT among patients with simple weaning [42]. As indicated above, approximately two thirds of patients require minimal to no weaning and after the first SBT is extubated without difficulty [4, 22]. The remaining one third require a more graduated approach to reducing the amount of ventilator support [4]. Both Ezingeard et al. and Cabello et al. found that a PSV trial immediately after a T-piece trial failure was successful in a number of patients, further reducing the "difficult-to-wean" pool [43, 44]. After a failed weaning effort, if evidence for fatigue is evident, then clinicians should provide 24 h of rest on full MV before proceeding with the next weaning effort [45]. If not, a repeated SBT should be encouraged.

9.2.3 Weaning Protocol

The wake-up and breathe protocol pairs daily spontaneous awakening trials (i.e., sedatives interruption) with daily SBT, produces better outcomes than historic approaches, and has been recommended as routine practice [46]. The general outline of the standard wake-up and wean process is displayed in Fig. 9.1 and although not specifically designed for patients with ARDS is the consensus view on the standard ventilator management [46].

There is insufficient evidence to evaluate the effectiveness of protocol-directed sedation regimes as results from the two randomized controlled trials were conflicting [51, 52]. Patients who are not immediately weaned need further immediate assessment to identify reversible factors and then usually undergo either a strategy of progressive reduction of level of assistance, such as pressure support ventilation, or progressively longer periods of spontaneous breathing, with or without CPAP [26, 27]. There are now a wide variety of alternative modes and strategy with apparent equivalence in weaning [53–56]. Partial ventilatory support mode in patients with ALI/ARDS is associated with physiological benefits, but evidence of an impact on clinical outcomes in ARDS is lacking [56, 57]. These are outlined below under adaptive ventilation.

9.2.4 Movement to Spontaneous Breathing

In severe ARDS, the value of neuromuscular blockade and prone positioning mean that spontaneous breathing cannot be recommended in early severe ARDS [58, 59].

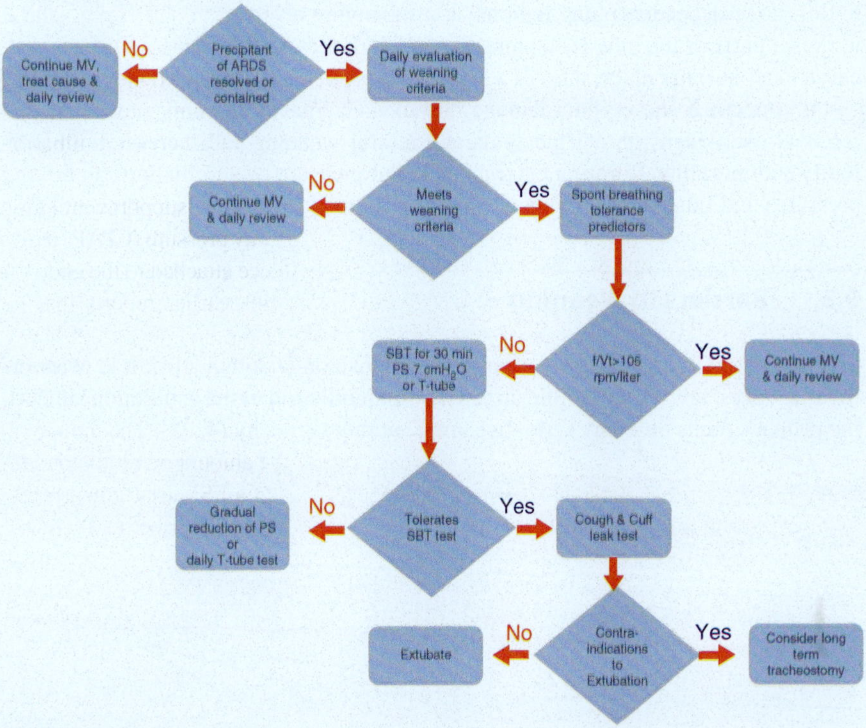

Fig. 9.1 Flow diagram for weaning in ARDS; derived from [26, 27, 34, 47–50]

After this initial period, spontaneous breathing supported by modes such as ASV, APRV, BIPAP, or pressure support has appealed [30]. In less severe ARDS and as lungs recover, spontaneous ventilation has potential to improve lung ventilation at lower levels of airway pressure and traditionally has been encouraged as it requires less sedation and improves cardiopulmonary function, presumably by recruiting non-ventilated lung units, requiring a shorter duration of ventilatory support [57, 30]. In animals with severe lung injury, spontaneous breathing could worsen lung injury, and muscle paralysis might be more protective for injured lungs by preventing injuriously high trans-pulmonary pressure and high driving pressure [60]. Inspiratory pressure support provided to match the demand for a higher minute ventilation can lead to large trans-pulmonary pressure swings and TV that exceed the recommended maximums, both of which are major contributing factors to ventilator-induced lung injury and possibly to weaning failure [31, 61].

Strong spontaneous efforts in animals increase lung injury [31]. In injured lungs, the lungs' normal fluidlike behavior is not universally present. With spontaneous breathing, the negative pleural pressures generated by diaphragmatic excursion are not uniformly transmitted across lung surfaces but concentrated in dependent regions. In the supine position, these dependent posterior regions are affected, but following prolonged prone positioning, this may also affect the ventral regions [62]. Locally increased pleural pressure variations cause underdiagnosed regional overstretching in dorsal (or dependent) lung regions, accompanying alveolar air shift from ventral to dorsal parts of the lung (i.e., pendelluft) [62]. Excessive spontaneous efforts may cause local overstretch because of a significant pendelluft effect [63].

Of concern is the cryptic damage due to high trans-pulmonary pressures, and regional overdistension will postpone successful weaning and increase both morbidity and mortality. Limiting the trans-alveolar pressure by strictly limiting driving pressures and tidal volumes generated is important [31].

9.3 Barriers to Weaning

The barriers to immediate easy weaning are shown on Diagram 2 [4]. It is noteworthy that only a few are reversible directly by manipulation of the ventilation support, the primary focus on many early "weaning" attempts.

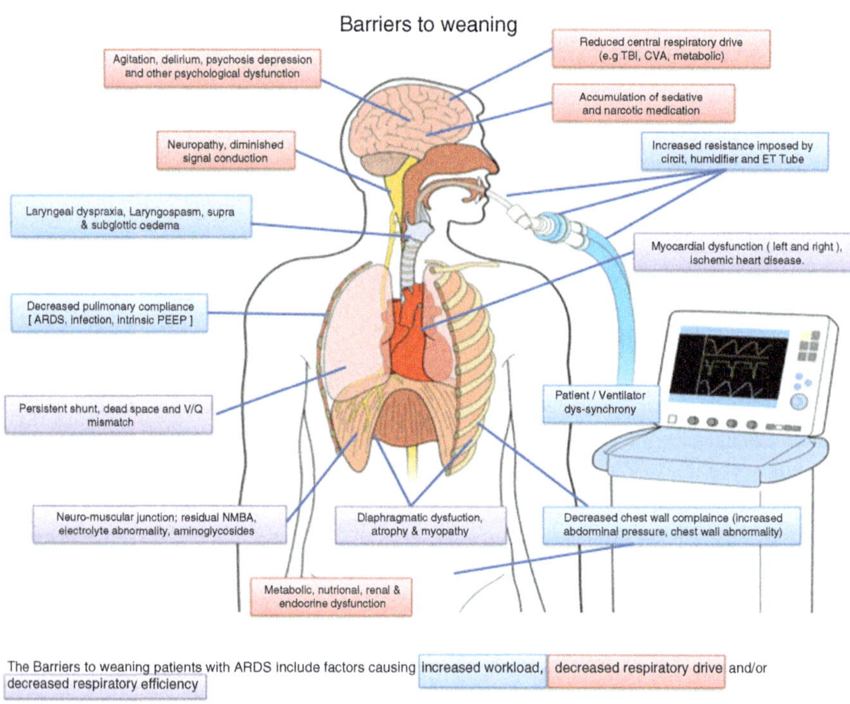

9.3.1 Increased Respiratory Load

With ARDS the residual shunt, increased dead space, and ongoing poor ventilation-perfusion matching does not resolve immediately [64]. Weaning patients have supranormal minute ventilation requirements, increased airway resistance, decreased pulmonary and/or chest wall compliance changes, and thus a greater work of breathing [65]. Decreased pulmonary compliance can arise from reversible causes like pleural effusions and pulmonary edema. Drainage or diuretics may improve compliance and oxygenation, decrease trans-pulmonary pressure, and shorten weaning time [66, 67].

After a week of ventilation, one third of intensive care patients have impaired inspiratory muscle endurance after successful weaning [68]. Although inspiratory muscle training improves tidal volumes, it appears to be of no overall benefit [68–70].

9.3.2 Decreased Respiratory Drive

A central respiratory drive is necessary for ventilatory activity to continue once the ventilator support is removed. Commonly, there is a reduced respiratory drive with an inadequate response to either hypercarbia or hypoxemia. Carbon dioxide responsiveness is seldom tested formally, although ventilatory response to reduction in pressure support is used as part of the weaning algorithm. Responsiveness to carbon dioxide assessed from the 100 ms occlusion pressure has been shown to predict weaning [71].

9.3.3 Excess Sedation and Analgesia

The triad of adequate analgesia, control of delirium, and optimal sedation to facilitate tolerable MV is never more important than during weaning [72]. Early sedation depth predicts delayed extubation [73, 74]. This association is confounded by severity of illness, and with neuromuscular blockade and prone positioning in severe ARDS, both precipitating deeper sedation, being recommended therapy for severe ARDS, it is not surprising that ARDS patients are deeply sedated [58, 59]. Kress demonstrated that daily interruption of sedative infusions reduced the duration of MV, but less than one third of the studied group had ARDS or pulmonary edema [75]. Protocol-directed sedation is controversial as results from the two randomized controlled trials were conflicting [51, 52].

Prolonged weaning can be a complication of inappropriate dosing sedative/hypnotic medication, with delayed clearance in multi-organ failure, a common feature of ARDS patients [6, 76]. Increased understanding of sedation goals by attending staff principles may further reduce ventilation duration [77]. Change in sedation choice may contribute to shorter weaning periods. A fivefold increase in propofol use and a 70% reduction in midazolam use over 8 years were associated with a decline in MV duration, tracheostomy rate, and ICU and hospital length of stay [78]. Sedation techniques, particularly those that include the use of benzodiazepines, may increase delirium, agitation, withdrawal, and other neuropsychiatric conditions, which either directly or indirectly delay weaning [79, 80].

Withdrawal syndromes were associated with high doses of analgesic, and sedative medications with neuromuscular blockade and prolonged MV means that patients with ARDS are at increased risk of withdrawal syndrome [81].

9.3.4 Cardiac Load

Cardiac dysfunction is among the most common barriers to weaning [82].

The onset of ARDS respiratory failure may be precipitated by, exacerbate or importantly mask, congestive and right heart failure. Positive pressure reduces pulmonary edema, provides increased alveolar pressures, and reduces afterload. With weaning, spontaneous breathing is reestablished; the process reverses with a negative pleural pressure during inspiration [83]. This decrease in intrathoracic pressure increases the systemic venous return pressure gradient, the right ventricular (RV) preload, the central blood volume, and subsequently the LV preload [84]. A second effect is a decrease of the LV ejection pressure gradient, increasing the LV afterload [85]. As a consequence, respiratory and cardiac failure may occur, associated with increased work of breathing and hypoxemia.

Diagnosis and monitoring, augmented by echocardiography, allow titration of treatment by diuretics, vasodilators, inotropes, and coronary angioplasty when indicated. Using diuretics guided by brain natriuretic peptide (BNP) measurements shortens weaning suggesting that negative fluid balance using diuretics could hasten extubation [16]. The use of a conservative fluid strategy shortened MV in patients with acute lung injury although poor longer-term cognitive outcomes are concerning [66, 86].

9.3.5 Muscle Atrophy and Weakness

Early muscle changes are driven by inflammation and disuse, with atrophy from increased protein degradation [28, 87]. Late-phase muscle weakness persists in many despite resolution of lung injury and cessation of ongoing acute inflammation [87]. Late-phase muscle dysfunction may reflect a failure of the musculoskeletal system to regain homeostatic balance. These differences may require different therapies. Electrical muscle stimulation for those that cannot exercise has been suggested although this novel technique in the ICU setting is scarce [88]. Denervation injuries, for which there are no specific therapies, may persist and delay weaning.

9.3.6 Metabolic Electrolyte and Endocrine Considerations

Metabolic alkalosis, a common disorder in ICU, impedes respiratory drive and can be caused by diuretic use, hypernatremia, and hypokalemia, all classically associated with ARDS management [89]. Increased serum bicarbonate is associated with increased ICU LOS, more days on MV, and higher hospital mortality [90]. Chloride-restrictive buffered solutions theoretically could increase metabolic alkalosis, but in an interventional trial, chloride restriction did not increase in ventilation time [91, 92]. Studies of "contraction alkalosis" and effect medications such as acetazolamide on weaning are needed [93].

Serum calcium, phosphate, magnesium, and potassium deficiency all cause muscle weakness [94]. Hypothyroidism, hypoadrenalism, and relative or absolute cortisol efficiency also contribute to weaning difficulty. Endogenous hormones, and the exogenous corticosteroids that are often used in critical illness for septic shock, directly for ARDS, or for other indications may also contribute [95]. The corticosteroids and steroid-based neuromuscular blocking agents are associated with muscular weakness, but their overall effect on weaning remains unclear [96]. Avoidance and, when present, early correction of electrolyte abnormality as routine care are crucial to successful weaning [94].

9.3.7 Psychological Dysfunction

Forty-two percent of patients weaning from prolonged MV have depression, and weaning failure is twice as common in patients with depression [97, 98]. Fatigue, excessive daytime somnolence, and associated depression also delay weaning [99].

Second-generation antipsychotic and stimulants such as donepezil, modafinil, and methylphenidate have been used in difficult-to-wean patient depression [99–103]. Whether their effect is through counteracting depression or anxiety or as a direct respiratory stimulus is unclear.

Up to 80% of patients in ICU have delirium and are associated with delayed weaning and higher 6-month mortality [72, 104]. Prevention strategies include an early and exercise/mobility. Patients exposed to an "ABCDE" bundle spent 3 more days breathing without assistance and experienced nearly half the delirium, than patients treated with usual care [77]. Haloperidol is most commonly used for ICU delirium although evidence is entirely anecdotal [72]. Dexmedetomidine is also recommended [105]. Olanzapine, risperidone, and quetiapine are also used and may have some advantages in the critically ill [72].

9.3.8 Consent, Compliance, and Comfort

Prolonged MV could produce suffering. While deeply sedated, with adequate analgesia and ventilatory support, it is unlikely that a patient "suffers." However, later, as patient "emerges," and weaning begins, "suffering" may manifest. Long-term outcomes from prolonged MV are worse than generally expected by relatives and physicians [106]. In a recent systematic review of studies reporting outcomes of patients requiring MV for more than 14 days, only half were successfully weaned, one in five were able to return home, and half were dead in 1 year [107]. ARDS is associated with exercise limitation, physical and psychological sequelae, decreased physical quality of life, increased costs, and the use of health-care services although there is a similar functional recovery in survivors who did and did not develop ARDS [3, 64]. Overly optimistic expectations do not encourage meaningful discussion surrounding weaning outcomes or end-of-life decision-making. Initiation of weaning is a timely juncture when the objectives of future treatments are considered.

9.4 Adjunctive Care

In addition to standard ventilation care, during weaning, some interventions need further consideration.

9.4.1 Monitoring

A venous CO_2 threshold of below 45 mmHg is sensitive enough to reliable enough to exclude hypercarbia in lieu of sequential arterial samples [108]. If hypercarbia is detected, venous samples are insufficient to determine the degree of hypercarbia. End-tidal monitoring is less reliable. For end-tidal CO_2 to accurately reflect arterial CO_2, lung perfusion levels and alveoli CO_2 must be consistent throughout the lung, and TV must be at least three times the 2.2 mL/kg anatomic dead space [109]. As TV of 6 mL/kg is recommended, and CO_2 is unevenly distributed, the utility of end-tidal CO_2 monitoring is limited.

Standard cardiac monitoring of vital signs and rhythm remains minimum requirements. More extensive cardiac monitoring is variable; many invasive processes to estimate cardiac performance have been withdrawn prior to weaning. Repeated echocardiograms may detect cardiac dysfunction during dys-synchrony, during weaning failure, or during the transition from controlled to spontaneous modes. Ultrasound may also detect undetected diaphragmatic dysfunction that contributes to delayed weaning [110].

9.4.2 Therapy and Mobilization

Early mobilization is beneficial, can be safely initiated, and should be incorporated into routine daily activities [111]. Active mobilization may improve muscle strength and the ability to wean by reducing disuse atrophy [111].

9.4.3 Tracheostomy

In some situations, tracheostomy may reduce the work of breathing, lower in-hospital mortality, and improve weaning [112, 113]. Systemic analysis of randomized controlled trials suggests that early tracheostomy generally achieved better outcomes, including more ventilator-free days, shorter ICU stays, shorter sedation, and reduced long-term mortality [114, 115].

While early tracheostomy may be desirable for weaning, timing is dependent upon having safe operating conditions, including low enough FiO_2 and PEEP settings to allow safe airway manipulation. With ARDS, both the decision to wean and the identification of a "difficult-to-wean" patient are important decision points, at which the longer-term prognosis and treatment strategy, including tracheostomy, should be considered [113, 116].

9.4.4 Extubation to Noninvasive Ventilation

Noninvasive ventilation (NIV) has been used both in an attempt to prospectively reduce "invasive ventilation" time, through "early extubation," and as a rescue therapy for patients on the threshold of failing an extubation attempt.

Early trials of NIV in post-extubation respiratory failure produced conflicting outcomes. Subsequent trials of "prophylactic" use of immediate post-extubation in patients who "fail" a SBT have been found to be beneficial [17, 117–125]. Systematic reviews have evaluated this technique and are support its clinical use in appropriate clinical circumstances [126, 127].

Extrapolating this data to ARDS requires considerable caution [128, 129]. Firstly, patients studied were predominantly suffering from chronic lung disease (CLD). Noninvasive ventilation has the capacity to reduce intubation rates and lower the length of stay and mortality, in patients with CLD when used before invasive MV. In contrast on patients with moderate to severe ARDS, NIV used prior to invasive ventilation had high intubation rates, had delivered high tidal volumes, and had a high mortality with NIV failure [61, 129].

With NIV, oxygenation is increased by a raised mean alveolar pressure, a reduction in tidal de-recruitment of alveoli, and/or a provision of high oxygen concentrations through a semi-closed system [130]. After extubation, a less than perfect NIV mask seal may produce air entrainment and airway pressures below airway "closing" pressure more frequently than during invasive ventilation [131].

While entrainment can be managed by mask adjustment, or increasing oxygen, the decreased airway pressure may result in small airway collapse with de-recruitment.

NIV may assist patients suffering from respiratory failure where work of breathing rather than hypoxia predominates. These patients are less sensitive to short periods of mask removal or leaks. In patient recovering from ARDS although NIV supports the work of breathing, there is a risk of tidal de-recruitment [130]. At lower levels of support requirement, high-flow nasal cannula (HFNC) is likely to provide better oxygenation than venturi mask and is as least effective as, and better tolerated than, NIV for treatment of post-extubation respiratory failure [19, 20]. HFNC role in ARDS is as yet undefined [21]. NIV is not recommended and if used for weaning must be used with caution [61, 128].

9.4.5 Adaptive and Automated Weaning Systems (AWS)

While transition to pressure support or T-piece has traditionally been used, more recently "adaptive modes" have been advocated for weaning. Available "adaptive modes" are listed in Table 9.1.

The first adaptive modes with feedback were volume-targeted pressure control modes such as "pressure-regulated volume control" which titrated pressures to achieve a TV. Subsequent iterations targeted MV. Adaptive support ventilation (ASV) is a partially automated mode available from Hamilton Medical. ASV targets

Table 9.1 Available advanced "adaptive" modes used in weaning

Name	Company	Principles	Ref.
Mandatory minute ventilation (MMV)	Dräger Medical, Lübeck, Germany	Closed loop control of the mandatory breath rate while considering the patient's spontaneous breath rate based on a prescribed minute ventilation	[132]
SmartCare/PSTM	Dräger Medical, Lübeck, Germany	Closed loop control of pressure support based on monitoring of respiratory rate, tidal volume, and end-tidal carbon dioxide. Tests for extubation readiness using a 1-h spontaneous breath trial adaptive	[12]
Adaptive support ventilation (ASV)	Hamilton Medical, Bonaduz, Switzerland	Closed loop control to maintain preset minimum minute ventilation by adjusting inspiratory pressure and mandatory breath rate on a breath-by-breath basis. Pressure support ventilation based on respiratory rate and tidal volume. Adjusts I:E ratio based on RC	[133]
IntelliVent-ASV®	Hamilton Medical, Rhäzüns, Switzerland	Extension of ASV that uses closed loop control to adjust minute ventilation using end-tidal carbon dioxide and oxygenation by adjusting PEEP and inspired O_2 concentration. Conducts automated SBT	[134]
Automode	Siemens, Solna, Sweden	PC, PRVC, or VC switches to a support mode such as (either VS or PS ventilation) on detection of patient-initiated ventilation of two consecutive breaths	[135]
Neurally adjusted ventilatory assist	Maquet, Solna, Sweden	Partial ventilatory support proportional to inspiratory diaphragmatic electrical activity measured via an esophageal catheter	[136]
Proportional assist ventilation (PAV)	The University of Manitoba, Canada	Adjusts airway pressure based on measurement of compliance and resistance throughout the inspiratory cycle to maintain an clinician selected % degree of support	[137]
Proportional pressure support (PPS)	Dräger Medical, Lübeck, Germany	Germany pressure support is provided proportionately to changes in airway resistance and lung compliance. PPS is based on the PAV algorithm	[137]
Mandatory rate ventilation (MRV)	Taema-Horus Ventilator® Air Liquide, France	Closed loop control to titrate pressure support based on a set respiratory rate target	[138]

minute ventilation with an algorithm using the "Otis equation," to target the least work of breathing. Studies comparing ASV weaning to standard care found that ASV could shorten weaning in post-cardiac surgery or chronic lung disease patient. When ASV was compared to assist control in patients with ARDS, no differences were found [133]. Of concern is that ASV allows TV of up to 22 mL/kg and in ARDS delivered median tidal volumes greater than the recommended 8 mL/kg [55, 133–135, 139, 140].

The most recent fully AWS incorporates feedback loops that titrate to ventilation and oxygenation targets and provides interesting opportunities. Two AWS are currently available the SmartCare® from Dräger Medical and IntelliVent from Hamilton Medical [141, 142].

While they differ slightly, the principles of the AWS are to establish ventilation through titration of adaptive ventilation: when stable, the sequential application of a SBT and then if successful conversion to titrated pressure support weaning. An early study of SmartCare® found that closed-loop weaning resulted in more rapid weaning, whereas a similar study carried out in an extremely well-staffed unit demonstrated no benefit [12, 142]. Differences in the nursing intensity and clinical governance may be explain this discrepancy. This development highlights two possibilities:

Firstly, a more consistent weaning system, which if calibrated correctly, could provide rapid weaning.

Compared to nonautomated weaning methods, these systems demonstrated positive advantages in weaning time, time to successful extubation, and possibly assisted in reducing ICU length of stay and the number of patients requiring prolonged MV [54, 143] However, most patients studied received relatively short-term ventilation after surgery or ventilation for exacerbation of COPD. Clinical evidence from patients who have suffered ARDS is scarce [144, 145].

Secondly, when skilled personnel are scarce, equivalent outcomes may be achieved with less clinician input. Adaptive weaning systems follow a computerized protocol and as such could be viewed as being identical to a "manual" weaning protocols, with more assured compliance. If "weaning protocols" are non-inferior to standard care, an automated form of these should also demonstrate at least equivalent outcomes.

While the automated weaning systems show promise and some evidence of efficacy, proprietary systems are generally available only on a single manufacturer's ventilator, and for multiple reasons, these systems have not been widely adopted [54].

9.5 Summary

Weaning patients with ARDS from ventilatory support present a challenge, with patient presenting disease, comorbidity, and severity of the ARDS all influencing the success rate. Most knowledge in the area is derived from trials in mixed populations or excluded ARDS patient; the evidence supporting the use of specific techniques is very rare. General attention to nutrition, physiotherapy, mobilization, and psychological support is pragmatically useful. Automated systems offer some promise, but clinical evidence of benefit in patients who have suffered from ARDS remains scarce.

References

1. Bellani G, Laffey JG, Pham T, Fan E, Brochard L, Esteban A et al (2016) Epidemiology, patterns of care, and mortality for patients with acute respiratory distress syndrome in intensive care units in 50 countries. JAMA 315(8):788–800

2. Cox CE, Carson SS, Govert JA, Chelluri L, Sanders GD (2007) An economic evaluation of prolonged mechanical ventilation. Crit Care Med 35(8):1918–1927
3. Herridge MS, Tansey CM, Matté A, Tomlinson G, Diaz-Granados N, Cooper A et al (2011) Functional disability 5 years after acute respiratory distress syndrome. N Engl J Med 364(14):1293–1304
4. Boles JM, Bion J, Connors A, Herridge M, Marsh B, Melot C et al (2007) Weaning from mechanical ventilation. Eur Respir J 29(5):1033–1056
5. Ambrosino N, Gabbrielli L (2010) The difficult-to-wean patient. Exp Rev Respir Med 4(5):685–692
6. Dhanireddy S, Altemeier WA, Matute-Bello G, O'Mahony DS, Glenny RW, Martin TR et al (2006) Mechanical ventilation induces inflammation, lung injury, and extra-pulmonary organ dysfunction in experimental pneumonia. Lab Investig 86(8):790–799
7. Blackwood B, Clarke M, McAuley DF, McGuigan PJ, Marshall JC, Rose L (2014) How outcomes are defined in clinical trials of mechanically ventilated adults and children. Am J Respir Crit Care Med 189(8):886–893
8. Contentin L, Ehrmann S, Giraudeau B (2014) Heterogeneity in the definition of mechanical ventilation duration and ventilator-free days. Am J Respir Crit Care Med 189(8):998–1002
9. Zilberberg MD, De Wit M, Pirone JR, Shorr AF (2008) Growth in adult prolonged acute mechanical ventilation: implications for healthcare delivery. Crit Care Med 36(5):1451–1455
10. MacIntyre NR, Epstein SK, Carson S, Scheinhorn D, Christopher K, Muldoon S (2005) Management of patients requiring prolonged mechanical ventilation: report of a NAMDRC consensus conference. Chest 128(6):3937–3954
11. Combes A, Costa MA, Trouillet JL, Baudot J, Mokhtari M, Gibert C et al (2003) Morbidity, mortality, and quality-of-life outcomes of patients requiring ≥14 days of mechanical ventilation. Crit Care Med 31(5):1373–1381
12. Rose L, Presneill JJ, Johnston L, Cade JF (2008) A randomised, controlled trial of conventional versus automated weaning from mechanical ventilation using SmartCare™/PS. Intensive Care Med 34(10):1788–1795
13. Schädler D, Engel C, Elke G, Pulletz S, Haake N, Frerichs I et al (2012) Automatic control of pressure support for ventilator weaning in surgical intensive care patients. Am J Respir Crit Care Med 185(6):637–644
14. Thomas NJ, Guardia CG, Moya FR, Cheifetz IM, Markovitz B, Cruces P et al (2012) A pilot, randomized, controlled clinical trial of lucinactant, a peptide-containing synthetic surfactant, in infants with acute hypoxemic respiratory failure. Pediatr Crit Care Med 13(6):646–653
15. Mehta S, Burry L, Cook D, Fergusson D, Steinberg M, Granton J et al (2012) Daily sedation interruption in mechanically ventilated critically ill patients cared for with a sedation protocol: a randomized controlled trial. JAMA 308(19):1985–1992
16. Dessap AM, Roche-Campo F, Kouatchet A, Tomicic V, Beduneau G, Sonneville R et al (2012) Natriuretic peptide-driven fluid management during ventilator weaning: a randomized controlled trial. Am J Respir Crit Care Med 186(12):1256–1263
17. Girault C, Bubenheim M, Abroug F, Diehl JL, Elatrous S, Beuret P et al (2011) Noninvasive ventilation and weaning in patients with chronic hypercapnic respiratory failure: a randomized multicenter trial. Am J Respir Crit Care Med 184(6):672–679
18. Kang BJ, Koh Y, Lim CM, Huh JW, Baek S, Han M et al (2015) Failure of high-flow nasal cannula therapy may delay intubation and increase mortality. Intensive Care Med 41(4):623–632
19. Yoo JW, Synn A, Huh JW, Hong SB, Koh Y, Lim CM (2016) Clinical efficacy of high-flow nasal cannula compared to noninvasive ventilation in patients with post-extubation respiratory failure. Korean J Intern Med 31(1):82–88
20. Maggiore SM, Idone FA, Vaschetto R, Festa R, Cataldo A, Antonicelli F et al (2014) Nasal high-flow versus venturi mask oxygen therapy after extubation: effects on oxygenation, comfort, and clinical outcome. Am J Respir Crit Care Med 190(3):282–288
21. Chiumello D, Coppola S, Froio S, Gregoretti C, Consonni D (2013) Noninvasive ventilation in chest trauma: systematic review and meta-analysis. Intensive Care Med 39(7):1171–1180

22. Funk GC, Anders S, Breyer MK, Burghuber OC, Edelmann G, Heindl W et al (2010) Incidence and outcome of weaning from mechanical ventilation according to new categories. Eur Respir J 35(1):88–94
23. Kao KC, Hu HC, Hsieh MJ, Tsai YH, Huang CC (2015) Comparison of community-acquired, hospital-acquired, and intensive care unit-acquired acute respiratory distress syndrome: a prospective observational cohort study. Crit Care. 19(1):384
24. Töpfer L, Menk M, Weber-Carstens S, Spies C, Wernecke KD, Uhrig A et al (2014) Influenza A (H1N1) vs non-H1N1 ARDS: analysis of clinical course. J Crit Care 29(3):340–346
25. Gracey DR, Viggiano RW, Naessens JM, Hubmayr RD, Silverstein MD, Koenig GE (1992) Outcomes of patients admitted to a chronic ventilator-dependent unit in an acute-care hospital. Mayo Clin Proc 67(2):131–136
26. Brochard L, Rauss A, Benito S, Conti G, Mancebo J, Rekik N et al (1994) Comparison of three methods of gradual withdrawal from ventilatory support during weaning from mechanical ventilation. Am J Respir Crit Care Med 150(4):896–903
27. Esteban A, Frutos F, Tobin MJ, Alía I, Solsona JF, Valverdú I et al (1995) A comparison of four methods of weaning patients from mechanical ventilation. N Engl J Med 332(6):345–350
28. Levine S, Nguyen T, Taylor N, Friscia ME, Budak MT, Rothenberg P et al (2008) Rapid disuse atrophy of diaphragm fibers in mechanically ventilated humans. N Engl J Med 358(13):1327–1335
29. Hussain SNA, Mofarrahi M, Sigala I, Kim HC, Vassilakopoulos T, Maltais F et al (2010) Mechanical ventilation-induced diaphragm disuse in humans triggers autophagy. Am J Respir Crit Care Med 182(11):1377–1386
30. Yoshida T, Papazian L (2014) When to promote spontaneous respiratory activity in acute respiratory distress patients? Anesthesiology 120(6):1313–1315
31. Freebairn R, Hickling K (2005) Spontaneous breathing during mechanical ventilation in ARDS. Crit Care Shock 8(3):61–66
32. Okamoto K, Iwamasa H, Dogomori H, Morioka T (1990) Evaluation of conventional weaning criteria in patients with acute respiratory failure. J Anesth 4(3):213–218
33. Jeganathan N, Kaplan CA, Balk RA (2015) Ventilator liberation for high-risk-for-failure patients: improving value of the spontaneous breathing trial. Respir Care 60(2):290–296
34. Frutos-Vivar F, Esteban A (2013) Weaning from mechanical ventilation: why are we still looking for alternative methods? Med Int 37(9):605–617
35. Tanios MA, Nevins ML, Hendra KP, Cardinal P, Allan JE, Naumova EN et al (2006) A randomized, controlled trial of the role of weaning predictors in clinical decision making. Crit Care Med 34(10):2530–2535
36. Walsh TS, Dodds S, McArdle F (2004) Evaluation of simple criteria to predict successful weaning from mechanical ventilation in intensive care patients. Br J Anaesth 92(6): 793–799
37. MacIntyre NR (2001) Evidence-based guidelines for weaning and discontinuing ventilatory support: a collective task force facilitated by the American college of chest physicians; the American association for respiratory care; and the American college of critical medicine. Chest 120(6 Suppl):375S–395S
38. De Souza LC, Guimarães FS, Lugon JR (2015) Evaluation of a new index of mechanical ventilation weaning: the timed inspiratory effort. J Intensive Care Med 30(1):37–43
39. Nemer SN, Barbas CSV, Caldeira JB, Cárias TC, Santos RG, Almeida LC et al (2009) A new integrative weaning index of discontinuation from mechanical ventilation. Crit Care. 13(5):R152
40. Meade M, Guyatt G, Cook D, Griffith L, Sinuff T, Kergl C et al (2001) Predicting success in weaning from mechanical ventilation. Chest 120(6 Suppl):400S–424S
41. Perren A, Brochard L (2013) Managing the apparent and hidden difficulties of weaning from mechanical ventilation. Intensive Care Med 39(11):1885–1895
42. Ladeira MT, Vital FM, Andriolo RB, Andriolo BN, Atallah AN, Peccin MS (2014) Pressure support versus T-tube for weaning from mechanical ventilation in adults. Cochrane Database Syst Rev 5:CD006056

43. Cabello B, Thille AW, Roche-Campo F, Brochard L, Gómez FJ, Mancebo J (2010) Physiological comparison of three spontaneous breathing trials in difficult-to-wean patients. Intensive Care Med 36(7):1171–1179
44. Ezingeard E, Diconne E, Guyomarc'h S, Venet C, Page D, Gery P et al (2006) Weaning from mechanical ventilation with pressure support in patients failing a T-tube trial of spontaneous breathing. Intensive Care Med 32(1):165–169
45. Laghi F, D'Alfonso N, Tobin MJ (1995) Pattern of recovery from diaphragmatic fatigue over 24 hours. J Appl Physiol 79(2):539–546
46. Girard TD, Kress JP, Fuchs BD, Thomason JW, Schweickert WD, Pun BT et al (2008) Efficacy and safety of a paired sedation and ventilator weaning protocol for mechanically ventilated patients in intensive care (Awakening and Breathing Controlled trial): a randomised controlled trial. Lancet 371(9607):126–134
47. Yang KL, Tobin MJ (1991) A prospective study of indexes predicting the outcome of trials of weaning from mechanical ventilation. N Engl J Med 324(21):1445–1450
48. Ely EW, Baker AM, Dunagan DP, Burke HL, Smith AC, Kelly PT et al (1996) Effect on the duration of mechanical ventilation of identifying patients capable of breathing spontaneously. N Engl J Med 335(25):1864–1869
49. Esteban A, Alía I, Gordo F, Fernández R, Solsona JF, Vallverdu I et al (1997) Extubation outcome after spontaneous breathing trials with T-Tube or pressure support ventilation. Am J Respir Crit Care Med 156(2 Pt 1):459–465
50. Esteban A, Alía I, Tobin MJ, Gil A, Gordo F, Vallverdú I et al (1999) Effect of spontaneous breathing trial duration on outcome of attempts to discontinue mechanical ventilation. Am J Respir Crit Care Med 159(2):512–518
51. Aitken LM, Bucknall T, Kent B, Mitchell M, Burmeister E, Keogh S (2016) Sedation protocols to reduce duration of mechanical ventilation in the ICU: a Cochrane Systematic Review. J Adv Nurs 72(2):261–272
52. Bucknall TK, Manias E, Presneill JJ (2008) A randomized trial of protocol-directed sedation management for mechanical ventilation in an Australian intensive care unit. Crit Care Med 36(5):1444–1450
53. Luo J, Wang MY, Liang BM, Yu H, Jiang FM, Wang T et al (2015) Initial synchronized intermittent mandatory ventilation versus assist/control ventilation in treatment of moderate acute respiratory distress syndrome: a prospective randomized controlled trial. J Thorac Dis 7(12):2262–2273
54. Rose L, Schultz MJ, Cardwell CR, Jouvet P, McAuley DF, Blackwood B (2014) Automated versus non-automated weaning for reducing the duration of mechanical ventilation for critically ill adults and children. Cochrane Database Syst Rev 6:CD009235
55. Sulzer CF, Chioléro R, Chassot PG, Mueller XM, Revelly JP (2001) Adaptive support ventilation for fast tracheal extubation after cardiac surgery: a randomized controlled study. Anesthesiology 95(6):1339–1345
56. McMullen SM, Meade M, Rose L, Burns K, Mehta S, Doyle R et al (2012) Partial ventilatory support modalities in acute lung injury and acute respiratory distress syndrome-a systematic review. PLoS ONE. 7(8):e40190
57. Putensen C, Zech S, Wrigge H, Zinserling J, Stüber F, Von Spiegel T et al (2001) Long-term effects of spontaneous breathing during ventilatory support in patients with acute lung injury. Am J Respir Crit Care Med 164(1):43–49
58. Guérin C, Reignier J, Richard JC, Beuret P, Gacouin A, Boulain T et al (2013) Prone positioning in severe acute respiratory distress syndrome. N Engl J Med 368(23):2159–2168
59. Papazian L, Forel JM, Gacouin A, Penot-Ragon C, Perrin G, Loundou A et al (2010) Neuromuscular blockers in early acute respiratory distress syndrome. N Engl J Med 363(12):1107–1116
60. Yoshida T, Uchiyama A, Matsuura N, Mashimo T, Fujino Y (2013) The comparison of spontaneous breathing and muscle paralysis in two different severities of experimental lung injury. Crit Care Med 41(2):536–545

61. Carteaux G, Millán-Guilarte T, De Prost N, Razazi K, Abid S, Thille AW et al (2016) Failure of noninvasive ventilation for de novo acute hypoxemic respiratory failure: role of tidal volume*. Crit Care Med 44(2):282–290
62. Yoshida T, Torsani V, Gomes S, Santis RRD, Beraldo MA, Costa ELV et al (2013) Spontaneous effort causes occult pendelluft during mechanical ventilation. Am J Respir Crit Care Med 188(12):1420–1427
63. Yoshida T, Roldan R, Beraldo MA, Torsani V, Gomes S, de Santis RR et al (2016) Spontaneous effort during mechanical ventilation: maximal injury with less positive end-expiratory pressure. Crit Care Med. 44(8):e678–e688
64. Biehl M, Kashyap R, Ahmed AH, Reriani MK, Ofoma UR, Wilson GA et al (2015) Six-month quality-of-life and functional status of acute respiratory distress syndrome survivors compared to patients at risk: a population-based study. Crit Care 19(1):356
65. Tobin MJ, Perez W, Guenther SM, Semmes BJ, Mador MJ, Allen SJ et al (1986) The pattern of breathing during successful and unsuccessful trials of weaning from mechanical ventilation. Am Rev Respir Dis 134(6):1111–1118
66. Dessap AM, Katsahian S, Roche-Campo F, Varet H, Kouatchet A, Tomicic V et al (2014) Ventilator-associated pneumonia during weaning from mechanical ventilation: role of fluid management. Chest 146(1):58–65
67. Razazi K, Thille AW, Carteaux G, Beji O, Brun-Buisson C, Brochard L et al (2014) Effects of pleural effusion drainage on oxygenation, respiratory mechanics, and hemodynamics in mechanically ventilated patients. Ann Am Thorac Soc 11(7):1018–1024
68. Bissett B, Leditschke IA, Neeman T, Boots R, Paratz J (2015) Weaned but weary: one third of adult intensive care patients mechanically ventilated for 7 days or more have impaired inspiratory muscle endurance after successful weaning. Heart Lung J Acute Crit Care 44(1): 15–20
69. Caruso P, Denari SD, Ruiz SA, Bernal KG, Manfrin GM, Friedrich C et al (2005) Inspiratory muscle training is ineffective in mechanically ventilated critically ill patients. Clinics (São Paulo, Brazil) 60(6):479–484
70. Condessa RL, Brauner JS, Saul AL, Baptista M, Silva ACT, Vieira SRR (2013) Inspiratory muscle training did not accelerate weaning from mechanical ventilation but did improve tidal volume and maximal respiratory pressures: a randomised trial. J Physiother 59(2): 101–107
71. Montgomery AB, Holle RHO, Neagley SR, Pierson DJ, Schoene RB (1987) Prediction of successful ventilator weaning using airway occlusion pressure and hypercapnic challenge. Chest 91(4):496–499
72. Reade MC (2010) Optimal sedation for the ventilation of critically ill patients. Curr Respir Med Rev 6(4):292–299
73. Shehabi Y, Bellomo R, Reade MC, Bailey M, Bass F, Howe B et al (2012) Early intensive care sedation predicts long-term mortality in ventilated critically ill patients. Am J Respir Crit Care Med 186(8):724–731
74. Tanaka LMS, Azevedo LCP, Park M, Schettino G, Nassar AP, Re'a-Neto A et al (2014) Early sedation and clinical outcomes of mechanically ventilated patients: a prospective multicenter cohort study. Critical Care. 18(4):R156
75. Kress JP, Pohlman AS, O'Connor MF, Hall JB (2000) Daily interruption of sedative infusions in critically ill patients undergoing mechanical ventilation. N Engl J Med 342(20):1471–1477
76. Valta P, Uusaro A, Nunes S, Ruokonen E, Takala J (1999) Acute respiratory distress syndrome: frequency, clinical course, and costs of care. Crit Care Med 27(11):2367–2374
77. Balas MC, Vasilevskis EE, Olsen KM, Schmid KK, Shostrom V, Cohen MZ et al (2014) Effectiveness and safety of the awakening and breathing coordination, delirium monitoring/management, and early exercise/mobility bundle. Crit Care Med 42(5):1024–1036
78. Jarman AM, Duke GJ, Reade MC, Casamento A (2013) The association between sedation practices and duration of mechanical ventilation in intensive care. Anaesth Intensive Care 41(3):311–315

79. Devlin J, Fraser G, Ely EW, Kress J, Skrobik Y, Dasta J (2013) Pharmacological management of sedation and delirium in mechanically ventilated ICU patients: remaining evidence gaps and controversies. Semin Respir Crit Care Med 34(2):201–215
80. Porhomayon J, El-Solh AA, Adlparvar G, Jaoude P, Nader ND (2016) Impact of sedation on cognitive function in mechanically ventilated patients. Lung 194(1):43–52
81. Cammarano WB, Pittet JF, Weitz S, Schlobohm RM, Marks JD (1998) Acute withdrawal syndrome related to the administration of analgesic and sedative medications in adult intensive care unit patients. Crit Care Med 26(4):676–684
82. Thille AW, Boissier F, Ghezala HB, Razazi K, Mekontso-Dessap A, Brun-Buisson C (2015) Risk factors for and prediction by caregivers of extubation failure in ICU patients: a prospective study. Crit Care Med 43(3):613–620
83. Lemaire F, Teboul JL, Cinotti L, Giotto G, Abrouk F, Steg G et al (1988) Acute left ventricular dysfunction during unsuccessful weaning from mechanical ventilation. Anesthesiology 69(2):171–179
84. Pinsky MR (2012) Breathing as exercise: the cardiovascular response to weaning from mechanical variation. In: Applied physiology in intensive care medicine 2: physiological reviews and editorials. Springer, Heidelberg, pp 323–325
85. Buda AJ, Pinsky MR, Ingels NB Jr, Daughters Iind GT, Stinson EB, Alderman EL (1979) Effect of intrathoracic pressure on left ventricular performance. N Engl J Med 301(9): 453–459
86. Mikkelsen ME, Shull WH, Biester RC, Taichman DB, Lynch S, Demissie E et al (2009) Cognitive, mood and quality of life impairments in a select population of ARDS survivors. Respirology 14(1):76–82
87. Files DC, Sanchez MA, Morris PE (2015) A conceptual framework: the early and late phases of skeletal muscle dysfunction in the acute respiratory distress syndrome. Crit Care 19(1):266
88. Edwards J, McWilliams D, Thomas M, Shah S (2014) Electrical muscle stimulation in the intensive care unit: an integrative review. J Intensive Care Soc 15(2):142–149
89. Mæhle K, Haug B, Flaatten H, Nielsen EW (2014) Metabolic alkalosis is the most common acid-base disorder in ICU patients. Crit Care 18(2):420
90. Libório AB, Noritomi DT, Leite TT, de Melo Bezerra CT, de Faria ER, Kellum JA (2015) Increased serum bicarbonate in critically ill patients: a retrospective analysis. Intensive Care Med 41(3):479–486
91. Krajewski ML, Raghunathan K, Paluszkiewicz SM, Schermer CR, Shaw AD (2015) Meta-analysis of high- versus low-chloride content in perioperative and critical care fluid resuscitation. Br J Surg 102(1):24–36
92. Young P, Bailey M, Beasley R, Henderson S, Mackle D, McArthur C et al (2015) Effect of a buffered crystalloid solution vs saline on acute kidney injury among patients in the intensive care unit: the SPLIT randomized clinical trial. JAMA 314(16):1701–1710
93. Mazur JE, Devlin JW, Peters MJ, Jankowski MA, Iannuzzi MC, Zarowitz BJ (1999) Single versus multiple doses of acetazolamide for metabolic alkalosis in critically ill medical patients: a randomized, double-blind trial. Crit Care Med 27(7):1257–1261
94. Barron R, Freebairn R (2010) Electrolyte disorders in the critically ill. Anaes Intensive Care Med 11(12):523–528
95. Peter JV, John P, Graham PL, Moran JL, George IA, Bersten A (2008) Corticosteroids in the prevention and treatment of acute respiratory distress syndrome (ARDS) in adults: meta-analysis. BMJ 336(7651):1006–1009
96. Hermans G, Van den Berghe G (2015) Clinical review: intensive care unit acquired weakness. Critical Care. 19(1):274
97. Myhren H, Tøien K, Ekeberg O, Karlsson S, Sandvik L, Stokland O (2009) Patients' memory and psychological distress after ICU stay compared with expectations of the relatives. Intensive Care Med 35(12):2078–2086
98. Jubran A, Lawm G, Kelly J, Duffner LA, Gungor G, Collins EG et al (2010) Depressive disorders during weaning from prolonged mechanical ventilation. Intensive Care Med 36(5): 828–835

99. Gajewski M, Weinhouse G (2016) The use of modafinil in the intensive care unit. J Intensive Care Med 31(2):142–145
100. Rothenhausler HB, Ehrentraut S, Von Degenfeld G, Weis M, Tichy M, Kilger E et al (2000) Treatment of depression with methylphenidate in patients difficult to wean from mechanical ventilation in the intensive care unit. J Clin Psychiatry 61(10):750–755
101. Johnson CJ, Auger WR, Fedullo PF, Dimsdale JE (1995) Methylphenidate in the 'hard to wean' patient. J Psychosom Res 39(1):63–68
102. Abbasi S, Farsaei S, Fazel K, Golzari SE, Mahmoodpoor A (2015) Can donepezil facilitate weaning from mechanical ventilation in difficult to wean patients? An interventional pilot study. DARU J Pharmaceut Sci 23(1):23
103. Rosenthal LJ, Kim V, Kim DR (2007) Weaning from prolonged mechanical ventilation using an antipsychotic agent in a patient with acute stress disorder. Crit Care Med 35(10):2417–2419
104. Jeon K, Jeong BH, Ko MG, Nam J, Yoo H, Chung CR et al (2016) Impact of delirium on weaning from mechanical ventilation in medical patients. Respirology 21(2):313–320
105. Shehabi Y, Botha JA, Ernest D, Freebairn RC, Reade M, Roberts BL et al (2010) Clinical application, the use of dexmedetomidine in intensive care sedation. Crit Care Shock 13(2):40–50
106. Cox CE, Martinu T, Sathy SJ, Clay AS, Chia J, Gray AL et al (2009) Expectations and outcomes of prolonged mechanical ventilation. Crit Care Med 37(11):2888–2894
107. Damuth E, Mitchell JA, Bartock JL, Roberts BW, Trzeciak S (2015) Long-term survival of critically ill patients treated with prolonged mechanical ventilation: a systematic review and meta-analysis. Lancet Respir Med 3(7):544–553
108. McCanny P, Bennett K, Staunton P, McMahon G (2012) Venous vs arterial blood gases in the assessment of patients presenting with an exacerbation of chronic obstructive pulmonary disease. Am J Emerg Med 30(6):896–900
109. Downs JB (2011) PaCO2, PETCO2, and gradient. In: Capnography, vol 2nd. Cambridge University Press, New York, pp 225–230
110. Kim WY, Suh HJ, Hong SB, Koh Y, Lim CM (2011) Diaphragm dysfunction assessed by ultrasonography: influence on weaning from mechanical ventilation. Crit Care Med 39(12):2627–2630
111. Li Z, Peng X, Zhu B, Zhang Y, Xi X (2013) Active mobilization for mechanically ventilated patients: a systematic review. Arch Phys Med Rehabil 94(3):551–561
112. Lin WC, Chen CW, Wang JD, Tsai LM (2015) Is tracheostomy a better choice than translaryngeal intubation for critically ill patients requiring mechanical ventilation for more than 14 days? A comparison of short-term outcomes. BMC Anesthesiol 15:181
113. Lim CK, Ruan SY, Lin FC, Wu CL, Chang HT, Jerng JS et al (2015) Effect of tracheostomy on weaning parameters in difficult-to-wean mechanically ventilated patients: a prospective observational study. PLoS ONE. 10(9):e0138294
114. Hosokawa K, Nishimura M, Egi M, Vincent J-L (2015) Timing of tracheotomy in ICU patients: a systematic review of randomized controlled trials. Crit Care 19(1):1–12
115. Szakmany T, Russell P, Wilkes AR, Hall JE (2015) Effect of early tracheostomy on resource utilization and clinical outcomes in critically ill patients: meta-analysis of randomized controlled trials. Br J Anaesth 114(3):396–405
116. Bice T, Nelson JE, Carson SS (2015) To trach or not to trach: uncertainty in the care of the chronically critically ill. Semin Respir Crit Care Med 36(6):851–858
117. Su CL, Chiang LL, Yang SH, Lin HI, Cheng KC, Huang YCT, Wu CP (2012) Preventive use of noninvasive ventilation after extubation: A prospective, multicenter randomized controlled trial Respiratory Care, 57(2):204–210.
118. Du LL, Han H, Zhang XJ, Wei L (2009) Randomized control study of sequential non-invasive following short-term invasive mechanical ventilation in the treatment of acute respiratory distress syndrome as a result of existing pulmonary diseases in elderly patients. Chinese Crit Care Med 21(7):394–396
119. Fauroux B, Leboulanger N, Roger G, Denoyelle F, Picard A, Garabedian EN et al (2010) Noninvasive positive-pressure ventilation avoids recannulation and facilitates early weaning from tracheotomy in children*. Pediatr Crit Care Med 11(1):31–37

120. Ferrer M, Sellarés J, Valencia M, Carrillo A, Gonzalez G, Badia JR et al (2009) Non-invasive ventilation after extubation in hypercapnic patients with chronic respiratory disorders: randomised controlled trial. Lancet 374(9695):1082–1088
121. Hess DR (2012) The role of noninvasive ventilation in the ventilator discontinuation process. Respir Care 57(10):1619–1625
122. Laiq N, Khan RA, Malik A (2013) Non-invasive positive pressure ventilation facilitates early extubation in post operative cardiac patients. J Postgradu Med Inst 27(4):361–365
123. Plant N, Walker R (2009) Immediate extubation to noninvasive ventilation can reduce postoperative morbidity and need for PICU in children with neuromuscular disorders. Paediatr Anaesth 19(5):549–550
124. Samra T, Borthakur B, Pawar M, Deepak D, Yadav A (2010) Non-invasive ventilation is helpful in early weaning and early extubation in H1N1 infected, ventilated patients: a case series. Anaes Pain Intensive Care 14(1):35–37
125. Trevisan CE, Vieira SR (2008) Noninvasive mechanical ventilation may be useful in treating patients who fail weaning from invasive mechanical ventilation: a randomized clinical trial. Crit Care 12(2):R51
126. Burns KE, Meade MO, Premji A, Adhikari NK (2013) Noninvasive positive-pressure ventilation as a weaning strategy for intubated adults with respiratory failure. Cochrane Database Syst Rev 12:CD004127
127. Glossop AJ, Shepherd N, Bryden DC, Mills GH (2012) Non-invasive ventilation for weaning, avoiding reintubation after extubation and in the postoperative period: a meta-analysis. Br J Anaesth 109(3):305–314
128. Agarwal R, Aggarwal AN, Gupta D (2010) Role of noninvasive ventilation in acute lung injury/acute respiratory distress syndrome: a proportion meta-analysis. Respir Care 55(12):1653–1660
129. Antonelli M, Conti G, Esquinas A, Montini L, Maggiore SM, Bello G et al (2007) A multiple-center survey on the use in clinical practice of noninvasive ventilation as a first-line intervention for acute respiratory distress syndrome. Crit Care Med 35(1):18–25
130. Freebairn R (2008) Noninvasive ventilation, a thing of beauty! Crit Care Med 36(2): 630–631
131. Vignaux L, Vargas F, Roeseler J, Tassaux D, Thille AW, Kossowsky MP et al (2009) Patient-ventilator asynchrony during non-invasive ventilation for acute respiratory failure: a multicenter study. Intensive Care Med 35(5):840–846
132. Davis S, Potgieter PD, Linton DM (1989) Mandatory minute volume weaning. Anaesth Intensive Care 17(2):170–174
133. Agarwal R, Srinivasan A, Aggarwal AN, Gupta D (2013) Adaptive support ventilation for complete ventilatory support in acute respiratory distress syndrome: a pilot, randomized controlled trial. Respirology 18(7):1108–1115
134. Arnal JM, Garnero A, Novonti D, Demory D, Ducros L, Berric A et al (2013) Feasibility study on full closed-loop control ventilation (IntelliVent-ASV™) in ICU patients with acute respiratory failure: a prospective observational comparative study. Crit Care. 17(5):R196
135. Gruber PC, Gomersall CD, Leung P, Joynt GM, Ng SK, Ho KM et al (2008) Randomized controlled trial comparing adaptive-support ventilation with pressure-regulated volume-controlled ventilation with automode in weaning patients after cardiac surgery. Anesthesiology 109(1):81–87
136. Carteaux G, Cordoba-Izquierdo A, Lyazidi A, Heunks L, Thille AW, Brochard L (2016) Comparison between neurally adjusted ventilatory assist and pressure support ventilation levels in terms of respiratory effort. Crit Care Med 44(3):503–511
137. Bosma KJ, Read BA, Bahrgard Nikoo MJ, Jones PM, Priestap FA, Lewis JF (2016) A pilot randomized trial comparing weaning from mechanical ventilation on pressure support versus proportional assist ventilation. Crit Care Med. 44(6):1098–1108
138. Taniguchi C, Eid RC, Saghabi C, Souza R, Silva E, Knobel E et al (2009) Automatic versus manual pressure support reduction in the weaning of post-operative patients: a randomised controlled trial. Crit Care. 13(1):R6

139. Veelo DP, Dongelmans DA, Binnekade JM, Paulus F, Schultz MJ (2010) Adaptive support ventilation: a translational study evaluating the size of delivered tidal volumes. Int J Artif Organs 33(5):302–309
140. Dongelmans DA, Veelo DP, Paulus F, De Mol BAJM, Korevaar JC, Kudoga A et al (2009) Weaning automation with adaptive support ventilation: a randomized controlled trial in cardiothoracic surgery patients. Anesth Analg 108(2):565–571
141. Sulemanji DS, Marchese A, Wysocki M, Kacmarek RM (2013) Adaptive support ventilation with and without end-tidal CO2 closed loop control versus conventional ventilation. Intensive Care Med 39(4):703–710
142. Lellouche F, Mancebo J, Jolliet P, Roeseler J, Schortgen F, Dojat M et al (2006) A multicenter randomized trial of computer-driven protocolized weaning from mechanical ventilation. Am J Respir Crit Care Med 174(8):894–900
143. Burns KE, Lellouche F, Nisenbaum R, Lessard MR, Friedrich JO (2014) Automated weaning and SBT systems versus non-automated weaning strategies for weaning time in invasively ventilated critically ill adults. Cochrane Database Syst Rev 9:CD008638
144. Dojat M, Harf A, Touchard D, Laforest M, Lemaire F, Brochard L (1996) Evaluation of a knowledge-based system providing ventilatory management and decision for extubation. Am J Respir Crit Care Med 153(3):997–1004
145. Antonelli M, Bonten M, Chastre J, Citerio G, Conti G, Curtis JR et al (2012) Year in review in Intensive Care Medicine 2011: III. ARDS and ECMO, weaning, mechanical ventilation, noninvasive ventilation, pediatrics and miscellanea. Intensive Care Med 38(4):542–556

Lung Imaging in ARDS

10

Silvia Coppola, Sara Froio, and Davide Chiumello

10.1 Introduction

The definition of acute respiratory distress syndrome (ARDS) has been recently revised with the new Berlin definition [1]. According to this latest definition, the diagnosis is based on the onset of the hypoxemia and of bilateral radiological opacities within 1 week. Three mutually exclusive categories of ARDS based on the degree of hypoxemia were identified (mild, $\leq$300 mmHg $PaO_2/FiO_2 > 200$ mmHg; moderate, $\leq$200 mmHg $PaO_2/FiO_2 > 100$ mmHg; severe, $PaO_2/FiO_2 \leq 100$ mmHg with a positive end-expiratory pressure $\geq$5 cmH_2O) associated with increased mortality and associated with median length of mechanical ventilation in survivors. The new definition updated the following concepts:

- The specific time frame identifying the acute onset as "ARDS developing within 1 week of a known clinical insult or new/worsening respiratory symptoms"
- The origin of edema judging ARDS, a respiratory failure not fully explained by cardiac failure or fluid overload
- The chest radiological criterion specifying that it should include bilateral opacities not fully explained by effusion, lobar lung collapse on chest radiograph, or on CT scan if available

S. Coppola • S. Froio
Dipartimento di Anestesia, Rianimazione ed Emergenza Urgenza, Fondazione IRCCS Ca' Granda–Ospedale Maggiore Policlinico, Milan, Italy
e-mail: sara.froio@hotmail.it

D. Chiumello (✉)
Director of Anaesthesia and Intensive Care Services, ASST Santi Paolo e Carlo, Department of Scienze della Salute, University of Milan, Milan, Italy
e-mail: chiumello@libero.it

D. Chiumello (ed.), *Acute Respiratory Distress Syndrome (ARDS)*,
DOI 10.1007/978-3-319-41852-0_10

Table 10.1 Lung imaging techniques: clinical role and technical limitations

Imaging technique	Clinical role	Technical limitations
X-ray	Lung assessment	Poor contrast diagnostic resolution Quality of the exam affected by ICU conditions Radiation exposure
Computed tomography	Lung assessment Lung recruitment Overdistension evaluation Lung perfusion analysis	Risk of critically ill patient's transport Radiation exposure
Lung ultrasound	Lung assessment Lung recruitment	Operator-dependent technique Physical shape such as obesity, subcutaneous emphysema, large rib cage
Positron emission tomography	Lung assessment	Risk of critically ill patient's transport Time-consuming Short half-life of tracers
Electrical impedance tomography	Lung assessment Lung recruitment Lung perfusion analysis	Indirect acquisition Detection of relative changes in functionally active structure
Magnetic resonance imaging	Lung assessment	Risk of critically ill patient's transport Required dedicated assistance, monitoring, and devices Time-consuming

From a pathophysiological point of view, ARDS can be considered an acute, diffuse inflammatory lung injury that leads to increased pulmonary vascular permeability, increased lung weight, and loss of aerated lung tissue. In this context of parenchymal abnormalities, lung imaging plays a role in the diagnosis and follow-up and can provide prognostic information.

Therefore, the aim of this chapter is to summarize the role of the different imaging techniques that have been developed throughout the years to better understand ARDS and to monitor ARDS patients. In particular we would focus on the role of each lung imaging technique in the diagnosis and in the evaluation over the time of lung recruitment, overdistension, and perfusion (Table 10.1).

10.2 Diagnostic Assessment

10.2.1 Chest X-Ray

For almost 20 years, chest X-ray has represented the main tool to evaluate the extension and the distribution of ARDS lung opacities.

However, in the first 24 h following the insult, chest X-ray can be quite normal. During the following 2–3 days, the chest X-ray can show bilateral opacities due to exudation of inflammatory fluid into the interstitium and air spaces independent of its etiology [2, 3]. It has been demonstrated that chest radiography can be insufficient to detect lung alteration in the initial stages of the disease; in fact up to 50% of patients with acute respiratory failure within the first 3 days do not present any lung abnormalities on chest X-ray [4]. Currently, it has been also reported a lower accuracy in detecting pleural effusions, alveolar consolidation, and alveolar-interstitial syndrome compared to lung ultrasound [5]. In fact a recent meta-analysis concluded that a systematic but unselective daily routine chest radiographs might probably be eliminated without increasing adverse outcomes in ICU adult patients [6].

10.2.2 Computed Tomography

Computed tomography (CT) scan has substantially improved our understanding of the inhomogeneous pattern of ARDS. Differently from chest X-ray, it avoids the superimposition of different structures and also allows accurate measurement of the extent of the abnormalities and of their density [7].

The classical morphological CT description includes the recognition of normally aerated lung, poorly inflated areas, characterized by increased density but with still recognizable vessels (ground-glass opacifications) and not-inflated areas with increased density and no recognizable vessels (consolidation) [8]. The increase in lung tissue and the reduction in lung gas volume due to the combination of alveolar flooding (edema), interstitial inflammation, and compression atelectasis are typical of the acute phase of ARDS.

In the early phase, ground-glass opacity has quite a distribution over the entire lung field, whereas consolidation is more prevalent in the dependent ones. In the late phase, over 2 weeks after the first insult, the reticular pattern is the single most frequent pattern and is more represented in the nondependent regions [9]. More than 70% of patients present with CT abnormalities at 6 months follow-up, characterized by fibrosis, air cysts, and bullae mainly located in the ventral, nondependent regions. They are more evident at CT scan than at chest radiography [10].

Furthermore, differences in pathophysiology between ARDS secondary to direct pulmonary insult and ARDS secondary to extrapulmonary disease reflect different CT morphological patterns. The former presents asymmetrical focal areas of consolidation, while extrapulmonary ARDS shows a symmetrical pattern with prevalence of ground-glass areas [11].

In the past decades, the CT quantitative analysis of poorly/normally aerated lung regions has led to the discovery that the ARDS lung is not stiff but "small" (the "baby lung") and that the residual inflated lung is nearly normal. Moreover, it was showed that ARDS lung is very heavy, weighing 2–3 times that of a normal lung with a content of air decreased to values 20–30% of normal [12].

Then, CT proved that the acute exudative lesions in ARDS have a gravitationally dependent gradient of distribution, with more consolidation in the posterobasal regions, as a result of compressive gravitational forces [13]. In conclusion regional analysis of CT scan has allowed to demonstrate a nonhomogeneous distribution of densities since the gas content progressively decreases from top to bottom because each alveolus is compressed by the weight of the superimposed structures [14]. Accordingly this physical model, in order to inflate the collapsed lung regions and to maintain open these regions, mechanical ventilation should overcome the superimposed pressure generated by the lung mass and pleural pressure.

10.2.3 Lung Ultrasound

Nowadays there is a great interest in the application of lung ultrasound in intensive care unit (ICU). In particular lung ultrasound (LUS) is a reproducible noninvasive bedside technique [15]. It has been shown to be superior to auscultation and chest radiography in the detection of the main ARDS pathology entities (alveolar-interstitial syndrome, pleural effusions, and lung consolidation) when considering CT scan as the reference method for a correct diagnosis [5]. Recently, evidence-based and expert consensus recommendations for LUS with a focus on emergency and ICU settings were provided [16]. To summarize, four patterns corresponding to various degrees of lung aeration can be described [16]:

1. Artifactual horizontal A lines parallel to the pleural line that characterize normal pulmonary aeration
2. Multiple and well-separated hyperechoic vertical lines, arising from pleural line (B lines) corresponding to moderate decrease in lung aeration resulting from interstitial syndrome
3. Coalescent B lines less than 3 mm apart corresponding to more severe decrease in lung aeration resulting from partial filling of alveolar spaces by pulmonary edema or confluent bronchopneumonia [17]
4. Lung consolidation containing white points characterized by dynamic bronchograms corresponding to complete loss of lung aeration with persisting aeration of distal bronchioles

Alveolar-interstitial syndrome (moderate or severe) and consolidation are present in all ultrasound examinations of ARDS patients. In fact the heterogeneous LUS pattern including well-separated or coalescent B lines and the presence of posterior lung consolidations with dynamic bronchograms is typical of ARDS [18, 19] and allows its early distinction from acute cardiogenic pulmonary edema [20].

10.2.4 Positron Emission Tomography

Positron emission tomography (PET) is a functional imaging technique based on the administration of a molecule labeled with a radioactive isotope, which decays with the emission of a positron. Any molecule virtually can be labeled without altering its properties so that PET scan can be useful to investigate any physiological process characterized by the kinetics of a given molecule. Hundreds of tracers have been developed and applied, and depending on which tracer is used, we can study the in vivo imaging of several organic functions. PET with 18-fluoride-2-deoxy-D-glucose (18-FDG) has been used to study cellular metabolic activity, reflecting the activity of inflammatory cells [21, 22]. In fact, 18-FDG is an analogue of glucose that is taken up by cells at the same rate of the glucose, so its accumulation is proportional to the intensity of the glycolytic metabolism of the cells. The uptake of 18-FDG is principally related to the activation of neutrophils [21, 22].

In patients with ARDS, PET with 18-FDG revealed an increased metabolic activity; however, the inflammation is not confined to regions with parenchymal abnormalities at CT scan but also involved normally aerated regions, suggesting that no pulmonary region is spared from inflammatory process [23]. It was demonstrated that in subjects who subsequently developed ARDS, a diffuse 18-FDG uptake was identified 1–3 days before the clinical manifestation of disease [24].

Moreover, recent studies focused on the possible influence of ventilation strategies on metabolic activity. Bellani et al. found that the metabolic activity (i.e., FDG uptake) of normally aerated regions was higher at an airway plateau pressure higher than 26 cmH_2O, whereas no association was found between cyclic recruitment/derecruitment and increased metabolic activity [25].

In conclusion, although its role in the daily clinical practice is not feasible, it represents a precious tool to better understand the relationship between lung imaging and lung injury and the link between ventilator-induced lung injury and ventilatory strategies and to measure the effect of anti-inflammatory interventions [26].

10.2.5 Electrical Impedance Tomography

Electrical impedance tomography (EIT) is a noninvasive, radiation-free, bedside lung imaging technique, which tracks changes in regional electrical resistivity of the lung tissue, corresponding to changes in regional gas content in relation to a reference state. Only functionally active lung structures are displayed, whereas structures – either normal or pathological (e.g., stable pneumothoraces or pleural effusions) – that do not change over time are functionally mute and cannot be represented as an image [27].

10.2.6 Magnetic Resonance Imaging

Magnetic resonance imaging (MRI) is a functional technique that can provide information about ventilation-perfusion heterogeneity, pulmonary end-capillary diffusion of oxygen, and lung microstructure. According to the physical properties of the noble gas used as contrast agent, it can provide different information; in fact ^{3}helium remains into the airways and alveolar spaces, and ^{129}xenon follows the diffusion pathway of oxygen. An experimental study showed the redistribution of alveolar gas due to the application of recruitment maneuvers and PEEP using [3] helium in mechanically ventilated rats with atelectasis [28]. At now, MRI data on ICU patients are limited; however, this technique could offer the possibility to match information about regional lung microstructure, function, and ventilation [27].

10.3 Recruitment

Lung recruitment is the amount of lung-collapsed tissue that can be reopened by applying high transpulmonary pressure for an adequate period of time. The decrease of the lung gas volume with the development of non-aerated regions mainly in the more dependent part is typical of the ARDS because of the increase of lung edema and of lung weight.

10.3.1 Computed Tomography

Quantitative CT scan analysis is the reference method for computing lung recruitment. It requires dedicated software and manual delineation of the perimeter of the lungs in each CT image.

It can be computed as the amount of non-inflated tissue that regains inflation [29], or as the increase in gas volume in the poorly and non-aerated tissue [30] at two different levels of pressures (Fig. 10.1). However, these two methods are not interchangeable; in fact the first method underestimated lung recruitment compared to the second one probably because it did not take into account lung recruitment in the poorly aerated lung regions. Due to the different amount of lung edema, the lung recruitability, estimated by lung CT scan, was found in whole population of ARDS patients, to range from 0% up to 70% of the total lung weight [19].

In clinical practice, to quantify lung recruitability may be important for assessing the severity of ARDS, planning recruitment maneuvers, and setting adequate PEEP levels during mechanical ventilation. In fact, lung recruitability affects the response to the applied PEEP levels: the higher is the lung recruitability, the higher will be the end-expiratory alveolar collapse that PEEP can prevent.

Recently Chiumello et al. compared CT scan-based and respiratory mechanics-based methods to assess the lung recruitment, and they found that they measure different phenomena related to the pressure increase: the CT scan measures the amount collapsed tissue which regains inflation, while the respiratory mechanics-based methods measure gas entering in already open pulmonary units which improve their mechanical properties at higher PEEP that is the overall improvement of inflation [31].

Obviously, quantitative analysis of the whole lung is labor-intensive and time-consuming. To increase the feasibility of the use of CT, Chiumello and colleagues demonstrated that visual anatomical analysis of lung CT had a good accuracy in detecting patients with high or low recruitability, although this method is unable to estimate the hyperinflation [32].

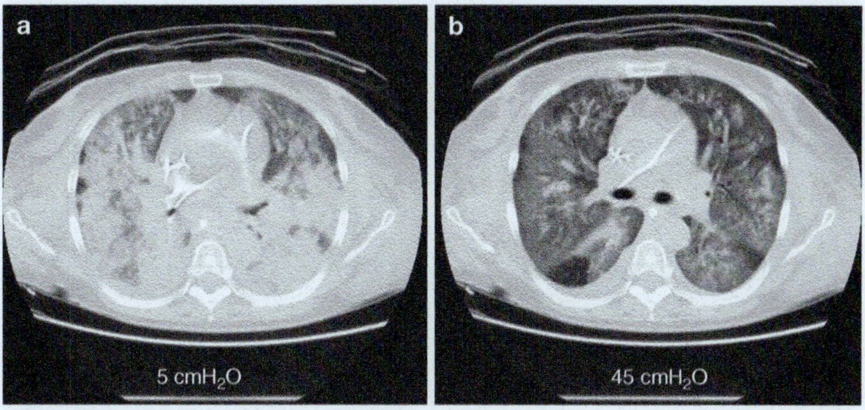

Fig. 10.1 Computed tomography and lung recruitment. The use of computed tomography scanning to identify potential for lung recruitment. Differences in aerated and non-aerated tissue at different pressure levels are presented. Panel (**a**) shows CT scan performed at end-expiration at 5 cmH_2O of PEEP; Panel (**b**) shows the CT scan of the same lung slice performed at inspiratory plateau pressure of 45 cmH_2O

10.3.2 Lung Ultrasound

It was demonstrated that an improvement in lung aeration might be detected by corresponding changes in LUS patterns. If the whole lung is examined, LUS using scores based on number of B lines can monitor extension of pulmonary edema, the amount of extravascular lung water, and the corresponding decrease in lung aeration.

Stefanidis and colleagues [33] estimated the size of non-aerated tissue in dependent lung regions at different PEEP levels, considering only not-inflated regions. Moreover, Bohaemad et al. realized a reaeration score to quantify the PEEP-induced lung recruitment that was demonstrated reliable as the pressure-volume curve method [34].

The LUS reaeration score should be performed on 12 regions of interest, including upper and lower posterior regions. In each region examined, changes in ultrasound pattern following the application of PEEP are detected, and numbers are attributed as follows:

- One point from multiple B lines to normal, from coalescent B lines to multiple B lines, and from consolidation to coalescent B lines
- Three points from coalescent B lines to normal or from consolidation to multiple B lines
- Five points from consolidation to normal

Interestingly in this study, the essential of recruitment results from the reaeration of poorly aerated lung regions. It means that coalescent B lines are transformed into separated B or A lines, and separated B lines are transformed into A lines. The reaeration of non-aerated lung regions remains marginal; in fact consolidations transformed into coalescent or separated B lines, or A lines, are a rarely observed event, occurring mostly in the lower parts of anterior, lateral, and posterior lung regions.

A high correlation was found between LUS reaeration score and CT reaeration. However, further studies using CT of the whole lung as gold standard are required to evaluate ability of LUS to reliably estimate PEEP-induced lung recruitment [35].

10.3.3 Electrical Impedance Tomography

In ARDS patients, the amount of potentially recruitable lung volume and the difference between the open, fully recruited, and the not recruited lung volume at 40 cmH_2O was computed as 26% ± 11% (range 11–47%) using EIT [36]. Thanks to its dynamic analysis, EIT has also allowed to identify alveolar opening of collapsed regions, the overdistension of opened areas, the collapse of previously opened regions, and the recovery of previously overdistended alveoli, during stepwise changes of mean airway pressure [37]. In particular, it was used to further study the regional intratidal gas distribution during the lung recruitment at different PEEP levels. For these purposes, EIT image can be divided in four anteroposterior quadrants (dorsal and ventral regions for the left and right lungs), and a regional analysis can be performed for each quadrant.

The study of the dynamic behaviors of the lung during slow recruitment maneuvers, in particular the delay time needed for the regional impedance in each quadrant to reach a certain threshold value of the maximal local impedance change, has allowed to construct maps of regional delays in ventilation that correlate with the amount of recruited lung and lung inhomogeneity and showed that distribution of gas started in the nondependent lung regions and ended in the dependent lung regions [38, 39].

The advantage of EIT is that the image might change following recruitment maneuvers, physiotherapy, or prone positioning, indicating a response to such treatments. In this context, EIT can open new scenarios to guide the PEEP titration strategy aimed at a decrease of the regional ventilation inhomogeneity, minimizing tidal collapse and hyperinflation.

10.4 Overdistension

10.4.1 Computed Tomography

The application of high levels of PEEP in patients with low lung recruitability can lead to overdistention of regions that are already aerated without opening the collapsed tissue (i.e., strain) [19]. CT scan is a unique tool to differentiate between recruitment and hyperinflation. Overdistension is defined by quantitative lung CT analysis as lung regions with a density threshold below – 900 Hounsfield units [18]. However, the quantitative computation of lung overdistension can be affected by the size of the voxel or the CT section thickness and by the type of reconstruction filter. In fact, a thick CT section (10 mm) underestimates the overinflated lung volume by 3–5% compared to thin CT sections (1.5 mm) [18]. The evaluation of hyperinflation can give information about the safety of our mechanical ventilation. In fact Terragni et al. have found that one-third of ARDS patients with large not aerated lung regions presented a substantial tidal hyperinflation, even when airway plateau pressure was between 28 and 30 cmH_2O [40].

Recently Cressoni et al. have quantified the lung inhomogeneities by CT scan. They found that the extent of lung inhomogeneities increased with the severity of ARDS, correlated with the physiologic dead space, and it was associated with overall mortality. Interestingly they also demonstrated that in most of the patients, lung inhomogeneities decrease by increasing PEEP or airway pressure, suggesting a more homogeneous lung at higher pressure. However, in a small part of patients, lung inhomogeneity extent increased, instead of decreased while increasing PEEP or plateau pressure. This was due to the increase of poorly aerated tissue and increasing pressures, while in most patients where lung inhomogeneities decreased increasing pressure, the poorly aerated tissue also decreased [41].

Once again CT scan has provided physiological information to better understand the complex interaction between mechanical ventilation and ventilator-induced lung injury.

10.5 Lung Perfusion

As known, arterial oxygenation results from the coupling between alveolar ventilation and perfusion. In fact in ARDS patients, hypoxemia is closely related to the consolidation or collapse of lung regions, which increases the intrapulmonary shunt. Accordingly, an important objective in the setting of mechanical ventilation is to optimally match ventilation with lung perfusion in order to improve gas exchange [27, 42]. Different imaging techniques such as computed tomography and electrical impedance tomography have been used to investigate the distribution of aeration and/or ventilation in ARDS. The understanding of the regional lung perfusion can be useful for the daily clinical practice for different reasons. Firstly, the response in oxygenation to different ventilatory strategies can be due to redistribution of lung perfusion and not to lung recruitment or derecruitment. Consequently, the level of PEEP should be titrated on respiratory mechanics changes and not on oxygenation. Then intravenous antibiotics cannot reach the affected regions because of the unpredictable distribution of blood flow.

10.5.1 Computed Tomography

CT scan studies have allowed analyzing the distribution of parenchymal consolidation and tissue perfusion in healthy and ARDS patients [43]. While in healthy subjects lung perfusion shows a gravitational bias, in ARDS patients it has an inhomogeneous distribution, and a great proportion of blood was directed toward collapsed areas. Obviously this shunt was related to the severity of hypoxemia. Unfortunately, CT scan does not provide real-time information [42].

10.5.2 Electrical Impedance Tomography

A promising method to quantify lung perfusion (pulsatile and non-pulsatile components) is by the injection of hypertonic saline that causes a decrease in the impedance signal as it travels through the right heart and the lungs to the left heart during a 10 s breath-hold. Through mathematical calculations of first-pass kinetics of the impedance-time dilution curve, it has been possible to estimate regional lung perfusion by electrical impedance tomography in a piglet model of lung collapse [44]. Although this is a real-time method, the evaluation of perfusion cannot happen continuously but only during the injection of a bolus of saline at high concentration. Moreover, the frequency of the measurements is limited by the potential side effects caused by the use of saline at high concentration.

10.6 Technical Advantages and Limitations

10.6.1 Chest X-Ray

Chest X-ray represents an inexpensive imaging technique, routinely and ubiquitously applied. The role of chest radiography is still actual, radiological findings are integral part of the diagnostic process, and X-ray images are still useful to detect malposition of tubes, catheters, and associated complications [10]. All patients admitted to an ICU receive at least one chest X-ray.

Nevertheless, the ICU features and the mandatory bedside application of radiography in these patients affect the quality of images. This technique has poor contrast diagnostic resolution, and in addition to this, the anterior-posterior view, the noncooperation of patients, and the presence of several lines in the field (e.g., endotracheal tube, arterial and central venous catheter, electrocardiogram monitoring, nasogastric tube, etc.) affect the quality of final imaging (Fig. 10.2).

10.6.2 Computed Tomography

Computed tomography represents the gold standard technique for the management of ARDS patients and provides several advantages: since from the 1980s, it has been used to study the inhomogeneous pattern of lung abnormalities in ARDS [45].

As described before, computed tomography allows to investigate the response to different types of ventilation in terms of lung morphology, lung recruitment, and overdistention.

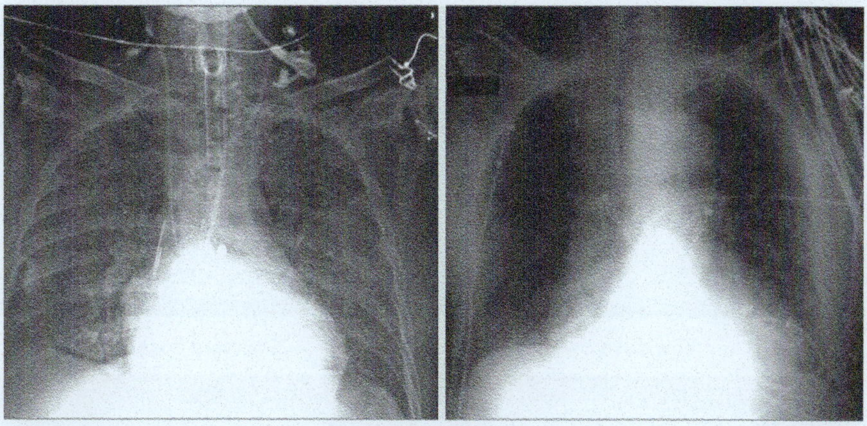

Fig. 10.2 Bedside application of chest X-ray in intensive care unit patients

Moving from these considerations, the use of CT scan analysis has spread in spite of risks of transferring critically ill patients outside the ICU to radiological department and of the risk of X-ray radiation exposure.

The radiation dose applied to perform a CT exam is related to image definition; the higher the dose, the lower the image noise; nevertheless, it is known that exposure to radiation could be associated with an increased incidence of cancer [46–49]. Moreover, a dose-effect relationship was observed [50], and the exposure to radiation during CT scans even if not able to cause immediate damage could be associated with subsequent sequelae [51].

Currently, no consensus for optimal acquisition is available; in the literature, a wide range of radiation dose is reported (tube current-time products from 100 to 350 mAs). Since from the 1990s, the use of low-dose chest CT was described to underline the possibility to visualize lung parenchyma reducing the effective mAs [52]. Recently Chiumello et al. aimed to evaluate the accuracy of quantitative analysis and the accuracy of visual anatomical analysis using low-dose chest CT to estimate lung recruitability in 45 ARDS patients [46]. Of note, the reduction of radiation dose (up to 30 mAs of the applied tube current-time product) did not affect the accuracy of quantitative analysis, and visual anatomical evaluation of lung recruitability was sufficiently accurate (Fig. 10.3). This study can open the prospective to potentially monitor ARDS patients by CT scan with a substantial reduction of radiation exposure.

10.6.3 Lung Ultrasound

The main advantages of lung ultrasonography include the possibility of avoiding patient's transport to the radiological department, of guiding lifesaving emergency procedures, and of decreasing radiation exposure [10]. Certainly, performing and interpreting ultrasound images require training to acquire the necessary skills and

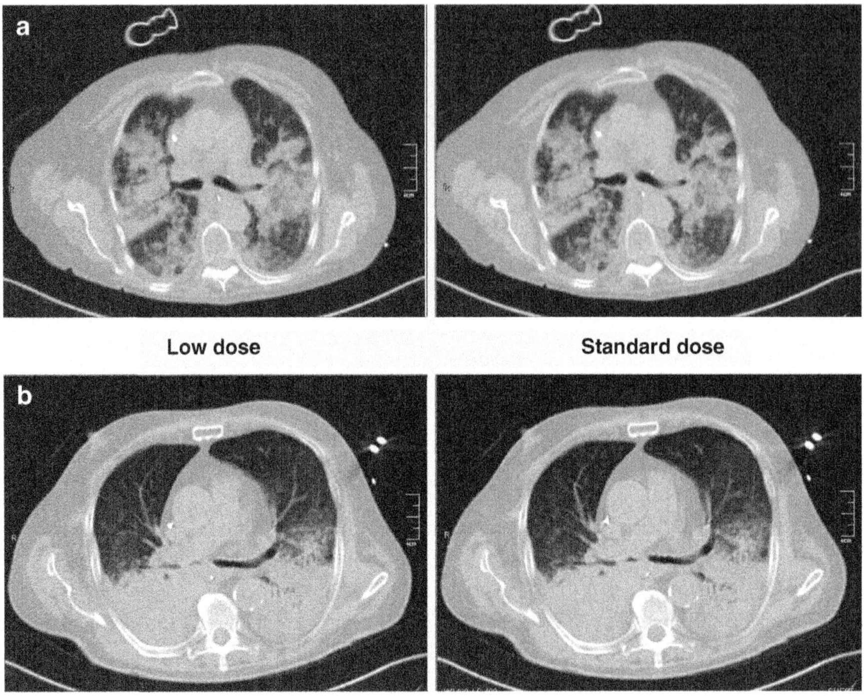

Fig. 10.3 Different radiation dose applied to perform chest computed tomography
Two consecutive scans of the lung are presented, performed during the same breath-hold in two ARDS patients (Panel **a**, patient 1; Panel **b**, patient 2). For couple of scans, two different mAs (tube current-time product) were applied. Panel (**a**) shows the image obtained with a reduced dose of 60 mAs (*left*), and the same image obtained with a standard dose of 110 mAs (*right*). Panel (**b**) shows the image obtained with a reduced dose of 60 mAs (*left*) and the same image obtained with a standard dose of 110 mAs (*right*). All other parameters of the CT scanner were kept unaltered during scan acquisition

knowledge. In addition to this operator-dependent limitation, some ultrasound patient-dependent limitations exist. Obese patients and patients with subcutaneous emphysema or large thoracic dressing are frequently difficult to examine. These features preclude the propagation of ultrasound beams to the lung periphery.

10.6.4 Positron Emission Tomography

One of the most relevant advantages of PET analysis concerns the detection of functional information. In fact, it is a flexible technique that allows the in vivo imaging of organic functions [21]. PET usefulness is further increased when associated with CT scan analysis, in order to provide an accurate anatomical localization of the functional studied process.

Depending of which tracer is selected, different pulmonary functions could be investigated, for example, regional blood volume [53], glycolytic metabolic activity and neutrophils' activation during inflammation [23, 54], regional perfusion and gas exchange [21], and endothelial permeability [55].

Unfortunately technical and clinical limitations exist in using this technique in daily clinical practice. The application of PET analysis is rather complex, tracers have short half-life, and patients should stay away from ICU for the length of the study procedure (hours), requiring dedicated assistance during transport and during permanence in the PET facility.

10.6.5 Electrical Impedance Tomography

Electrical impedance tomography provides bedside and noninvasive lung images available for continuous monitoring in daily ICU practice. However, EIT data can only indirectly quantify relative changes in lung impedance, and only structures that are functionally active are visualized (e.g., ventilated lung structures). Of note, EIT has a restricted spatial resolution (10–20 cm^3).

Finally, even if changes in end-expiratory lung impedance detected with EIT technique seem to correlate with changes in end-expiratory lung volume, this linear correlation is definitely dependent on electrode position.

10.6.6 Magnetic Resonance Imaging

MRI of the lung could offer the advantage of a functional technique and could be a valuable technique when radiation exposure or iodinated contrast is contraindicated. In spite of this, it is rarely used in ICU daily practice, because it is time-consuming, expensive, and limited by the low proton density of aerated lung tissue [10]. In addition, it requires patient's transport outside ICU, dedicated assistance and proper monitoring, and other patient-support devices during MRI procedures.

10.6.7 From Bedside to the Radiology Department: Risks of Patient's Transport

Among all described techniques, CT, PET, and MRI cannot be provided in the ICUs and require the transport of patients to the radiologic department. Critically ill patients that require transfer within the hospital are at risk of deterioration and at risk of adverse events caused by transfer. Although tube or line displacements are uncommon, they represent potentially serious events. Transfers are associated with small but significant rare adverse events, often related to deterioration of clinical condition or problems with equipment or patient's devices. Still today, adverse events have been found to occur from 8% to 68% [56]. Cases of major events such as major physiological derangement (15%) or cardiac arrest (3%) are uncommon but still described [57].

Therefore, risk of transport must be assessed, the possible benefits obtained by the diagnostic information should be higher compared to the possible adverse events caused by transfer, and finally patients should be transferred by an appropriately trained team with appropriated equipment [58, 59].

As recommended in the "transfer medicine" section of the recent Guidelines for Provision of Intensive Care Services 2015, the reason for transfer should be well documented and patients, where possible, must be informed [58]. Staff members of appropriate experience, with dedicated equipment and accurate monitoring to cope with any deterioration in clinical conditions, should transfer critically ill patients, especially when intubated and ventilated.

A recent study showed an occurrence of life-threatening adverse events of 6.7% in critically ill patients during intra-hospital transport required to perform CT scans [60]. Despite significant improvement in intra-hospital transport, the equipment failure, the lack of supervision, and the severity of patient's illness [60] are significant predictors for the occurrence of adverse events during transfer from ICU to radiology department.

References

1. Ranieri VM, Rubenfeld GD, Thompson BT, Ferguson ND, Caldwell E, Fan E, Camporota L, Slutsky AS (2012) Acute respiratory distress syndrome: the Berlin Definition. JAMA 307:2526–2533
2. Dushianthan A, Grocott MP, Postle AD, Cusack R (2011) Acute respiratory distress syndrome and acute lung injury. Postgrad Med J 87:612–622
3. Aberle DR, Brown K (1990) Radiologic considerations in the adult respiratory distress syndrome. Clin Chest Med 11:737–754
4. Endo S, Shibata S, Sato N, Hashiba E, Tajimi K, Saito K, Kawamae K, Nakane M, Murakawa M (2010) A prospective cohort study of ALI/ARDS in the Tohoku district of Japan (second report). J Anesth 24:351–358
5. Lichtenstein D, Goldstein I, Mourgeon E, Cluzel P, Grenier P, Rouby JJ (2004) Comparative diagnostic performances of auscultation, chest X-ray, and lung ultrasonography in acute respiratory distress syndrome. Anesthesiology 100:9–15
6. Oba Y, Zara T (2010) Abandoning daily routine chest radiography in the intensive care unit: meta-analysis. Radiology 255(2):386–395
7. Pesenti A, Tagliabue P, Patroniti N, Fumagalli R (2001) Computerised tomography scan imaging in acute respiratory distress syndrome. Intensive Care Med 27(4):631–639
8. Gattinoni L, Caironi P, Pelosi P, Goodman LR (2001) What has computed tomography taught us about the acute respiratory distress syndrome? Am J Respir Crit Care Med 164:1701–1711
9. Desai SR, Wells AU, Rubens MB, Evans TW, Hansell DM (1999) Acute respiratory distress syndrome: CT abnormalities at long-term follow-up. Radiology 210(1):29–35
10. Zompatori M, Ciccarese F, Fasano L (2014) Overview of current lung imaging in acute respiratory distress syndrome. Eur Respir Rev 23(134):519–530
11. Goodman LR, Fumagalli R, Tagliabue P, Tagliabue M, Ferrario M, Gattinoni L, Pesenti A (1999) Adult respiratory distress syndrome due to pulmonary and extrapulmonary causes: CT, clinical and functional correlations. Radiology 213(2):545–552
12. Gattinoni L, Pesenti A, Bombino M, Baglioni S, Rivolta M, Rossi F, Rossi G, Fumagalli R, Marcolin R, Mascheroni D (1988) Relationships between lung computed tomographic density, gas exchange, and PEEP in acute respiratory failure. Anesthesiology 69(6):824–832

13. Gattinoni L, Pesenti A (2005) The concept of "baby lung". Intensive Care Med 31(6):776–784
14. Pelosi P, D'Andrea L, Vitale G, Pesenti A, Gattinoni L (1994) Vertical gradient of regional lung inflation in adult respiratory distress syndrome. Am J Respir Crit Care Med 149:8–13
15. Constantin JM, Cayot-Constantin S, Roszyk L, Futier E, Sapin V, Dastugue B, Bazin JE, Rouby JJ (2007) Response to recruitment maneuver influences net alveolar fluid clearance in acute respiratory distress syndrome. Anesthesiology 106:944–951
16. Volpicelli G, Elbarbary M, Blaivas M, Lichtenstein DA, Mathis G, Kirkpatrick AW, Melniker L, Gargani L, Noble VE, Via G, Dean A, Tsung JW, Soldati G, Copetti R, Bouhemad B, Reissig A, Agricola E, Rouby JJ, Arbelot C, Liteplo A, Sargsyan A, Silva F, Hoppmann R, Breitkreutz R, Seibel A, Neri L, Storti E, Petrovic T (2012) International evidence-based recommendations for point-of- care lung ultrasound. Intensive Care Med 38:577–591
17. Bouhemad B, Liu ZH, Arbelot C, Zhang M, Ferarri F, Le Guen M, Girard M, Lu Q, Rouby JJ (2010) Ultrasound assessment of antibiotic-induced pulmonary reaeration in ventilator- associated pneumonia. Crit Care Med 38:84–92
18. Vieira SR, Puybasset L, Richecoeur J, Lu Q, Cluzel P, Gusman PB, Coriat P, Rouby JJ (1998) A lung computed tomographic assessment of positive end-expiratory pressure- induced lung overdistension. Am J Respir Crit Care Med 158:1571–1577
19. Gattinoni L, Caironi P, Cressoni M, Chiumello D, Ranieri VM, Quintel M, Russo S, Patroniti N, Cornejo R, Bugedo G (2006) Lung recruitment in patients with the acute respiratory distress syndrome. N Engl J Med 354:1775–1786
20. Copetti R, Soldati G, Copetti P (2008) Chest sonography: a useful tool to differentiate acute cardiogenic pulmonary edema from acute respiratory distress syndrome. Cardiovasc Ultrasound 6:16
21. Bellani G, Amigoni M, Pesenti A (2011) Positron emission tomography in ARDS: a new look at an old syndrome. Minerva Anestesiol 77:439–447
22. Musch G (2011) Positron emission tomography: a tool for better understanding of ventilator-induced and acute lung injury. Curr Opin Crit Care 17:7–12
23. Bellani G, Messa C, Guerra L, Spagnoli E, Foti G, Patroniti N, Fumagalli R, Musch G, Fazio F, Pesenti A (2009) Lungs of patients with acute respiratory distress syndrome show diffuse inflammation in normally aerated regions: a [18F]-fluoro-2-deoxy-D-glucose PET/CT study. Crit Care Med 37:2216–2222
24. Rodrigues RS, Miller PR, Bozza FA, Marchiori E, Zimmerman GA, Hoffman JM, Morton KA (2008) FDG-PET in patients at risk for acute respiratory distress syndrome: a preliminary report. Intensive Care Med 34:2273–2278
25. Bellani G, Guerra L, Musch G, Zanella A, Patroniti N, Mauri T, Messa C, Pesenti A (2011) Lung regional metabolic activity and gas volume changes induced by tidal ventilation in patients with acute lung injury. Am J Respir Crit Care Med 183:1193–1199
26. Chen DL, Bedient TJ, Kozlowski J, Rosenbluth DB, Isakow W, Ferkol TW, Thomas B, Mintun MA, Schuster DP, Walter MJ (2009) [18F]fluorodeoxyglucose positron emission tomography for lung antiinflammatory response evaluation. Am J Respir Crit Care Med 180:533–539
27. Chiumello D, Froio S, Bouhemad B, Camporota L, Coppola S (2013) Clinical review: lung imaging in acute respiratory distress syndrome patients – an update. Crit Care 17:243–255
28. Cereda M, Emami K, Kadlecek S, Xin Y, Mongkolwisetwara P, Profka H, Barulic A, Pickup S, Mansson S, Wollmer P, Ishii M, Deutschman CS, Rizi RR (2011) Quantitative imaging of alveolar recruitment with hyperpolarized gas MRI during mechanical ventilation. J Appl Physiol 110:499–511
29. Gattinoni L, Pelosi P, Crotti S, Valenza F (1995) Effects of positive end-expiratory pressure on regional distribution of tidal volume and recruitment in adult respiratory distress syndrome. Am J Respir Crit Care Med 151:1807–1814
30. Malbouisson LM, Muller JC, Constantin JM, Lu Q, Puybasset L, Rouby JJ (2001) Computed tomography assessment of positive end-expiratory pressure- induced alveolar recruitment in patients with acute respiratory distress syndrome. Am J Respir Crit Care Med 163:1444–1450
31. Chiumello D, Marino A, Brioni M, Cigada I, Menga F, Colombo A, Crimella F, Algeri I, Cressoni M, Carlesso E, Gattinoni L (2015) Lung recruitment assessed by respiratory mechan-

ics and by CT scan: what is the relationship? Am J Respir Crit Care Med 193(11):1254–1263. PMID: 26699672
32. Chiumello D, Marino A, Brioni M, Menga F, Cigada I, Lazzerini M, Andrisani MC, Biondetti P, Cesana B, Gattinoni L (2012) Visual anatomical lung CT scan assessment of lung recruitability. Intensive Care Med 39:66–73
33. Stefanidis K, Dimopoulos S, Tripodaki ES, Vitzilaios K, Politis P, Piperopoulos P, Nanas S (2011) Lung sonography and recruitment in patients with early acute respiratory distress syndrome: a pilot study. Crit Care 15:R185
34. Bouhemd B, Brisson H, Le-Guen M, Arbelot C, Lu Q, Rouby JJ (2011) Bedside ultrasound assessment of positive end-expiratory pressure-induced lung recruitment. Am J Respir Crit Care Med 183:341–347
35. Chiumello D, Froio S, Coppola S (2013) Update on lung imaging to select ventilatory management in ARDS patients. In: Practical issues in anesthesia and intensive care. Springer, Milan
36. Lowhagen K, Lindgren S, Odenstedt H, Stenqvist O, Lundin S (2011) A new non- radiological method to assess potential lung recruitability: a pilot study in ALI patients. Acta Anaesthesiol Scand 55:165–174
37. Grychtol B, Wolf GK, Adler A, Arnold JH (2010) Towards lung EIT image segmentation: automatic classification of lung tissue state from analysis of EIT monitored recruitment manoeuvres. Physiol Meas 31:S31–S43
38. Muders T, Luepschen H, Zinserling J, Greschus S, Fimmers R, Guenther U, Buchwald M, Grigutsch D, Leonhardt S, Putensen C, Wrigge H (2012) Tidal recruitment assessed by electrical impedance tomography and computed tomography in a porcine model of lung injury. Crit Care Med 40:903–911
39. Wrigge H, Zinserling J, Muders T, Varelmann D, Gunther U, von der GC, Magnusson A, Hedenstierna G, Putensen C (2008) Electrical impedance tomography compared with thoracic computed tomography during a slow inflation maneuver in experimental models of lung injury. Crit Care Med 36:903–909
40. Terragni PP, Rosboch G, Tealdi A, Corno E, Menaldo E, Davini O, Gandini G, Herrmann P, Mascia L, Quintel M, Slutsky AS, Gattinoni L, Ranieri VM (2007) Tidal hyperinflation during low tidal volume ventilation in acute respiratory distress syndrome. Am J Respir Crit Care Med 175:160–166
41. Cressoni M, Cadringher P, Chiurazzi C, Amini M, Gallazzi E, Marino A, Brioni M, Carlesso E, Chiumello D, Quintel M, Bugedo G, Gattinoni L (2014) Lung inhomogeneity in patients with acute respiratory distress syndrome. Am J Respir Crit Care Med 189:149–158
42. Pelosi P, de Abreu MG (2015) Acute respiratory distress syndrome: we can't miss regional lung perfusion! BMC Anesthesiol 15:35
43. Dakin J, Jones AT, Hansell DM, Hoffman EA, Evans TW (2011) Changes in lung composition and regional perfusion and tissue distribution in patients with ARDS. Respirology 16:1265–1272
44. Borges JB, Suarez-Sipmann F, Bohm SH, Tusman G, Melo A, Maripuu E, Sandstrom M, Park M, Costa EL, Hedenstierna G, Amato M (2012) Regional lung perfusion estimated by electrical impedance tomography in a piglet model of lung collapse. J Appl Physiol 112:225–236
45. Gattinoni L, Presenti A, Torresin A, Baglioni S, Rivolta M, Rossi F, Scarani F, Marcolin R, Cappelletti G (1986) Adult respiratory distress syndrome profiles by computed tomography. J Thorac Imaging 1:25–30
46. Chiumello D, Langer T, Vecchi V, Luoni S, Colombo A, Brioni M, Froio S, Cigada I, Coppola S, Protti A, Lazzerini M, Gattinoni L (2014) Low-dose chest computed tomography for quantitative and visual anatomical analysis in patients with acute respiratory distress syndrome. Intensive Care Med 40:691–699
47. Pearce MS, Salotti JA, Little MP, McHugh K, Lee C, Kim KP, Howe NL, Ronckers CM, Rajaraman P, Sir Craft AW, Paker L, Berrington de Gonzalez A (2012) Radiation exposure from CT scans in childhood and subsequent risk of leukaemia and brain tumours: a retrospective cohort study. Lancet 380:499–505

48. Sodickson A, Baeyens PF, Andriole KP, Prevedello LM, Nawfel RD, Hanson R, Kjorasani R (2009) Recurrent CT, cumulative radiation exposure, and associated radiation-induced cancer risks from CT of adults. Radiology 251:175–184
49. Rohner DJ, Bennett S, Samaratunga C, Jewell ES, Smith JP, Gaskill-Shipley M, Lisco SJ (2013) Cumulative total effective whole-body radiation dose in critically ill patients. Chest 144:1481–1486
50. Cardis E, Vrijheid M, Blettner M (2007) The 15-Country Collaborative Study of Cancer Risk among Radiation Workers in the Nuclear Industry: estimates of radiation-related cancer risks. Radiat Res 167:396–416
51. Shah DJ, Sachs RK, Wilson DJ (2012) Radiation-induced cancer: a modern view. Br J Radiol 85:e1166–e1173
52. Naidich DP, Marshall CH, Gribbin C, Arams RS, McCauley DI (1990) Low- dose CT of the lungs: preliminary observations. Radiology 175:729–731
53. Rhodes CG, Wollmer P, Fazio F, Jones T (1981) Quantitative measurement of regional extravascular lung density using positron emission and transmission tomography. J Comput Assist Tomogr 5:783–791
54. Chen DL, Schstes DP (2004) Positron emission tomography with [18F]fluorodeoxyglucose to evaluate neutrophil kinetics during acute lung injury. Am J Phys Lung Cell Mol Phys 286:L834–L840
55. Sandiford P, Province MA, Schuster DP (1995) Distribution of regional density and vasculare permeability in the adult respiratory distress syndrome. Am J Respir Crit Care Med 151:737–742
56. Fanara B, Manzon C, Barbot O, Desmettre T, Capellier G (2010) Recommendations for the intra-hospital transport of critically ill patients. Crit Care 14:R87
57. Beckmann U, Gillies DM, Berenholtz SM, Wu AW, Pronovost P (2004) Incidents relating to the intra-hospital transfer of critically ill patients. An analysis of the reports submitted to the Australian Incident Monitoring Study in Intensive Care. Intensive Care Med 30(8):1579–1585
58. http://www.ics.ac.uk Intensive Care Society: "Transfer medicine" in "Guidelines for the provision of intensive care services 2015"
59. http://www.ics.ac.uk 2011 Intensive Care Society: "Guidelines for the transport of the critically ill adult"
60. Aliaga M, Forel JM, de Bourmont S, Jung B, Thomas G, Mahul M, Bisbal M, Nougaret S, Hraiech S, Roch A, Chamuoitre K, Jaber S, Gainnier M, Papzian L (2015) Diagnostic yield and safety of CT scan in ICU. Intensive Care Med 41:436–443

Acute Respiratory Distress Syndrome: Metabolic Support

11

Michele Umbrello, Danilo Radrizzani,
and Gaetano Iapichino

11.1 Stress Response and Critically Ill Patients' Metabolic Requirements

Nutritional support to ARDS patients either shares metabolic concepts common to critically ill patients or generates particular concern due to the limitation of oxygen supply and the difficulties of carbon dioxide disposal. Metabolic response to injury and sepsis is characterized by the increased secretion of pro-inflammatory cytokines (IL-1, IL-6, and TNF) [1], catabolic hormones (cortisol, glucagon, and catecholamines) [2], as well as increased insulin resistance [3]. All these lead to glycogenolysis, increased gluconeogenesis and lipolysis, and enhanced muscle protein breakdown ensuring both energy and amino acids for wound repair and immune function.

Particularly, glucose is an indispensable substrate for host response in damaged tissues and immune cells. Endogenous glucose production from amino acids, lactate, and glycerol is necessary because glycogen stores are limited. Lipolysis is also necessary because of the energy required by gluconeogenesis. In fact this

M. Umbrello
Unità Operativa di Anestesia e Rianimazione, Ospedaliera San Paolo-Polo Universitario, ASST Santi Paolo e Carlo, Milan, Italy
e-mail: michele.umbrello@asst-santipaolocarlo.it

D. Radrizzani
Unità Operativa di Anestesia e Rianimazione, Ospedale Nuovo di Legnano, ASST Ovest Milanese, Legnano, Italy
e-mail: danilo.radrizzani@ao-legnano.it

G. Iapichino (✉)
Unità Operativa di Anestesia e Rianimazione, Ospedaliera San Paolo-Polo Universitario, ASST Santi Paolo e Carlo, Milan, Italy

Dipartimento di Fisiopatologia Medico-Chirurgica e dei Trapianti, Università degli Studi di Milano, Milan, Italy

D. Chiumello (ed.), *Acute Respiratory Distress Syndrome (ARDS)*,
DOI 10.1007/978-3-319-41852-0_11

cycling of substrates costs in terms of ATP and is responsible in part of the increased energy expenditure. Amino acid from muscle protein is in part converted to glutamine and alanine and then to glucose and urea. This is mainly the fate of branched chain amino acids. Despite the increased protein synthesis of acute phase protein, the dissimilarity of different amino acids' catabolism explains the large amount of wasted muscle tissue (500–1000 g per day) [4].

The stress response can only be reversed by resolution of the triggering event as infection control, wound healing, and so on. However, the rate of muscle tissue loss can be reduced by an adequate amount of energy and protein intake. This is important because body wasting impacts on tissue functions and hence on the recovery that can be delayed or even prevented by the loss of functional tissue.

For this reasons, metabolic support would comprise energy and protein/amino acids. Substrates can be administered either parenterally or by the enteral route. Parenteral nutrition can be given via the central or peripheral vein according to the osmolality; enteral tract can be accessed at the gastric or jejunal level either by nasal tubes or ostomies. Jejunal approach is preferred when the stomach fails to empty adequately. The relationship of gastric residual volume and diet tolerance is not completely understood; however, gastric residuals up to 500 mL can be tolerated, providing that in the end, the diet progresses to the jejunum [5]. Ostomies are indicated for long-term support.

Enteral nutrition is preferred because it maintains the absorptive function and the integrity of the intestinal barrier and leads to fewer complications, and also because it costs much less than parenteral nutrition. Enteral nutrition can be contraindicated (complete intestinal obstruction) or problematic (severe inflammation, high-output fistula) and sometimes is difficult to cover all the nutritional needs with the enteral administration. In these cases, it is necessary to substitute or integrate the enteral diet with parenteral nutrition in order to fulfill the requirements. The timing and the amount of this substitution/integration is a matter of debate [6, 7]; what is certain is that sooner or later, protein and energy deficits have negative effects on prognosis and that the negative effects are in some way proportional to the severity of the patient [8–10].

If some is good, more is not always better, and even if lack of energy and protein has negative effect, an excess of diet can be dangerous as well, both because of diet-induced thermogenesis (DIT) that furtherly increases energy expenditure and because excess substrates have to be stored or disposed giving way to waste product that can challenge organ functions of critically ill patients. For ARDS patients, energy excess can be particularly difficult to manage as will be explained ahead.

In the absence of the measurement of energy expenditure by indirect calorimetry, current guidelines suggest 20–30 kcal/kg/day [11–13]. The recommended protein/amino acid intake has increased in the last years up to 2 g/kg/day [14]. When nutritional support is administered enterally, the diet composition is predetermined. A standard diet is characterized by a ratio of 50:30:20 that represents the proportion of carbohydrates (CHO), fats, and protein in calories. Diets may differ for concentration (hypo- or hypercaloric) or composition. Differences in composition can depend upon relative quantity (high protein or fat) with respect to standard diet or upon quality of nutrients. Proteins' quality regards the source (casein, whey protein, soy, egg) and the degree of hydrolysis (from whole protein to single amino acid passing through oligopeptides). Lipid quality is represented by the length of chain and by the content of polyunsaturated fatty acid with double bond on carbon w3 or w6. CHO generally consist of maltodextrins, and their content varies to allow the variation of protein or lipid content.

The differences for parenteral nutrition are more or less the same; however, protein content consists of synthetic amino acids and, allowing chemical stability, can be varied in many ways. Lipid content can be really different comprising w9 polyunsaturated fatty acid. CHO are represented by glucose that as we have seen before is an indispensable substrate in critical illness.

Apart from the concentration that allows different water loads, detailed description of the indication of different diets is beyond the purpose of this chapter; however, any difference in composition of interest for ARDS patients will be discussed later.

Whichever the source of CHO, they are mainly metabolized to glucose that is the primary source of easily available energy for all tissues. However, stress hyperglycemia may have deleterious effect on outcome. For this reason, glycemic control, after many years of conflicting studies, stands yet as a significant target in critically ill patients. The key questions are the appropriate target ranges in different patients' population and the way to obtain it; both these goals should satisfy safety and feasibility. Glucose control is obtained by standardized i.v. insulin infusion. Protocols can either consist of intuitive rules or they can be paper-based or computerized algorithms; however, they generally do not take into account factors such as the degree of patient stress, i.e., insulin sensitivity, and the amount of nutritional support. Recently, a pathophysiology-based glucose control protocol which takes into account patient CHO load intake and patient insulin resistance has been proposed [15]. Computerization allows increasing complexity of the decisional tree, while diminishing the work effort; moreover, it performs better in terms of glucose control either as time in target or preventing hypoglycemia [16]. The more complex computer programs are able to react to or to anticipate glucose changes; future development in this field will probably be a closed-loop insulin infusion sustained by continuous glucose monitoring.

Critically ill patients receiving nutritional support may develop depletion of vitamins or trace elements; in some cases they can be already depleted. Usually, an adequate intake of calorie by the enteral route ensues the needs of microelements and vitamins; in case of inadequate intake or of parenteral support, trace elements and vitamins have to be supplemented.

Pharmakonutrition (i.e., nutritional support enriched with anti-inflammatory or immunomodulating substrates) is supported by many biochemical studies. It includes w3 polyunsaturated fatty acids, glutamine, arginine, and antioxidants. Larger clinical studies have demonstrated deleterious effect particularly of the amino acids glutamine and arginine as well as of antioxidants [17, 18]. These results have to be interpreted cautiously because of excessive dosage or due to different actions in different patient population (e.g., trauma vs septic shock patients). Particular effect of pharmakonutrients on ARDS patients will be discussed ahead.

11.2 Consequences of Acute Respiratory Failure on Patients' Stress Reaction

ARDS is a heterogeneous syndrome of acute onset of respiratory insufficiency, characterized by increased pulmonary permeability and subsequent pulmonary edema. Patients with ARDS typically have altered lung and respiratory system elastance and an increased shunt fraction and dead space; as a result, gas exchange is severely impaired, with refractory hypoxemia and hypercapnia [19]. The cause underlying the development of ARDS is generally infectious (pneumonia, sepsis with secondary development of pulmonary lesions), or infections can arise as a complication of the first diagnosis (trauma, pancreatitis, visceral sepsis).

From a metabolic point of view, ARDS is characterized by a pro-inflammatory response associated with hypercatabolism that could lead to significant nutritional deficits [20], which can modify respiratory muscle function, ventilatory drive, and lung defense mechanisms [21–23].

In these critically ill patients, elevated resting energy expenditure (REE), reaching up to 126% of that predicted by their body size, means increased oxygen consumption (VO_2) and carbon dioxide production (VCO_2), i.e., increased cardiac work and increased respiratory exchange demand, in spite of impaired lung and sometimes cardiac function.

11.3 Characteristic Features of Artificial Nutrition in Acute Respiratory Failure

Similar to other critically ill patients, some days of starving or hypoalimentation lead to caloric deficit; this is even more relevant in ARDS. Nutrition support is then necessary to prevent cumulative caloric deficits, malnutrition, loss of lean body mass, and deterioration of respiratory muscle strength [13, 24–26].

Several aspects of energy consumption physiology and of substrate supply, disposal and transformation, oxidation, or storage, generally not considered in the absence of respiratory failure, may have a relevant impact and have to be carefully taken into account when feeding critically ill patients with severe respiratory failure.

The human body extracts the energy that is needed to comply to processes requiring mechanical (muscular contraction), chemical (biosynthesis), and osmotic (active transport) work by oxidizing a mixture of CHO, lipids, and protein to produce carbon dioxide (CO_2), water, and nitrogen. Part of the energy packed in substrates is in fact utilized to generate adenosine triphosphate (ATP), while the remainder is converted to heat used to maintain body temperature. The energy ingested in excess to the expenditure is inevitably stored [27, 28]. As only small amounts of energy can be derived by phosphorylation at substrate level (glycolysis), energy is mainly released from substrate oxidation, so that VO_2 and REE are closely correlated.

11.3.1 Physiologic Effects of Substrate Metabolism

11.3.1.1 The Determinants of Energy Consumption

For a wider review of the present topic, see the paper by Iapichino et al. [27, 28].

The complete oxidation of one mole of CHO, lipids, or proteins requires very different amount of O_2 (134, 515, 114 L, respectively), so that to obtain 1 kcal oxidizing CHO, lipids, and proteins, we need 200, 212, and 239 mL of O_2, respectively. It means that cardiac work, demanded for oxygen supply, is greater burning lipids and minimal burning CHO. By contrast, 1 kcal from CHO produces 200 mL of CO_2, less from lipids (157 mL) and proteins (191 mL). It means that the respiratory work is minimal for lipids.

Moreover, each mole of produced ATP costs 3.7 L O_2 for CHO, 3.9 L O_2 for lipids, and 5 L O_2 for protein. Then, the ATP yield per liter of O_2 is maximal oxidizing CHO. Therefore, the most efficient way to use the available oxygen is burning CHO, while the most efficient way to reduce VCO_2 is lipid oxidation.

However, the energy released per gram of substrate oxidized is also different: 4.18 kcal/g for mixed CHO (3.72 kcal/g glucose, 4.31 kcal/g for glycerol); 9.44 kcal/g for mixed lipids (8.34 kcal/g for medium chain triglycerides (MCT)); 4.69 and 3.48 kcal/g for β-hydroxybutyric and acetoacetic acid, respectively [29]; and 4.7 kcal/g for protein oxidation.

11.3.1.2 Diet-Induced Termogenesis (DIT)

DIT refers to the amount of energy required to absorb, process and store nutrients and accounts for an increase in energy expenditure (EE) with respect to postabsorptive state [30]. Moreover, DIT depends upon the amount of substrate supply and disposal, and it is different among the different substrates. Jequier [30] investigated the thermic effect of nutrients. The authors found that when given intravenously, glucose (under euglycemic-hyperinsulinemic glucose clamp condition) induces an increase of EE of 7% of energy infused, whereas lipid infusion stimulates EE by 3% of energy infused. The stimulation of EE due to amino acid infusion in depleted patients is 30–40% of the energy infused as amino acids. The cost of nutrient storage for glucose was 12% of the energy content of the stored nutrient, while it was found to be 4% for lipids [30]. Eventually, as far as lipids are concerned, it has to be taken into account that the cost for the oxidation/storage of MCT is significantly higher when compared to palmitate [31], as the former need first to be elongated and then they can be oxidated.

11.3.1.3 Disposal, Transformation, and Storage of Nutrients

When CHO availability is increased by exogenous supply, endogenous and exogenous glucose have theoretically the same oxidation chances, i.e., in the presence of a total body glucose consisting of 50% infusion and 50% production, the net amount of the oxidized glucose (indirect calorimetry) will be constituted in equal parts by the two glucose pools. Only when hepatic glucose production is totally suppressed, the energy drawn by CHO totally comes from exogenous source.

Regarding fat oxidation, the nonprotein respiratory quotient (RQnp) does not indicate the source of the lipid that is oxidized (fat stores vs fat from diet). It is known that glucose availability reduces lipid oxidation. However, it is not sure whether the increased exogenous fat availability could result in a decrease of endo- or exogenous glucose oxidation. A further very interesting physiological aspect of fat disposal is whether the exogenous fat can supply an immediate energy need and, if any, the proportion between immediate oxidation and storage of an exogenous load.

The result is that the amount of oxidized exogenous substrates of either long-chain triglycerides (MCTs are a different story) or glucose (when hepatic neoglucogenesis is not suppressed) is less than that indicated by RQnp. The meaning is that to accomplish with REE, a part of exogenous substrates, equal or less than the need, are stored, and necessarily the oxidation of endogenous substrates continues even in feed state.

11.3.2 Resting Energy Expenditure

Despite the many predictive equations that have been proposed to estimate energy expenditure, their use fails to match the measured expenditure in >75% of patients [32, 33], and it tends to overestimate the needs [34]. Many factors are responsible for these errors in critically ill patients, and the use of predictive equation possibly leads to overnutrition and to its deleterious effects. The issue is relevant, as several studies reported an association between the amount of calories prescribed and a positive clinical outcome [8–10, 35, 36], as well as between protein intake and survival [37–40].

Nevertheless, measurement of energy expenditure is feasible using indirect calorimetry, a technique which relies on the principle that the amount of substrates involved in oxidative processes can be calculated on the basis of VO_2, VCO_2, and nitrogen excretion [27]. As matter of fact, energy production for a given time (i.e., REE) can be easily calculated by the simplified Weir equation [41]:

$$REE(\text{kcal}) = 3.9 * l\, O_2\text{consumed} + 1.1 * l\, CO_2\text{produced}$$

The correction due to protein catabolism is negligible (about 2.2 kcal for each g of excreted nitrogen) accounting for less than 1 kcal/kg/day in severely catabolic patients.

When patients are mechanically ventilated with $FiO_2 > 0.5$ or in ECMO, having measured cardiac output, and assuming a median RQnp of 0.94, $VO_2 \times 7$ yields the amount of kcal/24 h. Otherwise, measuring CO_2 production rate, and assuming a RQnp of 0.94, the formula gives kcal/24 h.

The lack of precision in the measurement of oxygen concentration above 60% [42] represents the main technical restriction to the use of this technique. Unsteady state is another limitation because of different transit time of oxygen and carbon dioxide. Further restrictions arise when the rates of gluconeogenesis or ketogenesis are elevated or net lipogenesis occurs; in these cases disappearance and oxidation of substrates follow different pathways [43]. Despite these restrictions, due to technical limits and basic assumption, indirect calorimetry is a sound method to estimate EE for the metabolic treatment of critically ill patients [28].

In summary, one should always keep in mind that the calculations adopted to estimate energy expenditure are far from being unbiased and precise independently from the complexity of the equations. To avoid any illusion of unrealistic accuracy, we suggest adopting the ESPEN guideline recommendation of 20–25 kcal/kg/day [11] that does not seem to differ in precision and, possibly, do better than more complex equations for patients' outcome [44, 45].

11.3.3 Possible Adverse Effects of Single Macronutrient on the Lung Tissue of Patients with ARDS

11.3.3.1 Carbohydrates and Lipids

High levels of intravenous CHO in TPN nutritional support increase body temperature [46], respiratory quotient, and VCO2, which in turn increase ventilatory demand, as seen in a small uncontrolled study [47] and in a small RCT [48]. It is nowadays becoming clearer that these effects are due to hyperalimentation, i.e., an excessive calorie load compared to metabolic needs (see later 11.4).

However, a prevalent CHO enteral feeding was associated with improved clinical outcomes [49] and with better muscle protein accretion compared with an isonitrogenous isocaloric high-fat feeding [50]. Then carbohydrates appear to be the preferential substrate in critical illness [51], because of a poor utilization of fat secondary to an impaired oxidation and inefficient transport between pools [52, 53].

Indeed, in healthy people, high-fat diets have been related to potential development of endotoxemia by causing changes to gastrointestinal barrier function or microbiota composition [54]. Hence, being patients with ARDS especially exposed to infectious complications, these considerations would argue against the use of high-fat diet in this population of patients.

Fatty acid chains differ by length, often categorized from short to long. Polyunsaturated fatty acids contain more than one double bond; depending on the location of the first double bond, they can be classified into w3, w6, or w9. Their relevance depends on their specific biological activity. More in details, long-chain w6 fatty acids (such as linoleic acid, LA, and gamma-linolenic acid, GLA) have been associated with pro-inflammatory phenotypes particularly dangerous in critically ill patients [55, 56]. Their supply also resulted in increased synthesis of vasodilating prostaglandins [57]; moreover, they can interfere with lung hemodynamics and with the V/Q regulation, which in turn may lead to worsened gas exchange due to resolution of hypoxic vasoconstriction in hypoventilated areas of a damaged lung [58, 59].

It has been reported that fatty acids from the w3 family (eicosapentaenoic, EPA, and docosahexaenoic acid, DHA), unlike w6, can modulate inflammatory processes [56]. Their use was associated with reduced availability of arachidonic acid, with a consequent shift in the production of cytokines from the highly pro-inflammatory four-series leukotrienes and dienoic prostaglandins to the less inflammatory five-series leukotrienes and trienoic prostaglandins [60]. Experimental w3 fatty acid supplementation was also associated with a restored permeability of injured alveolar-capillary membrane and with lower levels of tissue inflammation and apoptosis [61].

As for MCT, their higher DIT when compared to long-chain fats has already been mentioned, while we lack evidence as for any potential negative effect of w9 polyunsaturated fatty acids.

11.3.3.2 Proteins

Protein administration increases minute ventilation more than expected for the increase in REE, suggesting a specific activity on ventilatory drive [62] that has to be taken into account when dealing with a patient with limited possibilities to increase work of breathing. In case of development of severe sepsis, particular attention has to be given to the risks of an enhanced supply of arginine, due to its pro-inflammatory characteristics [18].

11.4 Peculiar Characteristics of Metabolic Control of Critically Ill Patients with ARDS

The goal of nutritional support remains to provide sufficient amount of calories to satisfy both the basal metabolic rate and the demands for the synthesis of protein to maintain lean body mass. National and international guidelines suggest administration of nutritional support to all patients suffering from ARDS and undergoing mechanical ventilation [11, 13]. An observational trial [37] and three RCTs [63–65] in critically ill mechanically ventilated patients tested the effect of energy prescription based on indirect calorimetry, and all reported clinical benefits.

However, all the abovementioned limitation needs to be considered when dealing with nutritional support in an ARDS scenario. As a result, adequate metabolic support of this category of patients is challenging. A first strategy is the reduction of REE that can be achieved in different ways.

At first, the reduction in the amount of physical activity (including the work of breathing), the control of body temperature, and the use of sedation are essential strategies.

Secondly, a daily amount of energy intake (EI) greater than needed need to be carefully avoided, as the impact of substrate disposal on REE (DIT increase) is certainly dangerous [27, 28, 66–68]. When circulatory function is suboptimal, this results in difficult heat dispersion, with hyperthermia [69], and in an increased ventilator and cardiocirculatory demand [22, 70]. Of interest, the increase in caloric provision per se, rather than excessive carbohydrate substrate, correlated more closely with VCO_2 [71]. Then, the recommended daily supply is 25 kcal/kg; however, when gas exchange is severely impaired, calorie load can be reduced to 20 kcal/kg, at least for the first phase of illness. In this scenario, be particularly aware of the likely development of an energy-protein deficit.

Third, the use of continuous feeding is protective. In fact, DIT is minimal during enteral feeding, both in health and disease [72, 73], provided that energy supply is less than 1–1.3 times the REE, while it increases to up to 20% of total EE when energy supply approaches two times the REE. This was interpreted as a lower energy cost of digestion and absorption of nutrients in comparison with the cost of nutrient storage. Indeed, oral administration of nutrients (i.e., as a bolus) induces a larger thermogenic response than continuous enteral administration [72, 73], due to the necessity of storing the ingested substrate until their utilization. During critical illness, moreover, VO_2 and VCO_2, and consequently DIT, are effectively blunted even with continuous TPN, provided that EI = REE [74].

Fourth, the composition of macronutrients can be altered. This can help minimize the requirements for mechanical ventilation, taking the pharmacological effect of nutrients into account and the possibility to manipulate DIT and VO_2/VCO_2. Indeed, macronutrient composition is much less likely to affect CO_2 production when the design of the nutrition support regimen approximates energy requirements [13, 67, 68, 71]. Then, the traditional suggestion that up to 50% of the nonprotein portion of caloric intake consists of lipid, to be able to limit VCO_2 and minute ventilation, should be abandoned. Instead, a more physiological composition (60% CHO/40% lipids) should be delivered, to allow the anabolic effects of insulin to take place. The use of EN formula can generally solve this problem, while careful attention should be paid to the nonprotein composition of the standardized commercially available PN formulas.

This said, a relevant issue is that of the type of lipids provided with artificial nutrition. Intravenous administration of high amounts of the w6 linoleic acid, even at slow rates of infusion, appears to be undesirable in patients with severe pulmonary failure [13, 75, 76], due to the pro-inflammatory effects and the interference with hypoxic pulmonary vasoconstriction.

To reduce this problem, several studies in patients with ARDS have shown that the use of w3 fatty acids, specifically EPA and GLA, possibly coupled with antioxidants, may confer biochemical and clinical advantage in ARDS by preventing oxidative cellular injury, modifying the metabolic stress response, and modulating immunity and inflammation [76–84]. Other authors [85, 86] and a recent meta-analysis [87] found that such an immunomodulatory diet did not show any significant reduction in the risk of all-cause mortality in ARDS patients, nor it increased the ventilator- and ICU-free days.

Actually, many of these studies have significant heterogeneity, and the majority share biases on the study design: the comparator diet provided in the control group often supplies a relatively high amount of w6 fatty acids, rather than the usual amount provided with commonly used balanced formulas, or they provide different amount of proteins among groups. As a consequence, the more-recently published guidelines on nutrition support [13] do not recommend the use of any enteral formula with an anti-inflammatory lipid profile and antioxidants in ARDS patients. Instead, the recommended strategy is the provision of an enteral/parenteral formula in which the w6 content is balanced by the presence of w3 and w9 long-chain fatty acids.

However, this strategy can often be vanished by the often underlooked issue of the energy contained in (w6) lipids used for sedation (i.e., propofol), which may represent up to 15% of the total energy administered and may lead to a profound unbalance in the composition of the diet [88]. The use of high-concentrated emulsion coupled with sedation strategies that use other compounds, such as enteral drugs [89], may give the advantage of reducing/eliminating this issue.

However, the sometimes necessary EI reduction during EN may result in a "caloric shortfall" and, even more dangerously, in a *protein shortfall* [37–40]. Bearing in mind that protein retention can improve by increasing either protein (main determinant) or even energy intake [90], if kidney function is normal, the protein shortfall can be limited by the use of a protein-strengthened enteral formula, yielding a supply of at least 0.8–1 g/kg. Still, under these circumstances, the early provision of adequate nutritional support is deeply relevant, so as to limit the unavoidable energy deficit. The role of enteral/parenteral glutamine supplementation is highly controversial [13], and in case of caloric shortfall, it should not be used at the expense of an optimal amount of proteins.

Fluid accumulation is a common and relevant issue in patients with ARDS. Restrictive fluid management can improve lung function and shorten the duration of mechanical ventilation and intensive care stay [91], so that water intake due to nutritional support has to be carefully considered. Fluid restriction is easier with PN solutions due to the calorie density of glucose (up to 2.8 kcal/mL) and lipids (up to 3 kcal/mL), but is feasible also with energy-dense enteral formulas (up to 2 kcal/mL). To adequately monitor the fluid status, daily and cumulative water and sodium balance and their relationship had to be monitored.

Conclusions

In summary, we suggest that nutritional support to patients with ARDS is provided early once patients are fluid resuscitated and hemodynamically stable (even if under vasoactive), and blood gas is acceptable.

Energy given in amounts equal to REE (possibly measured by indirect calorimetry) or not >25 kcal/kg with a balanced formula possibly coupled with insulin should be delivered. Indeed, if the kidney is normally functioning, an adequate (1–1.5 g/kg ideal body weight) amount of protein should be delivered, even if its cost in terms of VO_2/VCO_2 is significant.

This approach is not able to completely inhibit the utilization of endogenous stores and does not possess the same protein sparing action of diets with greater energy content; however, it significantly reduces the wasting of substrates as compared to starving condition, and it does not cause any dangerous increase in the cardiorespiratory demand. Such a strategy, mainly provided by continuous enteral mode, has successfully been employed even in the most severe ARDS patients under extracorporeal assistance for more than 30 years at our institution [92] and was recently confirmed as valid and feasible [93].

References

1. Armstrong L, Millar AB (1997) Relative production of tumour necrosis factor alpha and interleukin 10 in adult respiratory distress syndrome. Thorax 52(5):442–446
2. Nandi J, Meguid MM, Inui A, Xu Y, Makarenko IG, Tada T, Chen C (2002) Central mechanisms involved with catabolism. Curr Opin Clin Nutr Metab Care 5(4):407–418
3. Dungan KM, Braithwaite SS, Preiser JC (2009) Stress hyperglycaemia. Lancet 373(9677):1798–1807. doi:10.1016/S0140-6736(09)60553-5
4. Monk DN, Plank LD, Franch-Arcas G, Finn PJ, Streat SJ, Hill GL (1996) Sequential changes in the metabolic response in critically injured patients during the first 25 days after blunt trauma. Ann Surg 223(4):395–405
5. Montejo JC, Minambres E, Bordeje L, Mesejo A, Acosta J, Heras A, Ferre M, Fernandez-Ortega F, Vaquerizo CI, Manzanedo R (2010) Gastric residual volume during enteral nutrition in ICU patients: the REGANE study. Intensive Care Med 36(8):1386–1393. doi:10.1007/s00134-010-1856-y
6. Singer P, Pichard C (2013) Reconciling divergent results of the latest parenteral nutrition studies in the ICU. Curr Opin Clin Nutr Metab Care 16(2):187–193. doi:10.1097/MCO.0b013e32835c34be
7. Berger MM, Pichard C (2014) Development and current use of parenteral nutrition in critical care – an opinion paper. Crit Care 18(4):478. doi:10.1186/s13054-014-0478-0
8. Villet S, Chiolero RL, Bollmann MD, Revelly JP, Cayeux RNM, Delarue J, Berger MM (2005) Negative impact of hypocaloric feeding and energy balance on clinical outcome in ICU patients. Clin Nutr 24(4):502–509. doi:10.1016/j.clnu.2005.03.006
9. Dvir D, Cohen J, Singer P (2006) Computerized energy balance and complications in critically ill patients: an observational study. Clin Nutr 25(1):37–44. doi:10.1016/j.clnu.2005.10.010
10. Alberda C, Gramlich L, Jones N, Jeejeebhoy K, Day AG, Dhaliwal R, Heyland DK (2009) The relationship between nutritional intake and clinical outcomes in critically ill patients: results of an international multicenter observational study. Intensive Care Med 35(10):1728–1737. doi:10.1007/s00134-009-1567-4
11. Kreymann KG, Berger MM, Deutz NE, Hiesmayr M, Jolliet P, Kazandjiev G, Nitenberg G, van den Berghe G, Wernerman J, Ebner C, Hartl W, Heymann C, Spies C (2006) ESPEN guidelines on enteral nutrition: intensive care. Clin Nutr 25(2):210–223. doi:10.1016/j.clnu.2006.01.021
12. Singer P, Berger MM, Van den Berghe G, Biolo G, Calder P, Forbes A, Griffiths R, Kreyman G, Leverve X, Pichard C, ESPEN (2009) ESPEN guidelines on parenteral nutrition: intensive care. Clin Nutr 28(4):387–400. doi:10.1016/j.clnu.2009.04.024
13. Taylor BE, McClave SA, Martindale RG, Warren MM, Johnson DR, Braunschweig C, McCarthy MS, Davanos E, Rice TW, Cresci GA, Gervasio JM, Sacks GS, Roberts PR, Compher C (2016) Guidelines for the provision and assessment of nutrition support therapy in the adult critically ill patient: Society of Critical Care Medicine (SCCM) and American Society for Parenteral and Enteral Nutrition (A.S.P.E.N.). Crit Care Med 44(2):390–438. doi:10.1097/CCM.0000000000001525
14. Hoffer LJ, Bistrian BR (2013) Why critically ill patients are protein deprived. JPEN J Parenter Enteral Nutr 37(3):300–309. doi:10.1177/0148607113478192
15. Umbrello M, Salice V, Spanu P, Formenti P, Barassi A, Melzi d'Eril GV, Iapichino G (2014) Performance assessment of a glucose control protocol in septic patients with an automated

intermittent plasma glucose monitoring device. Clin Nutr 33(5):867–871. doi:10.1016/j.clnu.2013.10.007

16. Eslami S, Abu-Hanna A, de Jonge E, de Keizer NF (2009) Tight glycemic control and computerized decision-support systems: a systematic review. Intensive Care Med 35(9):1505–1517. doi:10.1007/s00134-009-1542-0
17. Heyland D, Muscedere J, Wischmeyer PE, Cook D, Jones G, Albert M, Elke G, Berger MM, Day AG (2013) A randomized trial of glutamine and antioxidants in critically ill patients. N Engl J Med 368(16):1489–1497. doi:10.1056/NEJMoa1212722
18. Bertolini G, Iapichino G, Radrizzani D, Facchini R, Simini B, Bruzzone P, Zanforlin G, Tognoni G (2003) Early enteral immunonutrition in patients with severe sepsis: results of an interim analysis of a randomized multicentre clinical trial. Intensive Care Med 29(5):834–840. doi:10.1007/s00134-003-1711-5
19. Ranieri VM, Rubenfeld GD, Thompson BT, Ferguson ND, Caldwell E, Fan E, Camporota L, Slutsky AS (2012) Acute respiratory distress syndrome: the Berlin Definition. JAMA 307(23):2526–2533. doi:10.1001/jama.2012.5669
20. Krzak A, Pleva M, Napolitano LM (2011) Nutrition therapy for ALI and ARDS. Crit Care Clin 27(3):647–659. doi:10.1016/j.ccc.2011.05.004
21. Aubier M, Murciano D, Lecocguic Y, Viires N, Jacquens Y, Squara P, Pariente R (1985) Effect of hypophosphatemia on diaphragmatic contractility in patients with acute respiratory failure. N Engl J Med 313(7):420–424. doi:10.1056/NEJM198508153130705
22. Askanazi J, Weissman C, Rosenbaum SH, Hyman AI, Milic-Emili J, Kinney JM (1982) Nutrition and the respiratory system. Crit Care Med 10(3):163–172
23. Pingleton SK, Harmon GS (1987) Nutritional management in acute respiratory failure. JAMA 257(22):3094–3099
24. Wilson DO, Rogers RM, Sanders MH, Pennock BE, Reilly JJ (1986) Nutritional intervention in malnourished patients with emphysema. Am Rev Respir Dis 134(4):672–677. doi:10.1164/arrd.1986.134.4.672
25. Fraser IM (1986) Effects of refeeding on respiration and skeletal muscle function. Clin Chest Med 7(1):131–139
26. McClave SA (1997) The consequences of overfeeding and underfeeding. J Resp Care Pract 10:57–58
27. Iapichino G, Radrizzani D, Armani S, Noto A, Spanu P, Mistraletti G (2006) Metabolic treatment of critically ill patients: energy balance and substrate disposal. Minerva Anestesiol 72(6):533–541
28. Iapichino G, Radrizzani D, Giacomini M, Pezzi A, Zaniboni M, Mistraletti G (2006) Metabolic treatment of critically ill patients: energy expenditure and energy supply. Minerva Anestesiol 72(6):559–565
29. Cahill GF Jr (2006) Fuel metabolism in starvation. Annu Rev Nutr 26:1–22. doi:10.1146/annurev.nutr.26.061505.111258
30. Jequier E (1986) The influence of nutrient administration on energy expenditure in man. Clin Nutr 5(4):181–186
31. Chassard D, Guiraud M, Gauthier J, Gelas P, Berrada KR, Bouletreau P (1994) Effects of intravenous medium-chain triglycerides on pulmonary gas exchanges in mechanically ventilated patients. Crit Care Med 22(2):248–251
32. Fraipont V, Preiser JC (2013) Energy estimation and measurement in critically ill patients. JPEN J Parenter Enteral Nutr 37(6):705–713. doi:10.1177/0148607113505868
33. McClave SA, Lowen CC, Kleber MJ, Nicholson JF, Jimmerson SC, McConnell JW, Jung LY (1998) Are patients fed appropriately according to their caloric requirements? JPEN J Parenter Enteral Nutr 22(6):375–381
34. De Waele E, Opsomer T, Honore PM, Diltoer M, Mattens S, Huyghens L, Spapen H (2015) Measured versus calculated resting energy expenditure in critically ill adult patients. Do mathematics match the gold standard? Minerva Anestesiol 81(3):272–282

35. Wei X, Day AG, Ouellette-Kuntz H, Heyland DK (2015) The association between nutritional adequacy and long-term outcomes in critically ill patients requiring prolonged mechanical ventilation: a Multicenter Cohort Study. Crit Care Med 43(8):1569–1579. doi:10.1097/CCM.0000000000001000
36. Heyland DK, Cahill N, Day AG (2011) Optimal amount of calories for critically ill patients: depends on how you slice the cake! Crit Care Med 39(12):2619–2626. doi:10.1097/CCM.0b013e318226641d
37. Weijs PJ, Stapel SN, de Groot SD, Driessen RH, de Jong E, Girbes AR, Strack van Schijndel RJ, Beishuizen A (2012) Optimal protein and energy nutrition decreases mortality in mechanically ventilated, critically ill patients: a prospective observational cohort study. JPEN J Parenter Enteral Nutr 36(1):60–68. doi:10.1177/0148607111415109
38. Allingstrup MJ, Esmailzadeh N, Wilkens Knudsen A, Espersen K, Hartvig Jensen T, Wiis J, Perner A, Kondrup J (2012) Provision of protein and energy in relation to measured requirements in intensive care patients. Clin Nutr 31(4):462–468. doi:10.1016/j.clnu.2011.12.006
39. Hoffer LJ, Bistrian BR (2015) Energy deficit is clinically relevant for critically ill patients: no. Intensive Care Med 41(2):339–341. doi:10.1007/s00134-014-3518-y
40. Chapple LA, Chapman MJ, Lange K, Deane AM, Heyland DK (2016) Nutrition support practices in critically ill head-injured patients: a global perspective. Crit Care 20(1):6. doi:10.1186/s13054-015-1177-1
41. Weir JB (1949) New methods for calculating metabolic rate with special reference to protein metabolism. J Physiol 109(1–2):1–9
42. Brandi LS, Bertolini R, Calafa M (1997) Indirect calorimetry in critically ill patients: clinical applications and practical advice. Nutrition 13(4):349–358
43. Simonson DC, DeFronzo RA (1990) Indirect calorimetry: methodological and interpretative problems. Am J Physiol 258(3 Pt 1):E399–E412
44. Compher C, Nicolo M, Chittams J, Kang Y, Day AG, Heyland DK (2015) Clinical outcomes in critically ill patients associated with the use of complex vs weight-only predictive energy equations. JPEN J Parenter Enteral Nutr 39(7):864–869. doi:10.1177/0148607114533127
45. Radrizzani D, Iapichino G (2015) Every need is perfectly met if you do not measure it. Minerva Anestesiol 81(3):253–254
46. Askanazi J, Elwyn DH, Silverberg PA, Rosenbaum SH, Kinney JM (1980) Respiratory distress secondary to a high carbohydrate load: a case report. Surgery 87(5):596–598
47. Askanazi J, Nordenstrom J, Rosenbaum SH, Elwyn DH, Hyman AI, Carpentier YA, Kinney JM (1981) Nutrition for the patient with respiratory failure: glucose vs. fat. Anesthesiology 54(5):373–377
48. al-Saady NM, Blackmore CM, Bennett ED (1989) High fat, low carbohydrate, enteral feeding lowers PaCO2 and reduces the period of ventilation in artificially ventilated patients. Intensive Care Med 15(5):290–295
49. Garrel DR, Razi M, Lariviere F, Jobin N, Naman N, Emptoz-Bonneton A, Pugeat MM (1995) Improved clinical status and length of care with low-fat nutrition support in burn patients. JPEN J Parenter Enteral Nutr 19(6):482–491
50. Hart DW, Wolf SE, Zhang XJ, Chinkes DL, Buffalo MC, Matin SI, DebRoy MA, Wolfe RR, Herndon DN (2001) Efficacy of a high-carbohydrate diet in catabolic illness. Crit Care Med 29(7):1318–1324
51. Wolf SE, Shields BA, Wade CE (2009) Substrate utilization in the critically ill. JPEN J Parenter Enteral Nutr 33(1):111; author reply 112. doi:10.1177/0148607108319798
52. Cree MG, Aarsland A, Herndon DN, Wolfe RR (2007) Role of fat metabolism in burn trauma-induced skeletal muscle insulin resistance. Crit Care Med 35(9 Suppl):S476–S483. doi:10.1097/01.CCM.0000278066.05354.53
53. Aarsland A, Chinkes DL, Sakurai Y, Nguyen TT, Herndon DN, Wolfe RR (1998) Insulin therapy in burn patients does not contribute to hepatic triglyceride production. J Clin Invest 101(10):2233–2239. doi:10.1172/JCI200

54. Pendyala G, Want EJ, Webb W, Siuzdak G, Fox HS (2007) Biomarkers for neuroAIDS: the widening scope of metabolomics. J Neuroimmune Pharmacol Off J Soc NeuroImmune Pharmacol 2(1):72–80. doi:10.1007/s11481-006-9041-3
55. Battistella FD, Widergren JT, Anderson JT, Siepler JK, Weber JC, MacColl K (1997) A prospective, randomized trial of intravenous fat emulsion administration in trauma victims requiring total parenteral nutrition. J Trauma 43(1):52–58; discussion 58–60
56. Calder PC (2004) n-3 fatty acids, inflammation, and immunity – relevance to postsurgical and critically ill patients. Lipids 39(12):1147–1161
57. McKeen CR, Brigham KL, Bowers RE, Harris TR (1978) Pulmonary vascular effects of fat emulsion infusion in unanesthetized sheep. Prevention by indomethacin. J Clin Invest 61(5):1291–1297. doi:10.1172/JCI109046
58. Venus B, Smith RA, Patel C, Sandoval E (1989) Hemodynamic and gas exchange alterations during Intralipid infusion in patients with adult respiratory distress syndrome. Chest 95(6):1278–1281
59. Mathru M, Dries DJ, Zecca A, Fareed J, Rooney MW, Rao TL (1991) Effect of fast vs slow intralipid infusion on gas exchange, pulmonary hemodynamics, and prostaglandin metabolism. Chest 99(2):426–429
60. Khan SA, Ali A, Khan SA, Zahran SA, Damanhouri G, Azhar E, Qadri I (2014) Unraveling the complex relationship triad between lipids, obesity, and inflammation. Mediat Inflamm 2014:16. doi:10.1155/2014/502749
61. Cox R Jr, Phillips O, Fukumoto J, Fukumoto I, Parthasarathy PT, Arias S, Cho Y, Lockey RF, Kolliputi N (2015) Enhanced resolution of hyperoxic acute lung injury as a result of aspirin triggered resolvin D1 treatment. Am J Respir Cell Mol Biol 53(3):422–435. doi:10.1165/rcmb.2014-0339OC
62. Takala J, Askanazi J, Weissman C, Lasala PA, Milic-Emili J, Elwyn DH, Kinney JM (1988) Changes in respiratory control induced by amino acid infusions. Crit Care Med 16(5):465–469
63. Heidegger CP, Berger MM, Graf S, Zingg W, Darmon P, Costanza MC, Thibault R, Pichard C (2013) Optimisation of energy provision with supplemental parenteral nutrition in critically ill patients: a randomised controlled clinical trial. Lancet 381(9864):385–393. doi:10.1016/S0140-6736(12)61351-8
64. Singer P, Anbar R, Cohen J, Shapiro H, Shalita-Chesner M, Lev S, Grozovski E, Theilla M, Frishman S, Madar Z (2011) The tight calorie control study (TICACOS): a prospective, randomized, controlled pilot study of nutritional support in critically ill patients. Intensive Care Med 37(4):601–609. doi:10.1007/s00134-011-2146-z
65. Petros S, Horbach M, Seidel F, Weidhase L (2016) Hypocaloric vs normocaloric nutrition in critically ill patients: a prospective randomized pilot trial. JPEN J Parenter Enteral Nutr 40(2):242–249. doi:10.1177/0148607114528980
66. Wolfe RR, O'Donnell TF Jr, Stone MD, Richmand DA, Burke JF (1980) Investigation of factors determining the optimal glucose infusion rate in total parenteral nutrition. Metab Clin Exp 29(9):892–900
67. Radrizzani D, Iapichino G (1998) Nutrition and lung function in the critically ill patient. Clin Nutr 17(1):7–10
68. Iapichino G (1989) Nutrition in respiratory failure. Intensive Care Med 15(8):483–485
69. Askanazi J, Rosenbaum SH, Michelsen CB, Elwyn DH, Hyman AI, Kinney JM (1980) Increased body temperature secondary to total parenteral nutrition. Crit Care Med 8(12):736–737
70. Iapichino G, Gattinoni L, Solca M, Radrizzani D, Zucchetti M, Langer M, Vesconi S (1982) Protein sparing and protein replacement in acutely injured patients during TPN with and without amino acid supply. Intensive Care Med 8(1):25–31
71. Talpers SS, Romberger DJ, Bunce SB, Pingleton SK (1992) Nutritionally associated increased carbon dioxide production. Excess total calories vs high proportion of carbohydrate calories. Chest 102(2):551–555

72. Heymsfield SB, Head CA, McManus CB 3rd, Seitz S, Staton GW, Grossman GD (1984) Respiratory, cardiovascular, and metabolic effects of enteral hyperalimentation: influence of formula dose and composition. Am J Clin Nutr 40(1):116–130
73. Heymsfield SB, Hill JO, Evert M, Casper K, DiGirolamo M (1987) Energy expenditure during continuous intragastric infusion of fuel. Am J Clin Nutr 45(3):526–533
74. Radrizzani D, Iapichino G, Colombo A, Codazzi D, Pasetti G, Ronzoni G, Savioli M (1995) Effect of infusion and withdrawal of glucose and insulin on gas exchange in injured ventilated patients. J Crit Care 10(1):15–20
75. Suchner U, Katz DP, Furst P, Beck K, Felbinger TW, Senftleben U, Thiel M, Goetz AE, Peter K (2001) Effects of intravenous fat emulsions on lung function in patients with acute respiratory distress syndrome or sepsis. Crit Care Med 29(8):1569–1574
76. Pacht ER, DeMichele SJ, Nelson JL, Hart J, Wennberg AK, Gadek JE (2003) Enteral nutrition with eicosapentaenoic acid, gamma-linolenic acid, and antioxidants reduces alveolar inflammatory mediators and protein influx in patients with acute respiratory distress syndrome. Crit Care Med 31(2):491–500. doi:10.1097/01.CCM.0000049952.96496.3E
77. Heller AR, Rossler S, Litz RJ, Stehr SN, Heller SC, Koch R, Koch T (2006) Omega-3 fatty acids improve the diagnosis-related clinical outcome. Crit Care Med 34(4):972–979. doi:10.1097/01.CCM.0000206309.83570.45
78. Pontes-Arruda A, Aragao AM, Albuquerque JD (2006) Effects of enteral feeding with eicosapentaenoic acid, gamma-linolenic acid, and antioxidants in mechanically ventilated patients with severe sepsis and septic shock. Crit Care Med 34(9):2325–2333. doi:10.1097/01.CCM.0000234033.65657.B6
79. Pontes-Arruda A, Demichele S, Seth A, Singer P (2008) The use of an inflammation-modulating diet in patients with acute lung injury or acute respiratory distress syndrome: a meta-analysis of outcome data. JPEN J Parenter Enteral Nutr 32(6):596–605. doi:10.1177/0148607108324203
80. DeMichele SJ, Wood SM, Wennberg AK (2006) A nutritional strategy to improve oxygenation and decrease morbidity in patients who have acute respiratory distress syndrome. Respir Care Clin N Am 12(4):547–566 . doi:10.1016/j.rcc.2006.09.006vi
81. Mizock BA, DeMichele SJ (2004) The acute respiratory distress syndrome: role of nutritional modulation of inflammation through dietary lipids. Nutr Clin Pract Off Publ Am Soc Parenteral Enteral Nutrition 19(6):563–574
82. Gadek JE, DeMichele SJ, Karlstad MD, Pacht ER, Donahoe M, Albertson TE, Van Hoozen C, Wennberg AK, Nelson JL, Noursalehi M (1999) Effect of enteral feeding with eicosapentaenoic acid, gamma-linolenic acid, and antioxidants in patients with acute respiratory distress syndrome. Enteral Nutrition in ARDS Study Group. Crit Care Med 27(8):1409–1420
83. Singer P, Theilla M, Fisher H, Gibstein L, Grozovski E, Cohen J (2006) Benefit of an enteral diet enriched with eicosapentaenoic acid and gamma-linolenic acid in ventilated patients with acute lung injury. Crit Care Med 34(4):1033–1038. doi:10.1097/01.CCM.0000206111.23629.0A
84. Grau-Carmona T, Moran-Garcia V, Garcia-de-Lorenzo A, Heras-de-la-Calle G, Quesada-Bellver B, Lopez-Martinez J, Gonzalez-Fernandez C, Montejo-Gonzalez JC, Blesa-Malpica A, Albert-Bonamusa I, Bonet-Saris A, Herrero-Meseguer JI, Mesejo A, Acosta J (2011) Effect of an enteral diet enriched with eicosapentaenoic acid, gamma-linolenic acid and anti-oxidants on the outcome of mechanically ventilated, critically ill, septic patients. Clin Nutr 30(5):578–584. doi:10.1016/j.clnu.2011.03.004
85. Rice TW, Wheeler AP, Thompson BT, deBoisblanc BP, Steingrub J, Rock P (2011) Enteral omega-3 fatty acid, gamma-linolenic acid, and antioxidant supplementation in acute lung injury. JAMA 306(14):1574–1581. doi:10.1001/jama.2011.1435
86. Stapleton RD, Martin TR, Weiss NS, Crowley JJ, Gundel SJ, Nathens AB, Akhtar SR, Ruzinski JT, Caldwell E, Curtis JR, Heyland DK, Watkins TR, Parsons PE, Martin JM, Wurfel MM, Hallstrand TS, Sims KA, Neff MJ (2011) A phase II randomized placebo-controlled trial of omega-3 fatty acids for the treatment of acute lung injury. Crit Care Med 39(7):1655–1662. doi:10.1097/CCM.0b013e318218669d

87. Li C, Bo L, Liu W, Lu X, Jin F (2015) Enteral immunomodulatory diet (omega-3 fatty acid, gamma-linolenic acid and antioxidant supplementation) for acute lung injury and acute respiratory distress syndrome: an updated systematic review and meta-analysis. Nutrients 7(7):5572–5585. doi:10.3390/nu7075239
88. Pichard C, Oshima T, Berger MM (2015) Energy deficit is clinically relevant for critically ill patients: yes. Intensive Care Med 41(2):335–338. doi:10.1007/s00134-014-3597-9
89. Cigada M, Corbella D, Mistraletti G, Forster CR, Tommasino C, Morabito A, Iapichino G (2008) Conscious sedation in the critically ill ventilated patient. J Crit Care 23(3):349–353. doi:10.1016/j.jcrc.2007.04.003
90. Iapichino G, Radrizzani D, Solca M, Pesenti A, Gattinoni L, Ferro A, Leoni L, Langer M, Vesconi S, Damia G (1984) The main determinants of nitrogen balance during total parenteral nutrition in critically ill injured patients. Intensive Care Med 10(5):251–254
91. Wiedemann HP, Wheeler AP, Bernard GR, Thompson BT, Hayden D, deBoisblanc B, Connors AF Jr, Hite RD, Harabin AL (2006) Comparison of two fluid-management strategies in acute lung injury. N Engl J Med 354(24):2564–2575. doi:10.1056/NEJMoa062200
92. Iapichino G, Pesenti A, Radrizzani D, Solca M, Pelizzola A, Gattinoni L (1983) Nutritional support to long-term anesthetized and curarized patients under extracorporeal respiratory assist for terminal pulmonary failure. JPEN J Parenter Enteral Nutr 7(1):50–54
93. Ferrie S, Herkes R, Forrest P (2013) Nutrition support during extracorporeal membrane oxygenation (ECMO) in adults: a retrospective audit of 86 patients. Intensive Care Med 39(11):1989–1994. doi:10.1007/s00134-013-3053-2

12 Pharmacological Interventions: Neuromuscular Blocking Agents

Samuel Lehingue, Sami Hraiech, and Laurent Papazian

12.1 Introduction

Several pharmacological treatments have been tested and found to improve the prognoses of patients presenting with acute respiratory distress syndrome (ARDS). Among these treatments, only the use of neuromuscular blocking agents (NMBAs) has been proven to be associated with increased survival in a randomized controlled trial (RCT). However, considering the current lack of clear recommendations, the role and appropriate place of NMBAs in ARDS treatment deserve to be clarified. The aims of this chapter are therefore to summarize the evidence supporting their use in this indication, to present elements of the pathophysiology to increase understanding of their beneficial role and to precisely delineate for which patients and in what conditions NMBAs should be administered.

12.2 Clinical Practice and Historical Context

Despite their frequent use, the guidelines concerning NMBAs have not been revised since 2002 [1]. NMBAs are frequently used in intensive care units (ICUs) [2] , specifically during episodes of ARDS. From 25% to 85% of patients with ARDS enrolled in contemporary multicentre randomized controlled trials (RCTs) received NMBAs [3–6]. In a recent large survey [7], 37.8% of patients with severe ARDS were treated with continuous neuromuscular blockade.

S. Lehingue, MD • S. Hraiech, MD, PhD (✉) • L. Papazian, MD, PhD
Assistance Publique – Hôpitaux de Marseille, Hôpital Nord, Réanimation – Détresses Respiratoires et des Infections Sévères, Chemin des Bourrely, 13015 Marseille, France

Aix-Marseille Université, Faculté de Médecine de Marseille, 22 boulevard Jean Moulin, 13305 Marseille, France
e-mail: samuel.lehingue@ap-hm.fr; sami.hraiech@ap-hm.fr; laurent.papazian@ap-hm.fr

D. Chiumello (ed.), *Acute Respiratory Distress Syndrome (ARDS)*,
DOI 10.1007/978-3-319-41852-0_12

Indeed, protective ventilation objectives, i.e. the prevention and the treatment of patient/ventilator asynchronies and the use of prone positioning, often require neuromuscular blockade [6, 8, 9].

The accurate place of NMBAs in ARDS treatment has been clarified in the last decade. The first publications concerning NMBAs were case reports and small non-randomized studies that reported controversial results concerning improvements in oxygenation [10–12]. The absence of strong scientific evidence demonstrating a benefit to the prognosis and potential adverse events, especially ICU-acquired weakness, were often responsible for a distrust of paralytics. Lagneau opened the path towards the era of RCTs and demonstrated that the continuous infusion of NMBAs for 2 h improves the PaO_2/FiO_2 ratio in a study that included 102 patients who presented with moderate to severe ARDS [13].

12.3 Randomized Controlled Trials

Three multicentre prospective randomized controlled trials published in the "era of the low tidal volumes strategy" [3] have addressed the use of NMBAs in the early phase of ARDS. All of these studies used continuous infusion of cisatracurium over a 48-h period in addition to sedation that was titrated to obtain a Ramsay score of 6 with no spontaneous triggering activity.

In the first study [14], the authors evaluated the effects of 48 h of cisatracurium infusion on gas exchange as evaluated over a 120 h time period. A sustained improvement in the PaO_2/FiO_2 ratio was delayed in time and appeared only from the 48th hour after randomization to the end of the study observation period. This improvement was associated with a decrease in the plateau pressure over time. Notably, the investigators reported strong trends towards greater numbers of ventilator-free days and lower mortality rates at both days 28 and 60.

In a second study [15], the same group evaluated the effects of 48 h of cisatracurium infusion on pulmonary and systemic inflammation. Bronchoalveolar lavage (BAL) was performed, and blood samples were collected at inclusion and 48 h after randomization to analyse the tumour necrosis factor-α (TNF_α), interleukin (IL)-1β, IL-6 and IL-8 levels. At 48 h, the authors reported lower concentrations of IL-1β, IL-6 and IL-8 in the lung epithelial lining fluid in the patients in the NMBA group compared with the control group. The serum concentrations of IL-8 and IL-6 also decreased. The results accorded with those of a previous study [14] regarding the beneficial effects of NMBAs on the PaO_2/FiO_2 ratio and the decrease in plateau pressure. Again, the same trend towards a lower mortality rate was reported.

The trends towards lower mortality rates reported in these two studies were the rationale for the design of the ACURASYS study [16], which was a multicentre double-blinded randomized controlled trial involving 20 ICUs in France. To date, this is the only trial that has investigated the use of NMBAs on the survival of patients with ARDS.

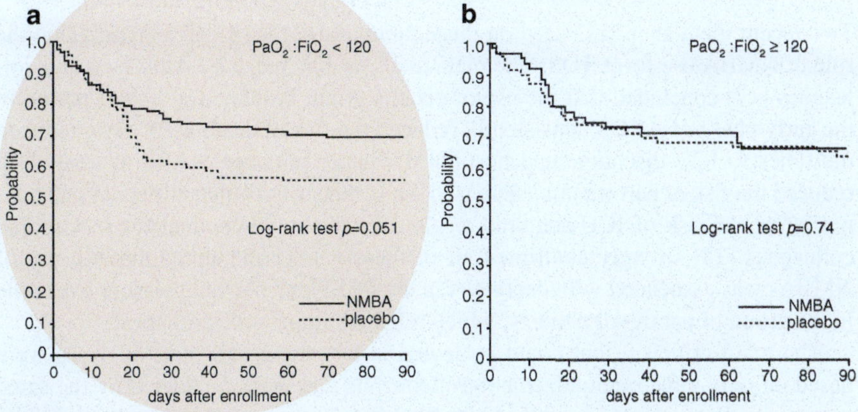

Fig. 12.1 Probability of survival according to the PaO_2/FiO_2 ratio in the ACURASYS study (Reproduced with permission from Papazian et al. [16], Appendix 2)

In this study, 339 adult patients who presented with ARDS with a PaO_2/FiO_2 ratio <150 (at a tidal volume of 6–8 mL/kg of ideal body weight and a positive end-expiratory pressure (PEEP) $\geq$ 5 cmH_2O) for less than 48 h were randomized into two groups; one group received a constant dose of 37.5 mg/h of cisatracurium besylate (177 patients), and the other group received a placebo (162 patients). Prior to either infusion, the patients were sedated to a Ramsay sedation score of 6. During the intervention period of 2 days, the volume-assisted controlled mode according to the low tidal volume strategy described in the ARDS Clinical Network Mechanical Ventilation Protocol was applied [3]. Open-label 20-mg boluses of cisatracurium (maximum of two per 24-h period) were allowed if the plateau pressures remained >32 cmH_2O despite increased sedation and despite decreased PEEP and decreased tidal volumes. The monitoring of paralysis via peripheral nerve stimulation was not permitted.

Notably, the weaning protocol was encouraged from day 3 after inclusion as soon as the FiO_2 reached $\leq$0.6.

Regarding mortality, the NMBA group exhibited an improvement in the adjusted 90-day survival rate compared with the placebo group. The hazard ratio for death after adjustments for the baseline PaO_2/FiO_2 ratio, SAPS II and plateau pressure was 0.68 (95% confidence interval [CI] 0.48–0.98; $p = 0.04$). The results suggested that the reduction in the 90-day mortality in the cisatracurium group was confined to the patients with a PaO_2/FiO_2 ratio <120 (Fig. 12.1). Additionally, the mortality rate at day 28 was 23.7% in the NMBA group versus 33.3% with the placebo ($p = 0.05$). The cisatracurium group also exhibited a significantly greater number of ventilator-free days, days outside the ICU and days free of organ failure (other than the lung). Pneumothorax also developed more often and earlier in the placebo group than in the cisatracurium group.

12.4 Summary of the Evidence-Based Data and Limitations

Two recent meta-analyses based on these three trials [17, 18] have investigated the role of NMBA use for ARDS. The meta-analysis conducted by Alhazzani and colleagues [17] concluded that the use of cisatracurium besylate for a short period in the early phase of ARDS consistently reduced the risk of death at 28 days, reduced the times to ICU discharge and hospital discharge (number needed to treat = 9), reduced the risk of barotrauma, increased the number of ventilator-free days and did not affect the risk of ICU-acquired weakness. The study conducted by Neto and colleagues [18] strongly confirmed all of these results and stated that the use of NMBAs was associated with decreases in the PEEP and plateau pressure over time in the group of paralysed patients, which reflected improved ventilation.

The main criticism that could be levied is that these two meta-analyses were based on only three randomized controlled trials that were conducted by the same group, which may have introduced bias into the conclusions. However, as noted by Neto and colleagues, the main study on which these meta-analyses were based included 20 different ICUs, which reduced the risk of bias.

12.5 Physiopathology

12.5.1 Short-Term Effects of NMBAs

The majority of the studies that have reported the effects of NMBA-induced paralysis were conducted in very short periods of time (<24 h) during anaesthesia (i.e. in "normal lungs") with muscle paralysis and mechanical ventilation without PEEP [19–21]. Tokics and colleagues demonstrated that patients displayed atelectasis. Shunt was placed in gravity-dependent lung regions that corresponded to the atelectatic areas. There were considerable $\dot{V}/\dot{Q}$ ventilation-to-perfusion mismatches that resulted in ventilation primarily of the ventral lung regions and perfusion of the dorsal lung regions [20]. Hedenstierna and colleagues demonstrated that due to the reduction of the cross-sectional chest area and the cephalic ascension of the diaphragm, the thoracic volume was reduced. This reduction was accompanied by a decrease in the functional residual capacity (FRC) that was attributed (at least in part) to the loss of muscular tone [21, 22] and was thought to be a major cause of post-operative hypoxaemia. However, few studies have reported the effects of anaesthesia and NMBA-induced paralysis on lung mechanics. In healthy subjects, Brismar and colleagues found no further reduction in FRC or modification of the elastic properties of the lung or the chest wall following the addition of paralysis to anaesthesia [23]. In the intensive care setting, Conti and colleagues conducted a study of 13 patients affected by diseases involving both lungs and the chest wall who required mechanical ventilation for acute respiratory failure and were heavily sedated (Ramsay scores of 5) and failed to demonstrate any further modification of either the chest wall or lung elastance following paralysis. CT scans and analysis of the pressure-volume curves revealed that derecruitment was reduced after the application of a

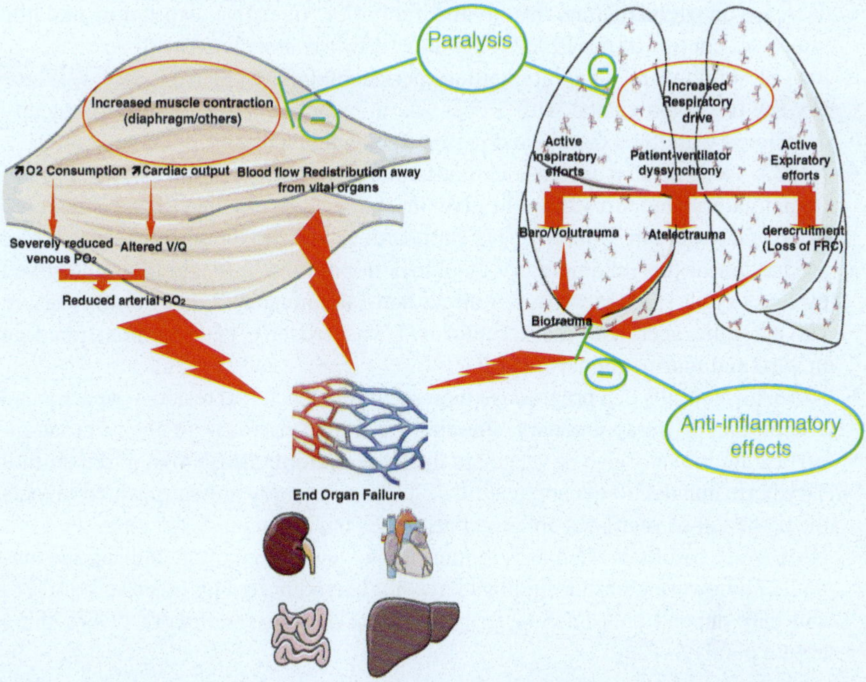

Fig. 12.2 Potential physiopathological effects that explain the benefits of NMBAs in the most severe forms of ARDS. *V/Q* ventilator/perfusion ratio, *FRC* functional residual capacity

PEEP of 10 cmH_2O [21, 24]. In summary, no data support any additional deleterious role of NMBAs in the onset of atelectasis in sedated ARDS patients.

12.5.2 Pathophysiological Hypothesis of the Beneficial Effects of NMBAs

The results of the three available RCTs about the use of NMBAs during the early phase of ARDS indicate that the effect of the treatment on oxygenation becomes significant after 24 h. Moreover, in the ACURASYS trial, the Kaplan-Meier survival curves did not separate until 18 days of treatment. These observations together with the available knowledge regarding the use of NMBAs for shorter periods in patients with healthy lungs raise hypotheses regarding the manners in which NMBAs could be beneficial (Fig. 12.2) during the acute phase of severe ARDS. Several mechanisms may be involved and are most likely interrelated. Slutsky [25] proposed a summary of the effects of NMBAs that included the following main points:

- Patient-to-ventilator dyssynchronies are reduced, and the control of tidal volume is improved, which leads to decreases in baro- and volutrauma as well as a decrease in atelectrauma due to the inhibition of active expiration and the improved control of the PEEP. This latter effect is associated with decreases in lung blood flow and alveolar-capillary permeability.

- NMBA use is associated with a decrease in respiratory drive that is classically associated with hypoxaemia and permissive hypercapnia.
- NMBA use leads to a decrease in biotrauma, an inhibition of the translocation of inflammatory mediators from the alveolar space to the circulation and a decrease in associated organ failure. These suppositions are supported by the decreased production of pro-inflammatory cytokines in both the lung and blood observed by Forel et al. [15]. Moreover, a direct anti-inflammatory role of cisatracurium via nicotinic acetylcholine receptor-α 1 has recently been demonstrated in in vitro and murine models [26].
- NMBA use results in a progressive increase in the functional residual capacity and a decrease in intrapulmonary shunting. The improvement in the ventilation-perfusion ratio may also be related to the more uniform distribution of the pulmonary perfusion due to the application of lower pulmonary pressure, which favours the perfusion of ventilated areas and decreases intrapulmonary shunting.
- NMBA use results in decreases in muscle oxygen consumption and cardiac output [27]; however, similar findings have not been reported by other authors [28] and may depend on ARDS severity, sedation deepness and work of breathing before paralysis [29].

12.5.3 Deleterious Effects of Spontaneous Breathing in the Acute Phase of ARDS

The beneficial effects of NMBAs in the most hypoxaemic patients in the initial phase of ARDS may also be due to the prevention of the deleterious role of spontaneous breathing (SB). In the early phase of ARDS, the high respiratory drive that results from hypoxaemia may result in elevated and uncontrolled transpulmonary pressure (TPP) with over-distension, particularly in the dependant vertebro-diaphragmatic zones, which results in major ventilator-induced lung injury (VILI) [30]. In these cases, the maintenance of a plateau pressure below 30 cmH_2O might not be sufficient to ensure protective ventilation, particularly in patients with the most severe forms of ARDS, as suggested by recent experimental work from Yoshida et al. [31]. In a rabbit model of ARDS, these authors demonstrated that the preservation of ventilatory effort lacked the same effects on oxygenation, pulmonary ventilation and lung injury depending on the severity of the ARDS (i.e. mild or severe). The preservation of SB induced improvements in pulmonary ventilation and oxygenation in mild ARDS subjects but resulted in increased TPP and VILI in a group of animals with severe ARDS. These deteriorations of the ventilatory and histological parameters were prevented by abolishing SB via the administration of NMBAs in the severe ARDS group.

In summary and in contrast to what occurs in patients with mild to moderate ARDS, in the initial phase of severe ARDS, the prevention of VILI and the optimization of alveolar recruitment appear to be based on controlled protective ventilation and the use of NMBAs and the consequent abolition of spontaneous ventilatory effort.

12.6 Adverse Events

12.6.1 NMBAS and ICU-Acquired Weakness (ICUAW)

NMBAs have been dispraised due to a supposed association with ICUAW.

ICUAW is defined by a generalized muscle weakness that develops during the course of an ICU admission and for which no cause other than the acute illness or its treatment can be identified [32]. ICUAW is present among approximately 60% of ARDS patients at the time of awakening [33] and 36% at the time of hospital discharge [34]. ICUAW is associated with prolonged ICU and hospital stays, prolonged mechanical ventilation duration and increased ICU and hospital mortalities [35–38]. Risk factors have been discussed widely in the literature, and independent risk factors, such as female sex, multiple organ dysfunctions (≥2), the duration of mechanical ventilation, hyperglycaemia [39] and the administration of corticosteroids [36], have been identified.

The prolonged use of neuromuscular blocking agents (more than 48 h) [40, 41], their simultaneous administration with corticosteroids [42] and steroid NMBAs may contribute to ICUAW [43, 44], but there is actually no evidence that non-steroid NMBAs increase the risk of ICUAW when used for short durations and without the simultaneous administration of corticosteroids [32]. In a meta-analysis [17] of RCTs evaluating the effects of the use of NMBAs during ARDS, the incidence of ICU-acquired paresis (assessed via clinical evaluations of quadriparesis or by the Medical Research Council (MRC) score at day 28 or at ICU discharge) was not higher among the treated patients than in the control group.

12.6.2 Insufficient Sedation and Memorizing

The continuous use of NMBA infusion highlights the problem of inadequate sedation. Hardin et al. [45] demonstrated that patients receiving NMBAs were awake for 22% of the sleep period over a time span of 24 h. Neuromonitoring via continuous electroencephalography or with a device such as the bispectral index (BIS, Aspect Medical Systems, Natick, MA, USA) can reduce the risk of consciousness in paralysed patients [46]. However, studies evaluating the reliabilities of such devices in the monitoring of the level of sedation of paralysed patients have found contradictory results [47, 48].

12.7 Perspectives: The Appropriate Place of NMBAs in ARDS Treatment

Clear recent recommendations concerning the use of NMBAs for ARDS are lacking. The most recent guidelines from 2002 [1] reduce the role of NMBAs to "facilitating mechanical ventilation when sedation alone is inadequate". These guidelines were created before the RCTs were conducted and appear to be obsolete. The recent data on the beneficial effects of NMBAs on mortality have modified their use. In a recent large international survey conducted in 50 countries, NMBAs were found to be the most frequently used adjunctive measure in severe ARDS [7]. NMBAs were also extensively used in the PROSEVA study, which demonstrated the beneficial effect of prone positioning on mortality [6]. Overall, that NMBAs have a crucial role in the management of ARDS seems to no longer be questionable. However, the available literature conveys the following "rules" with respect to the use of NMBAs:

- First, NMBAs should be used to paralyse patients in the early phase of the evolution of ARDS.
- Second, short courses of treatment should be administered to limit the occurrence of ICUAW. Forty-eight-hour treatments were used in the ACURASYS study [16], but shorter treatments (24 h) might be sufficient if the evolution is rapid and favourable. In contrast, in the most severe cases, a longer period may be required (72–96 h), particularly for patients who require several days of PP (as in the PROSEVA study) and those who require extracorporeal life support.
- Third, NMBAs should be reserved for the most hypoxaemic patients (including severe ARDS and the most hypoxaemic cases of moderate ARDS). A PaO_2/FiO_2 ratio cut-off of 120 can be proposed based on the ACURASYS study data [16], but a ratio of 150 might also be used. This cut-off is proposed in the most recent guidelines of the Surviving Sepsis Campaign, which support the use of short-course treatment with NMBAs during sepsis-related ARDS [49]. Moreover, NMBAs are almost always associated with PP [6], and PP has been demonstrated to be beneficial for patients with a PaO_2/FiO_2 ratio below 150. The Reevaluation Of Systemic Early Neuromuscular Blockade (ROSE study NCT02509078) study is currently recruiting patients with PaO_2/FiO_2 ratios below 150 and will hopefully help to form a conclusion.
- Fourth, NMBAs should be integrated into ventilatory strategies that allow for spontaneous ventilation as soon as the ventilatory parameters improve (Fig. 12.3). Indeed, in the ACURASYS study, following the initial 48-h period, NMBAs were discontinued, sedatives were reduced and pressure support ventilation was introduced in all patients with FiO_2 values less than or equal to 0.6. This concept was also present in the PROSEVA study; in this trial, when the PaO_2/FiO_2 ratio was $\geq$150 mmHg, the PEEP was $\leq$10 cmH_2O and the FiO_2 was $\leq$60%, the PP sessions, sedation and paralysis were stopped to allow for spontaneous efforts.

Adhering to these conditions might ensure the acquisition of the beneficial effects of NMBAs while preventing their deleterious side effects.

However, several questions remain to be answered. The potential anti-inflammatory properties of cisatracurium [15, 26] and the efficacies of other molecules need to be investigated, the appropriate dose needs to be identified (in the ACURASYS study, high and constant doses were used to preserve the blinding for both groups), NMBA efficacy needs to be examined with train-of-four monitors and the appropriate target paralysis depth needs to be clarified.

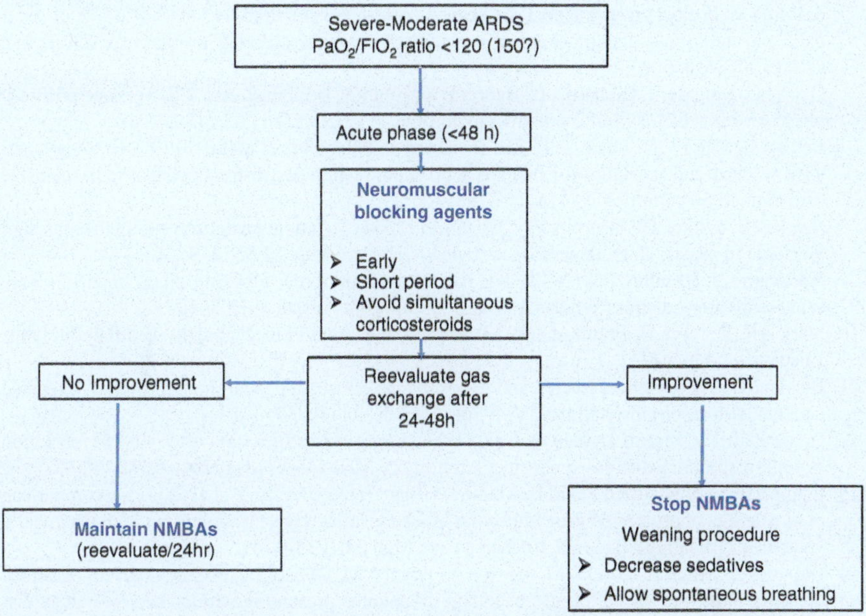

Fig. 12.3 The place of NMBAs in protective ventilation in ARDS. *NMBAs* neuromuscular blocking agents, *ARDS* acute respiratory distress syndrome

Conclusion

NMBAs are the most frequently used pharmacological treatment for ARDS. Recent strong evidence indicates that NMBAs improve survival in the most severe patients. Moreover, early and short-term administration is not associated with neuromuscular side effects and should be followed with a ventilator strategy that allows for spontaneous breathing as soon as gas exchange improves. Further studies will help to precisely identify the appropriate place of NMBAs in the treatment of moderate ARDS, the doses that should be used and the monitoring that must be performed.

References

1. Murray MJ, Cowen J, DeBlock H, Erstad B, Gray AW, Tescher AN et al (2002) Clinical practice guidelines for sustained neuromuscular blockade in the adult critically ill patient. Crit Care Med 30:142–156
2. Szakmany T, Woodhouse T (2015) Use of cisatracurium in critical care: a review of the literature. Minerva Anestesiol 81:450–460
3. Brower RG, Matthay MA, Morris A, Schoenfeld D, Thompson BT, Wheeler A et al (2000) Ventilation with lower tidal volumes as compared with traditional tidal volumes for acute lung injury and the acute respiratory distress syndrome. N Engl J Med 342:1301–1308
4. Brower RG, Lanken PN, MacIntyre N, Matthay MA, Morris A, Ancukiewicz M et al (2004) Higher versus lower positive end-expiratory pressures in patients with the acute respiratory distress syndrome. N Engl J Med 351:327–336

5. Arroliga A, Frutos-Vivar F, Hall J, Esteban A, Apezteguia C, Soto L et al (2005) Use of sedatives and neuromuscular blockers in a cohort of patients receiving mechanical ventilation. Chest J 128:496–506
6. Guérin C, Reignier J, Richard J-C, Beuret P, Gacouin A, Boulain T et al (2013) Prone positioning in severe acute respiratory distress syndrome. N Engl J Med 368:2159–2168
7. Bellani G, Laffey JG, Pham T, Fan E, Brochard L, Esteban A et al (2016) Epidemiology, patterns of care, and mortality for patients with acute respiratory distress syndrome in intensive care units in 50 countries. JAMA 315:788–800
8. Vender JS, Szokol JW, Murphy GS, Nitsun M (2004) Sedation, analgesia, and neuromuscular blockade in sepsis: an evidence-based review. Crit Care Med 32:S554–S561
9. Needham CJ, Brindley PG (2012) The role of neuromuscular blocking drugs in early severe acute respiratory distress syndrome. Can J Anesth Can Anesth 59:105–108
10. Stark AR, Bascom R, Frantz ID (1979) Muscle relaxation in mechanically ventilated infants. J Pediatr 94:439–443
11. Bishop MJ (1984) Hemodynamic and gas exchange effects of pancuronium bromide in sedated patients with respiratory failure. J Am Soc Anesthesiol 60:369–371
12. Coggeshall JW, Marini JJ, Newman JH (1985) Improved oxygenation after muscle relaxation in adult respiratory distress syndrome. Arch Intern Med 145:1718–1720
13. Lagneau F, D'honneur G, Plaud B, Mantz J, Gillart T, Duvaldestin P et al (2002) A comparison of two depths of prolonged neuromuscular blockade induced by cisatracurium in mechanically ventilated critically ill patients. Intensive Care Med 28:1735–1741
14. Gainnier M, Roch A, Forel J-M, Thirion X, Arnal J-M, Donati S et al (2004) Effect of neuromuscular blocking agents on gas exchange in patients presenting with acute respiratory distress syndrome*: Crit. Care Med 32:113–119
15. Forel J-M, Roch A, Marin V, Michelet P, Demory D, Blache J-L et al (2006) Neuromuscular blocking agents decrease inflammatory response in patients presenting with acute respiratory distress syndrome. Crit Care Med 34:2749–2757
16. Papazian L, Forel J-M, Gacouin A, Penot-Ragon C, Perrin G, Loundou A et al (2010) Neuromuscular blockers in early acute respiratory distress syndrome. N Engl J Med 363(12):1107–1116
17. Alhazzani W, Alshahrani M, Jaeschke R, Forel JM, Papazian L, Sevransky J et al (2013) Neuromuscular blocking agents in acute respiratory distress syndrome: a systematic review and meta-analysis of randomized controlled trials. Crit Care 17:R43
18. Neto AS, Pereira VGM, Espósito DC, Damasceno MCT, Schultz MJ (2012) Neuromuscular blocking agents in patients with acute respiratory distress syndrome: a summary of the current evidence from three randomized controlled trials. Ann Intensive Care 2:33
19. Rehder K, Sessler AD, Rodarte JR (1977) Regional intrapulmonary gas distribution in awake and anesthetized-paralyzed man. J Appl Physiol 42:391–402
20. Tokics L, Hedenstierna G, Svensson L, Brismar B, Cederlund T, Lundquist H et al (1996) $\dot{V}/\dot{Q}$ distribution and correlation to atelectasis in anesthetized paralyzed humans. J Appl Physiol 81:1822–1833
21. Brismar B, Hedenstierna G, Lundquist H, Strandberg Å, Svensson L, Tokics L (1985) Pulmonary densities during Anesthesia with muscular relaxation—a proposal of atelectasis. J Am Soc Anesthesiol 62:422–428
22. Hedenstierna G, Strandberg Å, Brismar B, Lundquist H, Svensson L, Tokics L (1985) Functional Residual Capacity, Thoracoabdominal Dimensions, and Central Blood Volume during General Anesthesia with Muscle Paralysis and Mechanical Ventilation. J Am Soc Anesthesiol 62:247–254
23. Westbrook PR, Stubbs SE, Sessler AD, Rehder K, Hyatt RE (1973) Effects of anesthesia and muscle paralysis on respiratory mechanics in normal man. J Appl Physiol 34:81–86
24. Sigurdsson S, Svantesson C, Larsson A, Jonson B (2000) Elastic pressure–volume curves indicate derecruitment after a single deep expiration in anaesthetised and muscle-relaxed healthy man. Acta Anaesthesiol Scand 44:980–984

25. Slutsky AS (2010) Neuromuscular blocking agents in ARDS. N Engl J Med 363:1176–1180
26. Fanelli V, Morita Y, Cappello P, Ghazarian M, Sugumar B, Delsedime L et al (2016) Neuromuscular blocking agent cisatracurium attenuates lung injury by inhibition of nicotinic acetylcholine receptor-α1. J Am Soc Anesthesiol 124:132–140
27. Marik PE, Kaufman D (1996) THe effects of neuromuscular paralysis on systemic and splanchnic oxygen utilization in mechanically ventilated patients. Chest 109:1038–1042
28. Putensen C, Mutz NJ, Putensen-Himmer G, Zinserling J (1999) Spontaneous breathing during ventilatory support improves ventilation–perfusion distributions in patients with acute respiratory distress syndrome. Am J Respir Crit Care Med 159:1241–1248
29. Freebairn RC, Derrick J, Gomersall CD, Young RJ, Joynt GM (1997) Oxygen delivery, oxygen consumption, and gastric intramucosal pH are not improved by a computer-controlled, closed-loop, vecuronium infusion in severe sepsis and septic shock. Crit Care Med 25:72–77
30. Hraiech S, Yoshida T, Papazian L (2015) Balancing neuromuscular blockade versus preserved muscle activity: Curr. Opin Crit Care 21:26–33
31. Yoshida T, Uchiyama A, Matsuura N, Mashimo T, Fujino Y (2013) The comparison of spontaneous breathing and muscle paralysis in two different severities of experimental lung injury. Crit Care Med 41:536–545
32. Hermans G, Van den Berghe G. Clinical review: intensive care unit acquired weakness. Crit Care [Internet]. 2015 [cité 28 janv 2016];19. Disponible sur: http://ccforum.com/content/19/1/274
33. Bercker S, Weber-Carstens S, Deja M, Grimm C, Wolf S, Behse F et al (2005) Critical illness polyneuropathy and myopathy in patients with acute respiratory distress syndrome. Crit Care Med 33:711–715
34. Fan E, Dowdy DW, Colantuoni E, Mendez-Tellez PA, Sevransky JE, Shanholtz C et al (2014) Physical complications in acute lung injury survivors: a two-year longitudinal prospective study. Crit Care Med 42:849–859
35. Ali NA, O'Brien JM, Hoffmann SP, Phillips G, Garland A, Finley JCW et al (2008) Acquired weakness, handgrip strength, and mortality in critically ill patients. Am J Respir Crit Care Med 178:261–268
36. De Jonghe B, Sharshar T, Lefaucheur J et al (2002) Paresis acquired in the intensive care unit: a prospective multicenter study. JAMA 288:2859–2867
37. De Jonghe B, Bastuji-Garin S, Durand M-C, Malissin I, Rodrigues P, Cerf C et al (2007) Respiratory weakness is associated with limb weakness and delayed weaning in critical illness. Crit Care Med 35:2007–2015
38. De Jonghe B, Bastuji-Garin S, Sharshar T, Outin H, Brochard L (2004) Does ICU-acquired paresis lengthen weaning from mechanical ventilation? Intensive Care Med 30: 1117–1121
39. Van den Berghe G, Schoonheydt K, Becx P, Bruyninckx F, Wouters PJ (2005) Insulin therapy protects the central and peripheral nervous system of intensive care patients. Neurology 64:1348–1353
40. Hermans G, Wilmer A, Meersseman W, Milants I, Wouters PJ, Bobbaers H et al (2007) Impact of intensive insulin therapy on neuromuscular complications and ventilator dependency in the medical intensive care unit. Am J Respir Crit Care Med 175:480–489
41. Hermans G, Casaer MP, Clerckx B, Güiza F, Vanhullebusch T, Derde S et al (2013) Effect of tolerating macronutrient deficit on the development of intensive-care unit acquired weakness: a subanalysis of the EPaNIC trial. Lancet Respir Med 1:621–629
42. Griffiths RD, Hall JB (2010) Intensive care unit-acquired weakness. Crit Care Med 38:779–787
43. Hansen-Flaschen J, Cowen J, Raps EC (1993) Neuromuscular blockade in the intensive care unit: more than we bargained for. Am Rev Respir Dis 147:234–236
44. Testelmans D, Maes K, Wouters P, Powers SK, Decramer M, Gayan-Ramirez G (2007) Infusions of rocuronium and cisatracurium exert different effects on rat diaphragm function. Intensive Care Med 33:872–879

45. Hardin KA, Seyal M, Stewart T, Bonekat HW (2006) Sleep in critically ill chemically paralyzed patients requiring mechanical ventilation. Chest 129:1468–1477
46. Ballard N, Robley L, Barrett D, Fraser D, Mendoza I (2006) Patients' recollections of therapeutic paralysis in the intensive care unit. Am J Crit Care 15:86–94
47. Inoue S, Kawaguchi M, Sasaoka N, Hirai K, Furuya H (2006) Effects of neuromuscular block on systemic and cerebral hemodynamics and bispectral index during moderate or deep sedation in critically ill patients. Intensive Care Med 32:391–397
48. Schuller PJ, Newell S, Strickland PA, Barry JJ (2015) Response of bispectral index to neuromuscular block in awake volunteers. Br J Anaesth 115:i95–103
49. The Surviving Sepsis Campaign Guidelines Committee including The Pediatric Subgroup, Dellinger RP, Levy MM, Rhodes A, Annane D, Gerlach H et al (2013) Surviving sepsis campaign: international guidelines for management of severe sepsis and septic shock, 2012. Intensive Care Med 39:165–228

13 Ventilator-Induced Lung Injury

Michele Umbrello and Paolo Formenti

13.1 Introduction

The vast majority of critically ill patients undergo invasive mechanical ventilation (MV) during their stay in the intensive care unit, and patients with ARDS are almost invariably managed by invasive mechanical ventilation. Despite extensive research over nearly half a century, no effective pharmacological therapies exist for ARDS, and supportive care with mechanical ventilation remains the cornerstone of treatment [1]. Indeed, mechanical ventilation, per se, does not substitute the function of the lungs: indeed, it is a substitute for the activity of respiratory muscles. Moreover, mechanical ventilation is a procedure that aims to improve the gas exchange, and, since it does not act either on the etiology or on the pathophysiology of ARDS, it is a measure to buy time for healing to take place [2]. On the other side, mechanical ventilation is not devoid of side effects and, namely, the hemodynamic instability secondary to the increased intrathoracic pressures and the mechanical trauma to the lung structure. Indeed, mechanical ventilation can further damage the lung, activating a biological inflammatory response and promoting the development of the so-called ventilator-induced lung injury (VILI). The present chapter will focus on the latter aspect, i.e., VILI. The classic distinction among factors related to the lung parenchyma, factors related to the mechanical ventilator, and extrapulmonary factors will be employed to classify the causes of VILI. The recently introduced theory of mechanical power, as a unifying hypothesis for all the mechanical ventilator-associated causes, will also be presented and discussed.

M. Umbrello (✉) • P. Formenti
Unità Operativa di Anestesia e Rianimazione, Ospedale San Paolo-Polo Universitario, ASST Santi Paolo e Carlo, Via A. Di Rudinì, 8, 20142 Milan, Italy
e-mail: michele.umbrello@asst-santipaolocarlo.it; paolo.formenti@asst-santipaolocarlo.it

D. Chiumello (ed.), *Acute Respiratory Distress Syndrome (ARDS)*,
DOI 10.1007/978-3-319-41852-0_13

13.2 The Concept of VILI

VILI arises from repeated application of high mechanical forces that either directly tear a weak tissue or initiate a signaling process that culminates in a pro-inflammatory state [3], in the context of an altered lung and in the presence of extrapulmonary factors which may potentially increase the damage. Soon after the times in which invasive mechanical ventilation was effectively introduced as a supportive therapy, i.e., the 1952 polio epidemic in Denmark, the potential harm from mechanical ventilation was noted and started to raise concerns, as the term "respirator lung syndrome" [4] was used to label the injury observed in ventilated patients. It was then discovered how mechanical ventilation itself could cause a structural damage to the lung, characterized by diffuse alveolar infiltrates and hyaline membranes that were found on postmortem examination [5], although the major factor causing injury was thought to be the high fractional concentrations of oxygen used in many ventilated patients.

Webb and Tierney [6] conducted one of the first comprehensive studies in intact animals, unambiguously demonstrating that mechanical ventilation can cause pulmonary edema. In their seminal investigation, the authors ventilated rats with very high peak airway pressures (and therefore overdistention) and zero positive end-expiratory pressure (PEEP). Hypoxemia developed in the animals, and postmortem examination revealed perivascular and alveolar edema. Edema did not develop in animals that underwent ventilation with the same peak airway pressure but with the addition of a PEEP of 10 cm of water, showing an interaction between overdistention and low end-expiratory lung volume with respect to lung injury.

Although the term used throughout this chapter is VILI, the mechanisms of injury are related to factors which can also occur during spontaneous ventilation. Indeed, in their proof-of-concept investigation, Mascheroni et al. [7] injected sodium salicylate into the cisterna magna of spontaneously breathing, otherwise healthy sheep, causing a marked increase in minute ventilation and alveolar overdistention with each breath. All the animals developed hypoxemia, along with an increased respiratory elastance and severe morphologic pulmonary alterations at postmortem examination, consistent with lung injury commonly observed during mechanical ventilation. Indeed, such effects did not develop in animals that were similarly treated with sodium salicylate, but underwent controlled ventilation which prevented unsafe lung stretching. Hence, a better term than VILI might be ventilation-induced lung injury. Nevertheless, experimental evidence provides consistent laboratory observations and clinical trials regarding the factors which, alone or in conjunction, lead to the development of VILI. As a consequence of adverse patterns of ventilation, both airway and alveolar injury occur, causing a damage that prevails in anatomically dependent zones. Indeed, VILI can resemble ARDS itself, and it is often difficult to diagnose in humans because its appearance can be similar to the underlying disease for which MV was instituted [8].

The consequences of our better understanding of the mechanisms related to VILI are significant in terms of lives saved. Indeed, the incidence and mortality of ARDS have declined steadily over the past decades. A pivotal study by Li et al. [9] found that the decline in the incidence was primarily due to a decrease in nosocomial

ARDS. Moreover, as documented by the first trial of extracorporeal membrane oxygenation, the mortality rate of patients with ARDS was close to 90% in the late 1970s [10]. Mortality in studies of ARDS has then fallen impressively from 48 to 59% between 1983 and 1991 to 25–26% since 2000 [11], and data from patients enrolled in the ARDS Network randomized controlled trials document a further significant trend toward improvement in mortality during the following period [12]. It is tempting to believe that, among the several major advances in critical care practice, the widespread use of lung-protective ventilation and a reduced incidence of VILI may significantly have contributed to this trend. Indeed, although it still remains unclear how inflammatory mediators exert their detrimental effects on distal organs, experimental studies and clinical trials in ARDS have shown that the application of protective ventilator strategies is associated with decreased serum cytokine levels [13], decreased extrapulmonary organ dysfunction [14], and decreased mortality [15].

13.3 Factors Related to Development of VILI

For an injury secondary to mechanical ventilation to develop, an interaction among different factors need to occur, in particular between what the ventilator delivers to the lung parenchyma and how the lung parenchyma accepts it, that is, the combined action of mechanical forces, lung pathoanatomy, and non-ventilatory characteristics [16]. In other words, one can identify factors related to the mechanical ventilator (i.e., the way that pressures and volumes are delivered), as well as factors related to the lung (such as decreased lung dimensions, increased lung inhomogeneity, presence of stress risers, and cyclic collapse and decollapse). Dynamic characteristics, such as respiratory frequency, flow rate, and strain rate, have recently been emphasized as key determinants of whether the "static" variables may or may not inflict injury [17, 18]. In addition to direct structural damage, mechanical stretch can trigger a complex array of inflammatory mediators associated with activation of the immune response, further adding to injury and potentially causing remote injury to other organs, which may result in multiple system organ dysfunction and ultimately in death; this is termed "biotrauma" [19]. Moreover, extrapulmonary factors such as perfusion, pH, gas tensions, and temperature may play a role in the development of VILI.

13.4 Lung-Dependent Factors of VILI: Stress, Strain, and Stress Raisers

The logical sequence of events in progression of VILI caused by inappropriate mechanical ventilation would seem to be mechanical damage to pulmonary tissue caused by excess stress- induced strain as the primary injury, followed by biotrauma in response to physical damage caused by excessive strain [20, 21]. Gattinoni's group applies engineering concepts as a novel approach to analyze the pathologic impact of mechanical ventilation on normal pulmonary tissue and to determine what adjustments in the mechanical breath can block progressive acute lung injury and thus reduce ARDS incidence [22, 23]. In their most recent paper, their goal was to identify the volumetric threshold for VILI and determine if PEEP was directly or indirectly protective in normal pigs [24]. Unlike many experiments in which the role of tidal volume (TV), plateau pressure (P_{plat}), and PEEP were correlated with VILI, the authors analyzed the mechanism of VILI under two main categories with two respective subcategories: (1) global strain (dynamic and static strain) and (2) energy load (dynamic and static) within the volumetric constraints of the lung, which is the inspiratory capacity.

Strain is the response to an applied stress, which in the case of the lung are TV and PEEP. Thus, global strain is the result of TV + PEEP volume. Dynamic strain is the amount the volume change caused by the TV over the functional residual capacity (FRC), and static strain is the volume change from PEEP over the FRC. Global energy load is a combination of the static component due to PEEP (conceptually equivalent to potential energy) and the dynamic cyclic component due to the driving pressure, defined as TV above PEEP (conceptually equivalent to kinetic energy).

Stress and strain are frequently used terms to describe the effect of external force acting on a subject. Stress is defined as the internal distribution of forces per unit of area of a specific material by an external force. The resulting change in shape of the material by the stress applied is called strain. Lung stress describes the distribution of forces due to PEEP and tidal volume, whereas strain describes the resulting change in lung volume. Calculations of strain require measurements of FRC. Traditional FRC measurements needed tracer gases such as helium, and expensive and bulky equipment [25] and modern device use the nitrogen multiple breath washout technique [26]. For the calculation of stress, the specific elastance should be known, or transpulmonary pressure measurements are required.

Ultimately, this mechanical insult results in the release of inflammatory mediators that exacerbate the primary mechanical damage resulting in a secondary biotrauma as mentioned above [27]. These studies are supported by physiological evidence that high static strain, which should be sufficient to cause overdistension-induced tissue damage, is benign unless this strain is dynamic [28]. However, if PEEP is reduced, thereby creating excessive dynamic strain, significant lung damage will occur at the identical peak static strain. Thus, it appears that dynamic strain, or atelectrauma, is the primary mechanical mechanism of injury to the pulmonary parenchyma. Volutrauma is also important because it can cause stress failure in small airways leading to pneumothoraces, but it does not cause pulmonary edema or histopathology to the pulmonary parenchyma.

More recently, another mechanical VILI mechanism has been identified. Evidence has shown that the damage to the pulmonary parenchyma can be caused by heterogeneous ventilation, which occurs at the junction between collapsed or edema-filled alveoli and air-inflated alveoli [29]. This heterogeneity causes stress concentrators that can significantly magnify the amount of alveolar and alveolar duct strain for any given stress and thus appears to be another mechanism of mechanical injury to the pulmonary tissue [30]. The main pathological cause for both heterogeneous ventilation and altered alveolar and small airway mechanics is airway flooding with edema fluid and altered surfactant function. Ventilator-induced loss of surfactant function exacerbates edema formation [31]. This leads to alveolar instability, which increments in vascular permeability, causing more edema and deactivating more surfactant in a cycle that repeats until established ARDS is recognized [32]. However, if a mechanical breath can be preemptively applied to maintain homogeneous lung ventilation (eliminate stress concentrators) and prevent alveolar collapse and reopening during ventilation (eliminate dynamic strain), it would ameliorate all components of the pathological tetrad and theoretically reduce ARDS incidence. Thus, physiological evidence suggests that progressive VILI may be blocked by applying a preemptive mechanical breath directed to maintain homogeneous lung inflation and not allowing alveoli to collapse during expiration.

13.5 Ventilator-Dependent Factors

It is now known, in general terms, that the mechanisms of VILI are alveolar overdistension (volutrauma), alveolar instability leading to alveolar collapse and reopening with each breath (atelectrauma), and the secondary inflammation caused by these mechanical injuries which is known as biotrauma [9].

Times ago, Lachmann [33] proposed that the optimal lung-protective strategy would be to "open the lung and keep it open." He hypothesized that heterogeneous lung inflation, which is a hallmark of ARDS pathology, plays a major role in driving mechanical ventilation-induced progressive acute lung injury. The corollary to this hypothesis is that keeping the lung open would result in a homogeneously ventilated lung, minimizing VILI and reducing ARDS mortality. If the approach of opening the ARDS lung and keeping it open can significantly reduce injury, then protective mechanical ventilation should be applied early in patients at a high risk of developing ARDS, in an attempt to "never let the lung collapse" and significantly reduce ARDS incidence [34]. As we will see in the next paragraphs, barotrauma, volutrauma, atelectrauma, and biotrauma are considered as undisputable truth and represent the background for the development and universal acceptance of the so-called lung-protective strategy.

13.5.1 Barotrauma and Volutrauma

Barotrauma was the first to be recognized as a form of stress at rupture, leading to pneumothorax, pneumoperitoneum, pneumomediastinum, and subcutaneous emphysema [35]. Although most frequently encountered in patients with the ARDS, it can occur in any patient receiving mechanical ventilation [14]. In addition, barotrauma can occur in patients with a wide range of underlying pulmonary conditions (i.e., asthma, chronic obstructive pulmonary disease, interstitial lung disease, pneumocystis pneumonia). In clinical medicine, barotrauma is used to describe the manifestations of extra-alveolar air during mechanical ventilation. Early descriptions of barotrauma refer to rupture of the lung after forceful exhalation against a closed glottis [27]. Although nonmechanically ventilated patients may have barotrauma, most cases occur in patients receiving mechanical ventilation.

The clinical presentation can vary, ranging from absent symptoms with the subtle radiographic findings of pulmonary (or perivascular) interstitial emphysema to respiratory distress or cardiac arrest due to a large tension pneumothorax [36]. Other manifestations include subcutaneous emphysema, pneumopericardium, pneumomediastinum, and even pneumoperitoneum, singly or in combination. Barotrauma was once the most frequent and easily recognized complication of mechanical ventilation. It is now evident, however, that barotrauma represents only one of the mechanisms underlying the broad category of VILI. As the term suggests, the lung injury associated with barotrauma is mediated by increased alveolar pressures.

It is important to recognize that lung involvement in persons with ARDS is heterogeneous and that some portions of the lungs are more adversely affected than others. This involvement can lead to misdistribution of mechanically delivered tidal volume, with some alveoli subjected to more distention than others. Pressures between adjacent alveoli may initially equilibrate, but alveolar pressures eventually increase, creating a pressure gradient between the alveoli and adjacent sheath. This gradient may result in rupture of the alveoli adjacent to the perivascular sheath and proximal dissection into the mediastinum (i.e., interstitial emphysema) [37]. In this circumstance, alveolar air is further decompressed by dissecting along lines of least resistance. These pathways include subcutaneous tissues, where the air produces subcutaneous emphysema, or along tissue planes, resulting in pneumopericardium, pneumoperitoneum, or subpleural air cysts. In the mediastinum, air can track along tissue planes, creating a pneumomediastinum, whereas increased pressures that rupture through the mediastinal pleura produce a pneumothorax. This is the most dreaded manifestation of barotrauma, and continued accumulation of air during mechanical ventilation can progress to a tension pneumothorax, sometimes with catastrophic consequences [38]. In view of the preceding description, alveolar overdistention is the key element in the development of barotrauma. In this sense, "barotrauma" is a misnomer, because the term suggests the presence of elevated pressures in its pathogenesis. Current concepts suggest that high tidal volume ventilation produces the alveolar disruption that triggers the aforementioned chain of events.

Therefore, VILI seen with high tidal volume is most accurately termed "volutrauma" [3], and it has been the basis for recent clinical trials that have established a low tidal volume approach to mechanical ventilation. On the other hand, transalveolar pressure, a measure of alveolar distention, provides another indication of the risk of barotrauma. The concept is the same, with overdistended alveoli leading to disruption in the alveolar epithelium and decompression of air as previously outlined. Although there has been some debate about the primary force that causes injury, both volume and pressure are two sides of the same coin – the transpulmonary pressure, the difference between airway pressure (P_{aw}) and pleural pressure (P_{pl}) [39]. In fact, the airway pressure is the pressure required to distend to the same extent not only the lung but also the chest wall. When the chest wall is free to expand, the pleural pressure is relatively low but high airway pressures are now associated with high transpulmonary pressures that may lead to a lung structural damage. In other words, for a given airway pressure, the development of VILI will depend on the resulting transpulmonary pressure. Chiumello et al. [20] recently demonstrated that a specific lung elastance is present in subjects with healthy lungs as well as in patients with ARDS. This means that even during lung injury, barotraumas (stress) and volutrauma (strain) bear the same constant relationship observed in normal subjects. The distinction between volutrauma and barotrauma then vanishes where at the cellular level, stretching the lung beyond its capacity ruptures alveolar cell membranes [40], and the resulting cell death induces inflammation. Moreover, subtler injuries to the cytoskeleton or extracellular matrix trigger inflammation through intracellular signals [41].

13.5.2 Atelectrauma and PEEP Effects

The second mechanism of injury, cyclic changes in non-aerated lung, was deduced from the observation of lung injury during ventilation with low end-expiratory lung volume (EELV) or in the absence of PEEP. In this case, the mechanisms at the cellular level are less clear. Air bubbles flowing through a collapsed or fluid-filled airway might induce damage to the epithelium by VILI consists of tissue damage and a biological response resulting from the application of inappropriate mechanical forces to the lung parenchyma [42].

Parenchymal stability resulting from the interplay of respiratory parameters such as tidal volume, PEEP, or respiratory rate can explain the results of different clinical trials and experimental studies that do not fit with the classic barotraumas/volutrauma model. A consequence of low EELV can be a heterogeneous lung where that the forces exerted on alveolar walls or septa in the interfaces between collapsed and aerated lung tissues can be amplified, leading to cell injury [43]. The application of PEEP is almost invariably associated with a decrease in VILI in different experimental models of lung injury, such as high TV ventilation or surfactant depletion [44, 45]. The focus of investigative attention regarding VILI has been on the individual tidal cycle – as defined by PEEP and tidal volume. However, it stands to reason that the number of damaging cycles delivered per unit time (closely correlated with minute ventilation, independently of mode) would accentuate the injury inflicted by the individual tidal cycle [46].

PEEP tends to reduce the number of lung units placed at high risk by critical junctional interfaces between expanding and reluctantly expanding tissues. For the same tidal volume, PEEP also elevates the mean airway pressure and with it the average tissue stress. In the absence of compensatory recruitment or reduction in tidal volume, PEEP therefore also tends to increase right ventricular afterload. Without a simultaneous reduction in driving pressure, raising PEEP will place the lung at higher risk for stretch-related injury. Tidal volume itself may not injure the ventilated lung, but rather, the causative variable relates to the ratio of the tidal volume to the capacity of the lung to accept it [47]. The transalveolar pressure and the swings of transalveolar pressure (transalveolar driving pressure) determine the damaging energy forces imparted to delicate tissue [48].

Experimental designs combining high PEEP with low TV make it impossible to clarify the contributions of each factor to the outcome. In intact lungs PEEP reduces VILI. One study showed that adding PEEP in intact rats ventilated with very high TV could reduce injury [44], and a randomized trial showed in patients without lung injury that ventilation with PEEP did not worsen outcome, but improved oxygenation and decreased the risk of ventilator-associated pneumonia [49]. The effect of TV on healthy lungs is also controversial. A classic experiment from Mascheroni and colleagues [7] demonstrated that, even in spontaneously breathing animals, chemically induced hyperventilation could trigger substantial lung damage. This work highlights the importance of tissue deformation, represented by increased transpulmonary pressures, even during negative pressure ventilation (absence of high alveolar pressure, more homogeneous inflation).

Low EELV has proved safe in both animals and patients, and this approach has sometimes been termed permissive atelectasis. In a recent study using an isolated lung model, Fanelli and colleagues [50] demonstrated that permissive atelectasis caused the same amount of lung injury as the open lung strategy and only subtle differences in apoptosis and ultrastructural changes favoring the open lung strategy. In the clinical setting, mortality rates in descriptive studies for patients managed with a low-pressure strategy are similar to those in clinical trials [51]. Taken together, these data contradict the volutrauma/atelectrauma model, suggesting that other mechanisms could be responsible for VILI.

13.5.3 Biotrauma

The concepts of VILI already discussed are based on the biophysical injury induced when applied forces cause mechanical destruction of the anatomical lung structure. Alveolar overdistention, lung strain (the associated deformation of a structure to an external load in relation to its resting state), and atelectasis are key inciting features of VILI. However, numerous studies have demonstrated that there can be a more subtle form of injury, with release of various mediators into the lung, pulmonary recruitment of leukocytes, and local initiation of inflammatory processes. This biological response to mechanical forces has been called "biotrauma" [19, 27]. The biotrauma hypothesis postulates that the circulating mediators can cause local lung injury, and if they translocate into the systemic circulation, they may lead to distal organ dysfunction and death [52]. One of the pioneristic papers that investigated the effects of mechanical ventilation in an animal model [13] found that isolated nonperfused rat lungs ventilated for 2 h with large tidal volumes without PEEP had large increases in lavage concentrations of tumor necrosis factor (TNF)-a, interleukin (IL)-1b, IL-6, and macrophage inflammatory peptide 2. The potential for ventilation-induced inflammation in humans was examined in patients with ARDS who were randomized to receive traditional or lung-protective ventilation [14]. BAL and plasma concentrations of several pro-inflammatory cytokines were lower in patients receiving protective ventilation, as were other indices of plasma and alveolar fluid inflammation, compared with patients receiving traditional tidal volumes and lower PEEP.

The main concept of these observations is that the healthy lung is a homogeneously ventilated organ that is structurally resistant to mechanical damage during ventilation. The shared walls of each alveolus with a two-fiber support system (i.e., the axial system anchored to the hilum and extending into the alveolar ducts and the peripheral system anchored to the visceral pleura distending into the central portion of the lung) are structurally very stable and resistant to either overdistension or collapse. As mentioned before, the concept of this alveolar interdependence was first introduced by Mead [43] and describes the structural mechanisms by which alveoli resist either collapse or hyperinflation. In addition, they also demonstrated how heterogeneous collapse of alveoli created stress concentrators in the areas between open and collapsed alveoli. These stress concentrators greatly amplify the mechanical damage to tissue in the transitional zone between open and collapsed or edema-filled alveoli [31].

Figure 13.1 summarizes the different pathophysiologic steps of lung injury developing as a consequence of barotrauma/volutrauma, atelectrauma, and biotrauma. Table 13.1 summarizes the most relevant studies which investigated the pathophysiology of VILI.

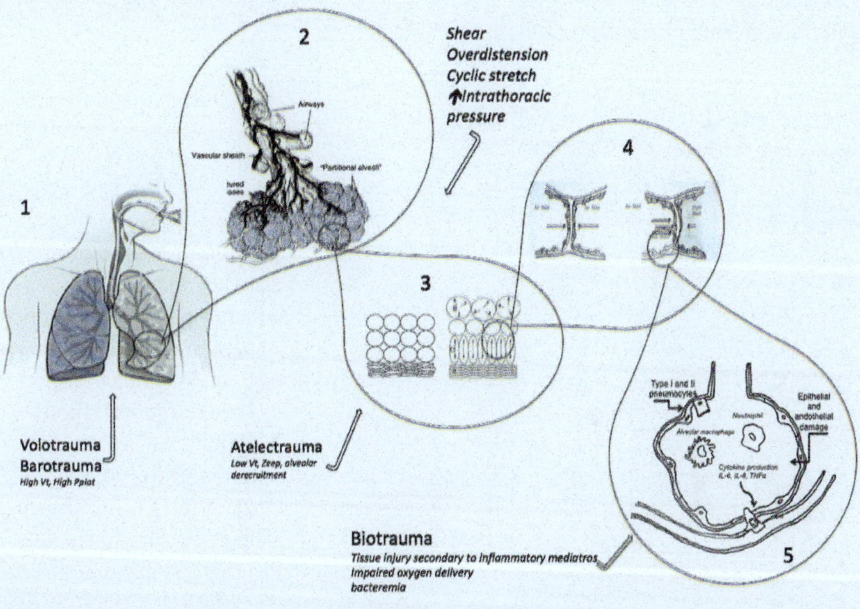

Fig. 13.1 From barotrauma/volutrauma to biotrauma. Ventilator-induced lung injury progresses from the primary mechanical injury to secondary atelectrauma, encouraged by both barotrauma and volutrauma. Atelectrauma resulting from alveolar interdependence is showed in *panel 3*, where at the interface between collapsed/consolidated (*A*) and overdistended lung units, the tissue may be injured by excessive shear stress and stretching caused by the uneven expansion of surrounding zone (*C*). *Panel 4* shows the stress concentration between an air-filled and edematous alveolus (a model of forces between air-filled and air-filled alveoli where all forces are in balance – *A*; a model of forces between an air-filled and edematous alveolus where a greater pressure drop across the alveolar interface causing and excessive strain). The progression of lung damage is seen through inflammatory mediators (*panel 5*), eventually resulting in distal tissue damage. Mechanical stretch impairs alveolar epithelial integrity, causing a loss of tight junction structure and cell attachment associated with a production of pro-inflammatory cytokines

Table 13.1 Summary of the most relevant studies regarding the ventilator-induced lung injury (VILI)

Concept	Author	Study type	Main thought
Barotrauma/volutrauma, atelectrauma	Kumar et al. 1973 [35]	Prospective	IPPV + PEEP vs IPPV at ZEEP and development of barotrauma. Major determinant a preexisting COPD
	Uhlig et al. 2012 [9]	Overview	Discussion of the forces generated by MV and how they may injure the lungs mechanically and through inflammation
	Lachmann et al. 1985 [33]	Experimental	A randomized study of five different ventilatory modes in a piglet model of severe respiratory distress
	Tremblay et al. 1998 [27]	Overview	Description of the mechanisms of VILI, including the involvement of cellular and inflammatory mediator-induced injury
	Ioannidis et al. 2015 [36]	Overview	Focus on barotrauma, from definition to treatment
	Dreyfuss et al. 1988 [3]	Experimental	Comparison of the consequences of normal tidal volume ventilation in mechanically ventilated rats at a high airway pressure with those of high tidal volume ventilation, including the effects of PEEP on both edema and lung ultrastructure
	Dos Santos et al. 1985 [39]	Overview	A perspective on ventilator-induced lung injury with a focus on mechanisms and clinical implications.
	Valenza et al. 2003 [44]	Experimental	Investigation on the protective role of PEEP with respect to the time needed to reach similar levels of lung injury
	Tremblay et al. 2005 [21]	Overview	From bench to bedside
	Fanelli et al. 2009 [50]	Observational	Useful for assessing diaphragmatic motion under resistive loading

Stress, strain, stress raisers	Mead et al. 1970 [43]	Observational	Pioneeristic description of lung stretching forces distribution.
	Chiumello et al. 2008 [20]	Prospective	Plateau pressure and tidal volume are inadequate surrogates for stress and strain; quantification of the stress to strain relationship
	Protti et al. 2011 [22]	Experimental	To identify a strain–stress threshold above which ventilator-induced lung damage can occur
	Protti t al 2013 [23]	Experimental	To clarify whether different combinations of dynamic and static strains, resulting in the same large global strain, constantly produce lung edema
	Protti et al. 2015 [24]	Experimental	To find the volumetric VILI threshold and see whether PEEP is protective per se or indirectly
	Nieman et al. 2016 [28]	Overview	Using engineering concepts to analyze the impact of the mechanical breath on the lung is a novel new approach to investigate VILI mechanisms and to help design the optimally protective breath
	Cressoni et al. 2014 [29]	Retrospective	To quantify lung inhomogeneities in patients with ARDS
	Chiumello et al. 2016 [47]	Prospective	Airway pressures and tidal volume normalized to body weight as surrogates for lung stress and strain in mild pediatric ARDS

(continued)

Table 13.1 (continued)

Concept	Author	Study type	Main thought
Biotrauma	Tremblay et al. 1997 [13]	Experimental	To study the effect of ventilation strategy on lung inflammatory mediators in the presence and absence of a preexisting inflammatory stimulus
	Muscedere et al. 1994 [42]	Experimental	To examine the hypothesis that ventilation at very low lung volumes can also worsen lung injury by repeated opening and closing of airway units as ventilation occurs from below to above the infection point as determined from the inspiratory pressure–volume curve
	Ridge et al. 2005 [41]	Experimental	To demonstrate that shear stress causes disassembly of keratin in lung alveolar epithelial cells
	Vlahakis et al. 2005 [40]	Overview	Experimental evidence for lung cells as injury targets and the relevance of these studies for human ventilator-associated lung injury

The table represents a summary of the most important studies regarding ventilator-induced lung injury, starting from the early evidence of barotrauma/volutrauma, ending to the concept of biotrauma and stress raisers

COPD chronic obstructive pulmonary disease, *ARDS* acute respiratory distress syndrome, *PEPP* positive end-expiratory pressure, *ZEEP* zero positive end-expiratory pressure

13.6 Mechanical Power

Very recently, a new way of looking at the ventilator side of VILI, i.e., the mechanical power, has been introduced [18] . According to this approach, every ventilator component already known to be associated with the development of VILI (tidal volume, driving pressure, respiratory rate, inspiratory-to-expiratory ratio and flow), with the addition of the effect of PEEP, contributes, each one to his proper extent, to the total amount of energy delivered to the respiratory system (and hence to the lung). The mechanical power concept does not introduce any new component to the field of ventilator-related causes of VILI; instead, it proposes and validates a mathematical description of machine power responsive to the relative contributions of its bedside-adjustable components. Starting from the classical equation of motion, an equation was developed that enables to calculate the mechanical power by some easily obtainable ventilator variables [53]. In fact, the initial trigger of stress and strain is the force applied to the lung extracellular matrix times its displacement, which equals the product of pressure times delta-volume. The cyclic energy loads applied at a given frequency (power) then triggers the development of VILI, which may be seen in this context as a sort of "fatigue" of the extracellular matrix [24]. If the lung is subject to an "excess" of energy, the unrecovered energy may be expected to be sufficient to break the molecular bonds of the polymers of the extracellular matrix [54, 55], to detach endothelial [56] and epithelial [57] cells from the basement membrane, and to fracture the capillary walls [58]. Alteration of the extracellular matrix, combined with capillary micro-fractures, may then activate an inflammatory reaction [59] and micro-hemorrhage, leading to the extracellular edema typical of VILI.

Indeed, the tidal change in lung volume is associated with a cyclic energy load delivered by the ventilator to the respiratory system. The energy load to the respiratory system (Fig. 13.2) is composed of a static component, due to PEEP and PEEP volume (conceptually equivalent to potential energy), and a dynamic cyclic component, due to driving pressure and tidal volume above PEEP (conceptually equivalent to kinetic energy), plus the additional, resistive and inertial component generated by the pressure spent for gas movement, the surface tension forces, and tissue resistances to motion. Energy is equal to the pressure applied times the change in volume, summed along the inspiratory volume-pressure curve. In contrast, once PEEP is applied, no further cyclic energy load is imposed on the system, as the volume is constant. As a matter of fact, PEEP plays a complex role in the context of the energy provided by the ventilator, as it provides increased continuous tension to the extracellular matrix which then accumulates potential energy. Further energy is added when cyclic tidal ventilation is superimposed to reach a given end-inspiratory volume. Therefore, if the end-inspiratory volume is the same, with or without PEEP, the energy is lower in the presence of PEEP than without it. Computed in this way, the energy/power load provided a single explanation of the different phenomena related to development of VILI.

In a recent paper, Gattinoni et al. [60] demonstrated how the "power equation," as derived from the classical equation of motion with the addition of PEEP (while

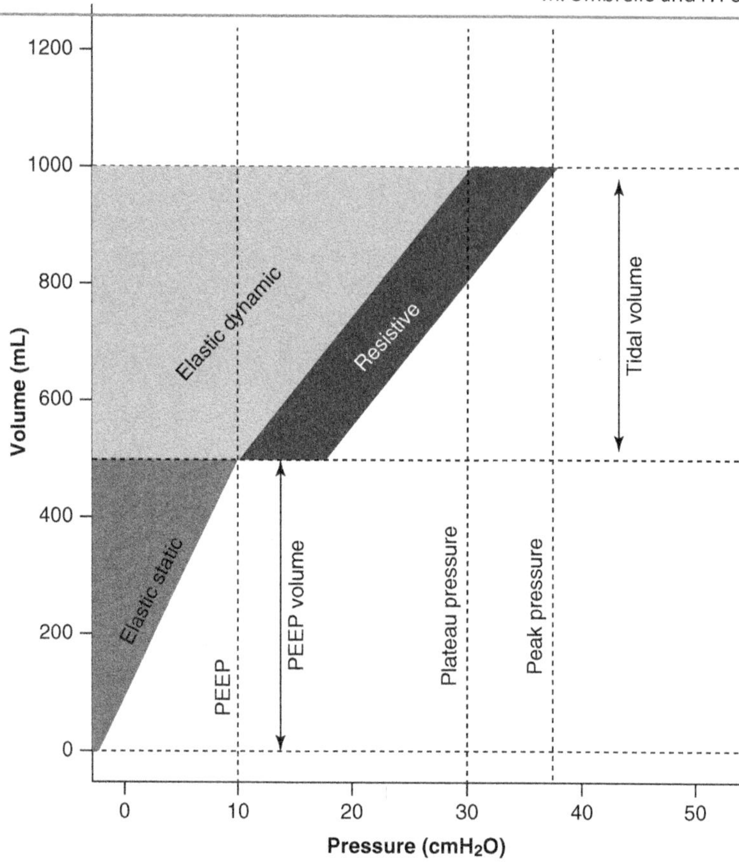

Fig. 13.2 Mechanical power and mechanical power equation. Mechanical energy provided during tidal ventilation and graphical representation of the power equation. The graphic is composed of a triangle on the lower left-hand side of the image, representing the elastic static component, i.e., the energy delivered just once when PEEP is applied, and of a larger trapezoid, representing the elastic dynamic component, whose area equals the elastic energy delivered at each tidal breath, to which a parallelogram is added on the right, representing the resistive component

inertial forces were neglected), proved to yield comparable values of mechanical power when compared to data obtained experimentally through the pressure–volume curve analysis. The advantage of such a mathematical description of the mechanical power is that it enables the quantification of the relative contribution of its different components, thus allowing to anticipate the effects of their changes.

As far as mechanical ventilation is provided with PEEP, the static energy to reach the PEEP volume corresponds to the triangle equal to 1/2 × PEEP × PEEP volume. However, this energy is provided only once (as long as the same amount of PEEP is maintained), since during tidal ventilation the PEEP volume equals zero. However, in the presence of PEEP, more energy is required to inflate the lung. The energy needed for TV to reach P_{plat} corresponds to the trapezoid equal to (peak pressure − PEEP) × TV/2 + (PEEP × TV).

From the classical equation of motion in which PEEP is also considered [61], at any given time, the pressure (P) in the whole respiratory system is equal to

$$P = \mathrm{TV} \cdot E_{rs} + R_{aw} \cdot V_{\mathrm{i}} + \mathrm{PEEP}$$

where E_{rs} is the respiratory system elastance, R_{aw} is the total respiratory system resistance, and V_{i} is the inspiratory flow.

The energy provided by the ventilator per breath can be calculated by multiplying each pressure in the motion equation by the volume variation (i.e., TV); after substituting V_{i} with $\mathrm{TV}/T_{\mathrm{insp}}$ (the inspiratory time) and then expressing T_{insp} as a function of respiratory rate (RR) and inspiratory-to-expiratory (I:E) ratio and converting the value to J/min, the following equation may be derived:

$$\mathrm{POWER} = 0.098 \cdot \mathrm{RR} \cdot \mathrm{TV}^2 \cdot \left(E_{rs} \cdot \frac{1}{2} + \mathrm{RR} \cdot \frac{(1 + \mathrm{I:E})}{60 \cdot \mathrm{I:E}} \cdot R_{aw} \right) + \mathrm{TV} \cdot \mathrm{PEEP}$$

In the same paper [60], the authors demonstrated how, both in patients with healthy lungs and in patients with ARDS, the mechanical power measured directly through the pressure–volume curve analysis was strictly correlated with the one computed via the power equation.

Recently, in a secondary analysis of patients enrolled in two previously published randomized controlled trials [62], Guerin and colleagues [63] found how mechanical power (computed as DP × TV × RR, where DP is the airway driving pressure) was higher in ARDS non-survivors than in survivors. A dose–response effect was found, with higher values of power associated with increased mortality, and a threshold of 12 J/min was identified, which was associated with significant distinct probabilities of survival. Despite the equation proposed by the authors is simpler than that derived from the equation of motion, it represents only the product of respiratory rate times twice the dynamic energy component due to tidal volume, thus neglecting both the role of PEEP and that of the resistive load.

Since VILI originates from the interaction between the mechanical power transferred to the ventilable lung parenchyma and the anatomo-pathological characteristics of the latter, it is possible that different combinations of the components of mechanical power, resulting in a value greater than a given threshold, may produce similar damage. This was recently confirmed by animal experiments in which different combinations of tidal volume and respiratory rate were applied to detect the threshold for VILI [18]. The authors found how up to a mechanical power of approximately 12 J/min, the computed tomography scans showed mostly isolated densities, whereas when mechanical power was above the 12 J/min threshold, all piglets developed whole-lung edema.

Since airway pressure represents the pressure applied to the respiratory system as a whole, its interpretation is influenced by alterations in the mechanical properties of the chest wall [20, 64]; a more informative parameter could be the computation of the mechanical power selectively applied to the lung, either via the transpulmonary pressure–volume curve analysis or via a rearrangement of the equation of motion. The mechanical power delivered to the lung ($\mathrm{POWER}_{\mathrm{l}}$) implies the use of the transpulmonary pressure (P_l) instead of airway pressure at P_{plat} and at PEEP. The relationship between P_l and P_{aw} (either P_{plat} or PEEP) is expressed by $P_l = P_{aw} \times (E_l/E_{rs})$, where E_l is the elastance of the lung [65].

Therefore, substituting in the equation:

$$\text{POWER}_l = 0.098 \cdot \text{RR} \cdot \left\{ \text{TV}^2 \left(\frac{1}{2} \cdot E_l \cdot + \text{RR} \cdot \frac{(1 + \text{I:E})}{60 \cdot \text{I:E}} \cdot R_{aw} \right) + \text{TV} \cdot \text{PEEP} \cdot \frac{E_l}{E_{rs}} \right\}$$

Eventually, it must be stressed that the mechanical power is just one part of the problem. The other part is represented by the lung's conditions. The same mechanical power may have different effects depending on dimensions of the lung, the presence of inhomogeneity, the extent of the stress risers, and the vessels' filling state, all factors which condition an uneven distribution of the delivered energy. Therefore, to be clinically meaningful, the mechanical power must be normalized, at least to the lung volume [66].

13.7 Extra-Parenchymal Factors

Nonmechanical background factors have repeatedly been proven important in the process of VILI generation, and, for any given ventilation pattern that applies potentially damaging stress, they may determine whether or not VILI is expressed [67]. These background factors, which may synergize with each other, include the preinjury and inflammatory state, the temperature at which ventilation occurs [68, 69], the amplitudes of vascular pressures and flows [56, 70], $PaCO_2$/pH [71, 72], and FiO_2 [73, 74].

In an experimental study aimed at investigating whether thermal stress could modulate the development of VILI, Suzuki et al. [68] randomized three groups of anesthetized rabbits to be ventilated for 2 h at core body temperatures of 33, 37, or 41° while ventilated with a noninjurious or a potentially injurious strategy. The hyperthermic group compared with the hypothermic animals developed a significantly higher degree of hypoxia and had increased lung edema and an altered pressure–volume relationship. To correct for potential effects arising from cardiac output fluctuations or from extrapulmonary organs, an isolated lung model was used for a confirmatory study, with similar findings. In a similarly designed study on rats, Akinci et al. [69] found how concomitant hyperthermia increased systemic inflammatory response, as assessed by higher levels of serum chemokines and cytokines, and a worse histology, during an injurious, high-pressure ventilation strategy.

Despite the great majority of studies of VILI which have specifically investigated the airspace mechanics, i.e., factors as tidal volume, plateau pressure, and PEEP, one must consider that the pulmonary alveolus is an interface between gas and blood. Indeed, because the intraluminal pressures applied to the airway epithelium also impact on the vascular endothelium, the potential for pressures and flows within blood vessels to influence the development and/or evolution of VILI has also been taken into account. The vascular structure of the pulmonary circulation is composed of both intra-alveolar and extra-alveolar vessels, whose behavior during lung inflation is fundamentally different. In fact, inflation compresses wall-embedded capillaries but dilates extra-alveolar microvessels. Under the high-permeability conditions of ARDS, even small increases in pulmonary microvascular pressure lead to increased edema formation. Moreover, unlike in health tissue in which the blood–gas barrier is intact, there is no clear pressure threshold for edema formation in the lung tissue of ARDS patients [75]. It is a well-known phenomenon that mechanical forces that tear the delicate alveolar–capillary membrane can originate on either side of the boundary, when the application of adverse ventilatory patterns to previously healthy lungs not only causes formation of proteinaceous edema, but it also stimulates neutrophil aggregation and hemorrhage [76]. The complementary issue, that is, the vascular contribution to VILI, was investigated in a series of studies conducted by the group of Marini using isolated, ventilated, and perfused lungs. When isolated rabbit lungs were exposed to perfusion levels that were equivalent to greater or less than the normal resting blood flow of in vivo animals, while ventilated with airway pressures that proved damaging in vivo, the authors demonstrated that perfusion amplitude contributed to the reduced lung compliance and promoted both lung edema and hemorrhage [77]. In a subsequent experiment [78], the authors found a significant relationship between the magnitude of pulmonary arterial pressure and the length of time over which it was sustained with the extent of VILI. Subsequent studies showed how lungs exposed to cyclic elevations in pulmonary artery pressure in the absence of ventilation formed less edema and exhibited less perivascular and alveolar hemorrhage than did ventilated lungs exposed to similar peak and mean pulmonary artery pressures and mean airway pressure [70]. Taken together, the studies demonstrated that when the mechanical stresses of the tidal cycle are high, an increase in precapillary vascular pressure or a reduction in postcapillary vascular pressure each could influence the severity of VILI inflicted by an unchanging adverse pattern of ventilation [56]. These observations imply that the gradient of transalveolar vascular pressure may be instrumental in inflicting damage when airway stresses are high. Figure 13.3 shows the possible mechanisms by which hemodynamic parameters may induce or exacerbate VILI.

In an attempt to reduce the total amount of stress delivered by the mechanical ventilator, a strategy of reduced minute ventilation has long ago been suggested [79], which was generally associated with increased carbon dioxide retention and hypercapnic acidosis. Indeed, experiments by Sinclair and coworkers [80] and by Broccard and colleagues [81] strongly indicate that the generation of hypercapnic acidosis may exert a protective effect on the severity of VILI. More recent preclinical data still confirm the protective effects of therapeutic hypercapnia initiated concurrently with injurious ventilation in an in vivo model of VILI [72]. The beneficial effects of such hypercapnic acidosis in reducing the extent of VILI are increasingly well understood and include attenuation of lung neutrophil recruitment, pulmonary and systemic cytokine and eicosanoid concentrations, cell apoptosis, and oxygen-derived and nitrogen-derived free radical injury [71].

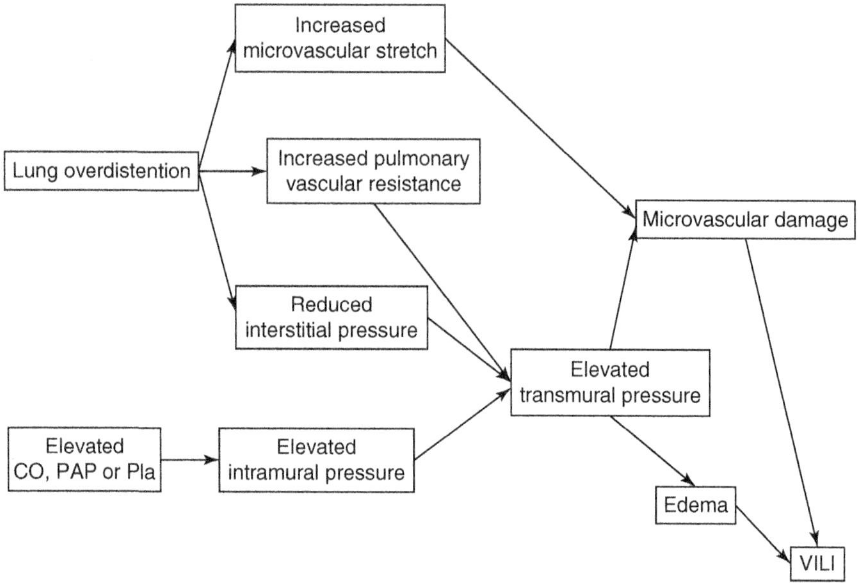

Fig. 13.3 Possible mechanisms by which pulmonary vascular hemodynamic parameters may incite or exacerbate ventilator-induced lung injury (VILI). Microvascular strain may be amplified at the junctions of open and closed lung units (*CO* cardiac output, *Pla* left atrial pressure, *PAP* pulmonary artery pressure)

The deleterious effects of hyperoxygenation are increasingly being recognized in several fields of intensive care medicine [82], to the extent that less aggressive approaches to oxygen supply have recently been suggested, even to not providing any supplemental oxygen, in several acute care settings, such as resuscitation of asphyxiated newborns, during acute myocardial infarction or after stroke or cardiac arrest [83]. Indeed, a recent trial showed how a conservative protocol for oxygen therapy vs conventional therapy resulted in lower mortality in a heterogeneous population of mechanically ventilated critically ill patients [84]. Experimental evidence points to the detrimental role of hyperoxia as a contributing factor to the development of VILI. In a laboratory investigation aimed at assessing whether hyperoxia could exacerbate lung injury caused by an injurious mechanical ventilation strategy, Sinclair and colleagues [73] found how hyperoxic animals, as compared to normoxic ones, had significantly reduced oxygenation and increased lung injury scores. Hyperoxia also significantly increased alveolar–capillary permeability and polymorphonuclear leukocytes and inflammatory mediator concentrations in bronchoalveolar lavage fluid. Similar results were found by Li et al. [74], who investigated the mechanisms regulating the interaction between injurious ventilation and hyperoxia. In their experiments, the authors found how the addition of hyperoxia to an unsafe ventilation strategy increased lung cytokine production, neutrophil infiltration by upregulation of the cytokine macrophage inflammatory protein-2, and apoptotic cell death through activation of the JNK and ERK1/2 pathways.

In conclusion, the vascular/metabolic/oxidative environment of the lung tissue at the onset of major mechanical stress has repeatedly shown to be influential in the VILI development process. Lowering ventilatory and cardiovascular demands – thereby reducing both minute ventilation and the vascular pressure gradient across the lung – are potentially important therapeutic targets when attempting to avoid VILI. It seems rational then to suggest a reduction in oxygen demand and ventilation requirement as a component of a comprehensive "lung-protective" strategy [67]. Indeed, reducing the ventilation requirement simultaneously allows reduction of driving pressures or ventilating frequencies. Because cardiac output also declines in response to lower oxygenation demands, the pulmonary microvascular blood flow gradient is lessened, thereby potentially reducing VILI risk.

References

1. Fan E, Needham DM, Stewart TE (2005) Ventilatory management of acute lung injury and acute respiratory distress syndrome. JAMA 294(22):2889–2896. doi:10.1001/jama.294.22.2889
2. Gattinoni L, Quintel M (2016) Is mechanical ventilation a cure for ARDS? Intensive Care Med 42(5):916–917. doi:10.1007/s00134-016-4266-y
3. Dreyfuss D, Soler P, Basset G, Saumon G (1988) High inflation pressure pulmonary edema. Respective effects of high airway pressure, high tidal volume, and positive end-expiratory pressure. Am Rev Respir Dis 137(5):1159–1164. doi:10.1164/ajrccm/137.5.1159
4. Nash G, Blennerhassett JB, Pontoppidan H (1967) Pulmonary lesions associated with oxygen therapy and artificial ventilation. N Engl J Med 276(7):368–374. doi:10.1056/NEJM196702162760702
5. Avignon PD, Lindahl J, Werneman H (1956) Causes of death. Acta Medica Scand Suppl 316:111–113
6. Webb HH, Tierney DF (1974) Experimental pulmonary edema due to intermittent positive pressure ventilation with high inflation pressures. Protection by positive end-expiratory pressure. Am Rev Respir Dis 110(5):556–565. doi:10.1164/arrd.1974.110.5.556
7. Mascheroni D, Kolobow T, Fumagalli R, Moretti MP, Chen V, Buckhold D (1988) Acute respiratory failure following pharmacologically induced hyperventilation: an experimental animal study. Intensive Care Med 15(1):8–14
8. Fan E, Villar J, Slutsky AS (2013) Novel approaches to minimize ventilator-induced lung injury. BMC Med 11:85. doi:10.1186/1741-7015-11-85
9. Uhlig U, Uhlig S (2011) Ventilation-induced lung injury. Compr Physiol 1(2):635–661. doi:10.1002/cphy.c100004
10. Zapol WM, Snider MT, Hill JD, Fallat RJ, Bartlett RH, Edmunds LH, Morris AH, Peirce EC 2nd, Thomas AN, Proctor HJ, Drinker PA, Pratt PC, Bagniewski A, Miller RG Jr (1979) Extracorporeal membrane oxygenation in severe acute respiratory failure. A randomized prospective study. JAMA 242(20):2193–2196
11. Bernard GR (2005) Acute respiratory distress syndrome: a historical perspective. Am J Respir Crit Care Med 172(7):798–806. doi:10.1164/rccm.200504-663OE
12. Erickson SE, Martin GS, Davis JL, Matthay MA, Eisner MD (2009) Recent trends in acute lung injury mortality: 1996-2005. Crit Care Med 37(5):1574–1579. doi:10.1097/CCM.0b013e31819fefdf
13. Tremblay L, Valenza F, Ribeiro SP, Li J, Slutsky AS (1997) Injurious ventilatory strategies increase cytokines and c-fos m-RNA expression in an isolated rat lung model. J Clin Invest 99(5):944–952. doi:10.1172/JCI119259

14. Ranieri VM, Suter PM, Tortorella C, De Tullio R, Dayer JM, Brienza A, Bruno F, Slutsky AS (1999) Effect of mechanical ventilation on inflammatory mediators in patients with acute respiratory distress syndrome: a randomized controlled trial. JAMA 282(1):54–61
15. Ventilation with lower tidal volumes as compared with traditional tidal volumes for acute lung injury and the acute respiratory distress syndrome. The acute respiratory distress syndrome network (2000). N Engl J Med 342(18):1301–1308. doi:10.1056/NEJM200005043421801
16. Marini JJ, Jaber S (2016) Dynamic predictors of VILI risk: beyond the driving pressure. Intensive Care Med 42(10):1597–1600. doi:10.1007/s00134-016-4534-x
17. Protti A, Maraffi T, Milesi M, Votta E, Santini A, Pugni P, Andreis DT, Nicosia F, Zannin E, Gatti S, Vaira V, Ferrero S, Gattinoni L (2016) Role of strain rate in the pathogenesis of ventilator-induced lung edema. Crit Care Med 44(9):e838–e845. doi:10.1097/CCM.0000000000001718
18. Cressoni M, Gotti M, Chiurazzi C, Massari D, Algieri I, Amini M, Cammaroto A, Brioni M, Montaruli C, Nikolla K, Guanziroli M, Dondossola D, Gatti S, Valerio V, Vergani GL, Pugni P, Cadringher P, Gagliano N, Gattinoni L (2016) Mechanical power and development of ventilator-induced lung injury. Anesthesiology 124(5):1100–1108. doi:10.1097/ALN.0000000000001056
19. Tremblay LN, Slutsky AS (2006) Ventilator-induced lung injury: from the bench to the bedside. Intensive Care Med 32(1):24–33. doi:10.1007/s00134-005-2817-8
20. Chiumello D, Carlesso E, Cadringher P, Caironi P, Valenza F, Polli F, Tallarini F, Cozzi P, Cressoni M, Colombo A, Marini JJ, Gattinoni L (2008) Lung stress and strain during mechanical ventilation for acute respiratory distress syndrome. Am J Respir Crit Care Med 178(4):346–355. doi:10.1164/rccm.200710-1589OC
21. Tremblay LN, Slutsky AS (2005) Pathogenesis of ventilator-induced lung injury: trials and tribulations. Am J Physiol Lung Cell Mol Physiol 288(4):L596–L598. doi:10.1152/ajplung.00438.2004
22. Protti A, Cressoni M, Santini A, Langer T, Mietto C, Febres D, Chierichetti M, Coppola S, Conte G, Gatti S, Leopardi O, Masson S, Lombardi L, Lazzerini M, Rampoldi E, Cadringher P, Gattinoni L (2011) Lung stress and strain during mechanical ventilation: any safe threshold? Am J Respir Crit Care Med 183(10):1354–1362. doi:10.1164/rccm.201010-1757OC
23. Protti A, Andreis DT, Monti M, Santini A, Sparacino CC, Langer T, Votta E, Gatti S, Lombardi L, Leopardi O, Masson S, Cressoni M, Gattinoni L (2013) Lung stress and strain during mechanical ventilation: any difference between statics and dynamics? Crit Care Med 41(4):1046–1055. doi:10.1097/CCM.0b013e31827417a6
24. Protti A, Andreis DT, Milesi M, Iapichino GE, Monti M, Comini B, Pugni P, Melis V, Santini A, Dondossola D, Gatti S, Lombardi L, Votta E, Carlesso E, Gattinoni L (2015) Lung anatomy, energy load, and ventilator-induced lung injury. Intensive Care Med Exp 3(1):34. doi:10.1186/s40635-015-0070-1
25. Hewlett AM, Hulands GH, Nunn JF, Minty KB (1974) Functional residual capacity during anaesthesia. I: methodology. Br J Anaesth 46(7):479–485
26. Olegard C, Sondergaard S, Houltz E, Lundin S, Stenqvist O (2005) Estimation of functional residual capacity at the bedside using standard monitoring equipment: a modified nitrogen washout/washin technique requiring a small change of the inspired oxygen fraction. Anesth Analg 101(1):206–212, table of contents. doi:10.1213/01.ANE.0000165823.90368.55
27. Tremblay LN, Slutsky AS (1998) Ventilator-induced injury: from barotrauma to biotrauma. Proc Assoc Am Physicians 110(6):482–488
28. Nieman GF, Satalin J, Andrews P, Habashi NM, Gatto LA (2016) Lung stress, strain, and energy load: engineering concepts to understand the mechanism of ventilator-induced lung injury (VILI). Intensive Care Med Exp 4(1):16. doi:10.1186/s40635-016-0090-5
29. Cressoni M, Cadringher P, Chiurazzi C, Amini M, Gallazzi E, Marino A, Brioni M, Carlesso E, Chiumello D, Quintel M, Bugedo G, Gattinoni L (2014) Lung inhomogeneity in patients with acute respiratory distress syndrome. Am J Respir Crit Care Med 189(2):149–158. doi:10.1164/rccm.201308-1567OC

30. Cressoni M, Gallazzi E, Chiurazzi C, Marino A, Brioni M, Menga F, Cigada I, Amini M, Lemos A, Lazzerini M, Carlesso E, Cadringher P, Chiumello D, Gattinoni L (2013) Limits of normality of quantitative thoracic CT analysis. Crit Care 17(3):R93. doi:10.1186/cc12738
31. Bilek AM, Dee KC, Gaver DP (1985) 3rd (2003) mechanisms of surface-tension-induced epithelial cell damage in a model of pulmonary airway reopening. J Appl Physiol 94(2):770–783. doi:10.1152/japplphysiol.00764.2002
32. Albert RK, Keniston A, Baboi L, Ayzac L, Guerin C (2014) Prone position-induced improvement in gas exchange does not predict improved survival in the acute respiratory distress syndrome. Am J Respir Crit Care Med 189(4):494–496. doi:10.1164/rccm.201311-2056LE
33. Lachmann B (1992) Open up the lung and keep the lung open. Intensive Care Med 18(6):319–321
34. Nieman GF, Gatto LA (1985) Habashi NM (2015) impact of mechanical ventilation on the pathophysiology of progressive acute lung injury. J Appl Physiol 119(11):1245–1261. doi:10.1152/japplphysiol.00659.2015
35. Kumar A, Pontoppidan H, Falke KJ, Wilson RS, Laver MB (1973) Pulmonary barotrauma during mechanical ventilation. Crit Care Med 1(4):181–186
36. Ioannidis G, Lazaridis G, Baka S, Mpoukovinas I, Karavasilis V, Lampaki S, Kioumis I, Pitsiou G, Papaiwannou A, Karavergou A, Katsikogiannis N, Sarika E, Tsakiridis K, Korantzis I, Zarogoulidis K, Zarogoulidis P (2015) Barotrauma and pneumothorax. J Thorac Dis 7(Suppl 1):S38–S43. doi:10.3978/j.issn.2072-1439.2015.01.31
37. Tagliabue M, Casella TC, Zincone GE, Fumagalli R, Salvini E (1994) CT and chest radiography in the evaluation of adult respiratory distress syndrome. Acta Radiol 35(3):230–234
38. Marini JJ, Culver BH (1989) Systemic gas embolism complicating mechanical ventilation in the adult respiratory distress syndrome. Ann Intern Med 110(9):699–703
39. Dos Santos CC (1985) Slutsky AS (2000) invited review: mechanisms of ventilator-induced lung injury: a perspective. J Appl Physiol 89(4):1645–1655
40. Vlahakis NE, Hubmayr RD (2005) Cellular stress failure in ventilator-injured lungs. Am J Respir Crit Care Med 171(12):1328–1342. doi:10.1164/rccm.200408-1036SO
41. Ridge KM, Linz L, Flitney FW, Kuczmarski ER, Chou YH, Omary MB, Sznajder JI, Goldman RD (2005) Keratin 8 phosphorylation by protein kinase C delta regulates shear stress-mediated disassembly of keratin intermediate filaments in alveolar epithelial cells. J Biol Chem 280(34):30400–30405. doi:10.1074/jbc.M504239200
42. Muscedere JG, Mullen JB, Gan K, Slutsky AS (1994) Tidal ventilation at low airway pressures can augment lung injury. Am J Respir Crit Care Med 149(5):1327–1334. doi:10.1164/ajrccm.149.5.8173774
43. Mead J, Takishima T, Leith D (1970) Stress distribution in lungs: a model of pulmonary elasticity. J Appl Physiol 28(5):596–608
44. Valenza F, Guglielmi M, Irace M, Porro GA, Sibilla S, Gattinoni L (2003) Positive end-expiratory pressure delays the progression of lung injury during ventilator strategies involving high airway pressure and lung overdistention. Crit Care Med 31(7):1993–1998. doi:10.1097/01.CCM.0000070401.65534.F9
45. Steinberg JM, Schiller HJ, Halter JM, Gatto LA, Lee HM, Pavone LA, Nieman GF (2004) Alveolar instability causes early ventilator-induced lung injury independent of neutrophils. Am J Respir Crit Care Med 169(1):57–63. doi:10.1164/rccm.200304-544OC
46. Hotchkiss JR Jr, Blanch L, Murias G, Adams AB, Olson DA, Wangensteen OD, Leo PH, Marini JJ (2000) Effects of decreased respiratory frequency on ventilator-induced lung injury. Am J Respir Crit Care Med 161(2 Pt 1):463–468. doi:10.1164/ajrccm.161.2.9811008
47. Chiumello D, Carlesso E, Brioni M, Cressoni M (2016) Airway driving pressure and lung stress in ARDS patients. Crit Care 20:276. doi:10.1186/s13054-016-1446-7
48. Chiumello D, Chidini G, Calderini E, Colombo A, Crimella F, Brioni M (2016) Respiratory mechanics and lung stress/strain in children with acute respiratory distress syndrome. Ann Intensive Care 6(1):11. doi:10.1186/s13613-016-0113-0

49. Manzano F, Fernandez-Mondejar E, Colmenero M, Poyatos ME, Rivera R, Machado J, Catalan I, Artigas A (2008) Positive-end expiratory pressure reduces incidence of ventilator-associated pneumonia in nonhypoxemic patients. Crit Care Med 36(8):2225–2231. doi:10.1097/CCM.0b013e31817b8a92
50. Fanelli V, Mascia L, Puntorieri V, Assenzio B, Elia V, Fornaro G, Martin EL, Bosco M, Delsedime L, Fiore T, Grasso S, Ranieri VM (2009) Pulmonary atelectasis during low stretch ventilation: "open lung" versus "lung rest" strategy. Crit Care Med 37(3):1046–1053. doi:10.1097/CCM.0b013e3181968e7e
51. Page B, Vieillard-Baron A, Beauchet A, Aegerter P, Prin S, Jardin F (2003) Low stretch ventilation strategy in acute respiratory distress syndrome: eight years of clinical experience in a single center. Crit Care Med 31(3):765–769. doi:10.1097/01.CCM.0000055402.68581.DC
52. Slutsky AS, Tremblay LN (1998) Multiple system organ failure. Is mechanical ventilation a contributing factor? Am J Respir Crit Care Med 157(6 Pt 1):1721–1725. doi:10.1164/ajrccm.157.6.9709092
53. Tonetti T, Cressoni M, Collino F, Maiolo G, Rapetti F, Quintel M, Gattinoni L (2017) Volutrauma, Atelectrauma, and mechanical power. Crit Care Med 45(3):e327–e328. doi:10.1097/CCM.0000000000002193
54. Parker JC, Breen EC (1985) West JB (1997) high vascular and airway pressures increase interstitial protein mRNA expression in isolated rat lungs. J Appl Physiol 83(5):1697–1705
55. Pelosi P, Rocco PR (2008) Effects of mechanical ventilation on the extracellular matrix. Intensive Care Med 34(4):631–639. doi:10.1007/s00134-007-0964-9
56. Marini JJ, Hotchkiss JR, Broccard AF (2003) Bench-to-bedside review: microvascular and airspace linkage in ventilator-induced lung injury. Crit Care 7(6):435–444. doi:10.1186/cc2392
57. Budinger GR, Sznajder JI (2006) The alveolar-epithelial barrier: a target for potential therapy. Clin Chest Med 27(4):655–669; abstract ix. doi:10.1016/j.ccm.2006.06.007
58. West JB (2013) Fragility of pulmonary capillaries. J Appl Physiol (1985) 115(1):1–15. doi:10.1152/japplphysiol.00229.2013
59. O'Neill LA (2005) TLRs play good cop, bad cop in the lung. Nat Med 11(11):1161–1162. doi:10.1038/nm1105-1161
60. Gattinoni L, Tonetti T, Cressoni M, Cadringher P, Herrmann P, Moerer O, Protti A, Gotti M, Chiurazzi C, Carlesso E, Chiumello D, Quintel M (2016) Ventilator-related causes of lung injury: the mechanical power. Intensive Care Med 42(10):1567–1575. doi:10.1007/s00134-016-4505-2
61. Marini JJ, Crooke PS 3rd (1993) A general mathematical model for respiratory dynamics relevant to the clinical setting. Am Rev Respir Dis 147(1):14–24. doi:10.1164/ajrccm/147.1.14
62. Papazian L, Forel JM, Gacouin A, Penot-Ragon C, Perrin G, Loundou A, Jaber S, Arnal JM, Perez D, Seghboyan JM, Constantin JM, Courant P, Lefrant JY, Guerin C, Prat G, Morange S, Roch A (2010) Neuromuscular blockers in early acute respiratory distress syndrome. N Engl J Med 363(12):1107–1116. doi:10.1056/NEJMoa1005372
63. Guerin C, Papazian L, Reignier J, Ayzac L, Loundou A, Forel JM (2016) Effect of driving pressure on mortality in ARDS patients during lung protective mechanical ventilation in two randomized controlled trials. Crit Care 20(1):384. doi:10.1186/s13054-016-1556-2
64. Cortes GA, Marini JJ (2013) Two steps forward in bedside monitoring of lung mechanics: transpulmonary pressure and lung volume. Crit Care 17(2):219. doi:10.1186/cc12528
65. Chiumello D, Cressoni M, Colombo A, Babini G, Brioni M, Crimella F, Lundin S, Stenqvist O, Gattinoni L (2014) The assessment of transpulmonary pressure in mechanically ventilated ARDS patients. Intensive Care Med 40(11):1670–1678. doi:10.1007/s00134-014-3415-4
66. Gattinoni L, Pesenti A (2005) The concept of "baby lung". Intensive Care Med 31(6):776–784. doi:10.1007/s00134-005-2627-z
67. Marini JJ (2015) Advances in the support of respiratory failure: putting all the evidence together. Crit Care 19(Suppl 3):S4. doi:10.1186/cc14722
68. Suzuki S, Hotchkiss JR, Takahashi T, Olson D, Adams AB, Marini JJ (2004) Effect of core body temperature on ventilator-induced lung injury. Crit Care Med 32(1):144–149. doi:10.1097/01.CCM.0000098857.14923.44

69. Akinci OI, Celik M, Mutlu GM, Martino JM, Tugrul S, Ozcan PE, Yilmazbayhan D, Yeldandi AV, Turkoz KH, Kiran B, Telci L, Cakar N (2005) Effects of body temperature on ventilator-induced lung injury. J Crit Care 20(1):66–73
70. Hotchkiss JR Jr, Blanch L, Naveira A, Adams AB, Carter C, Olson DA, Leo PH, Marini JJ (2001) Relative roles of vascular and airspace pressures in ventilator-induced lung injury. Crit Care Med 29(8):1593–1598
71. Curley G, Kavanagh BP, Laffey JG (2010) Hypocapnia and the injured brain: more harm than benefit. Crit Care Med 38(5):1348–1359. doi:10.1097/CCM.0b013e3181d8cf2b
72. Peltekova V, Engelberts D, Otulakowski G, Uematsu S, Post M, Kavanagh BP (2010) Hypercapnic acidosis in ventilator-induced lung injury. Intensive Care Med 36(5):869–878. doi:10.1007/s00134-010-1787-7
73. Sinclair SE, Altemeier WA, Matute-Bello G, Chi EY (2004) Augmented lung injury due to interaction between hyperoxia and mechanical ventilation. Crit Care Med 32(12):2496–2501
74. Li LF, Liao SK, Ko YS, Lee CH, Quinn DA (2007) Hyperoxia increases ventilator-induced lung injury via mitogen-activated protein kinases: a prospective, controlled animal experiment. Crit Care 11(1):R25. doi:10.1186/cc5704
75. Brigham KL, Woolverton WC, Blake LH, Staub NC (1974) Increased sheep lung vascular permeability caused by pseudomonas bacteremia. J Clin Invest 54(4):792–804. doi:10.1172/JCI107819
76. Dreyfuss D, Saumon G (1998) Ventilator-induced lung injury: lessons from experimental studies. Am J Respir Crit Care Med 157(1):294–323. doi:10.1164/ajrccm.157.1.9604014
77. Broccard AF, Hotchkiss JR, Kuwayama N, Olson DA, Jamal S, Wangensteen DO, Marini JJ (1998) Consequences of vascular flow on lung injury induced by mechanical ventilation. Am J Respir Crit Care Med 157(6 Pt 1):1935–1942. doi:10.1164/ajrccm.157.6.9612006
78. Broccard AF, Hotchkiss JR, Suzuki S, Olson D, Marini JJ (1999) Effects of mean airway pressure and tidal excursion on lung injury induced by mechanical ventilation in an isolated perfused rabbit lung model. Crit Care Med 27(8):1533–1541
79. Hickling KG, Henderson SJ, Jackson R (1990) Low mortality associated with low volume pressure limited ventilation with permissive hypercapnia in severe adult respiratory distress syndrome. Intensive Care Med 16(6):372–377
80. Sinclair SE, Kregenow DA, Lamm WJ, Starr IR, Chi EY, Hlastala MP (2002) Hypercapnic acidosis is protective in an in vivo model of ventilator-induced lung injury. Am J Respir Crit Care Med 166(3):403–408. doi:10.1164/rccm.200112-117OC
81. Broccard AF, Hotchkiss JR, Vannay C, Markert M, Sauty A, Feihl F, Schaller MD (2001) Protective effects of hypercapnic acidosis on ventilator-induced lung injury. Am J Respir Crit Care Med 164(5):802–806. doi:10.1164/ajrccm.164.5.2007060
82. Asfar P, Singer M, Radermacher P (2015) Understanding the benefits and harms of oxygen therapy: response to comments by Akca. Intensive Care Med 41(10):1875. doi:10.1007/s00134-015-3995-7
83. Sjoberg F, Singer M (2013) The medical use of oxygen: a time for critical reappraisal. J Intern Med 274(6):505–528. doi:10.1111/joim.12139
84. Girardis M, Busani S, Damiani E, Donati A, Rinaldi L, Marudi A, Morelli A, Antonelli M, Singer M (2016) Effect of conservative vs conventional oxygen therapy on mortality among patients in an intensive care unit: the oxygen-ICU randomized clinical trial. JAMA 316(15):1583–1589. doi:10.1001/jama.2016.11993

14 Monitoring of Respiratory Mechanics

Andrea Aliverti

14.1 Introduction

In the management of patients with ALI and ARDS, although the notion of ventilator-induced lung injury (VILI) is now well established [1] and the correlation between respiratory system mechanics and outcome have been clearly demonstrated [2, 3], the setting of mechanical ventilation is still based mostly on blood gases rather than assessment of respiratory mechanics.

Several reasons contribute to this anomaly. The limited knowledge of even simple models of respiratory system mechanics and the lack of recognition of the hidden assumptions which are often taken when assessing respiratory mechanics with different models and methods probably represent the most significant causes of the gap existing between research and clinical practice. These limitations include an incomplete awareness of the differences existing between static and dynamical procedures used to assess mechanical properties and between linear and nonlinear models of the respiratory system. In addition, there is still a limited familiarity with several measurements employed for a complete assessment of respiratory mechanics, such as airway opening pressure as an estimation of tracheal pressure and esophageal pressure in the supine position as an estimation of pressure in the pleural space.

This chapter is organized into four sections: (1) modeling of the respiratory mechanics, (2) methods of assessing respiratory mechanics in ARDS patients currently used in clinical practice, (3) methods for assessing active components of the respiratory system in ARDS, and (4) main issues related with measuring the variables necessary for the assessment of respiratory mechanics.

A. Aliverti (✉)
Dipartimento di Elettronica, Informazione e Bioingegneria, Politecnico di Milano, P.zza L. da Vinci, 32, 20133 Milan, Italy
e-mail: andrea.aliverti@polimi.it

D. Chiumello (ed.), *Acute Respiratory Distress Syndrome (ARDS)*,
DOI 10.1007/978-3-319-41852-0_14

14.2 Modeling Respiratory Mechanics

Studying the mechanics of the respiratory system means evaluating the parameters of a mathematical model that describes the position and motion of the respiratory system through a process called "inverse modeling" or "system identification" [4].

The models which are usually adopted are invariably rather simple, having few independent components and a small number of parameters. They do not consider detailed information of the structure of the airways, lung and chest wall, but only approximated versions, because such models have to be matched to experimental data, and usually only few variables can be measured.

Once the structure of an inverse model of the respiratory system has been defined, the so-called equations of motion are derived. These equations state how pressure is related to flow and volume within each component of the model and tell how the complete model will behave under every conceivable circumstance. The equations contain "variables", i.e., measurable parameters, which usually vary with time and are typically pressures, flows, and volumes. Equations also contain parameters that characterize the "mechanical properties" of the overall system and of its different components, typically including resistance and compliance. The process of finding those parameter values that cause the model to behave like a particular real respiratory system is known as parameter estimation.

The total pressure applied to the respiratory system (P_{RS}) is the pressure difference from airway opening (P_{AO}) to body surface (P_{BS}, usually equal to atmospheric pressure). In a ventilated patient, P_{RS} is given by the sum of the pressure generated by the mechanical ventilator (P_{VENT}) and the pressure developed by the respiratory muscles (P_{MUS}) (Fig. 14.1):

$$\begin{aligned} P_{RS} &= P_{AO} - P_{BS} = \\ &= P_{VENT} \pm P_{MUS} \end{aligned} \tag{14.1}$$

P_{VENT}, in turn, is the sum of the driving pressure necessary to move air into the thorax (ΔP) and the positive end-expiratory pressure (PEEP). P_{MUS} is the pressure generated by the respiratory muscles, with the inspiratory muscles producing a decrease in intrathoracic pressure and expiratory muscles an increase.

Considering a mechanical model of the respiratory system, the pulmonary system (composed of the airways and the lung) and the chest wall have to be considered as structures arranged in parallel, while if an electrical (or hydraulic) model is considered, like the one shown in the figures of the present chapter, they are in series. This means that, at least as a first approximation, the pulmonary system and the chest wall share the same volume (V) and volume variations (dV/dt), and the total pressure applied to the respiratory system (P_{RS}) is subdivided into the "transpulmonary" pressure (P_{TP}, i.e., the pressure difference from airway opening to pleural space) and the "thoracic" pressure (P_{CW}, i.e., the pressure difference from pleural space to body surface) (Fig. 14.2).

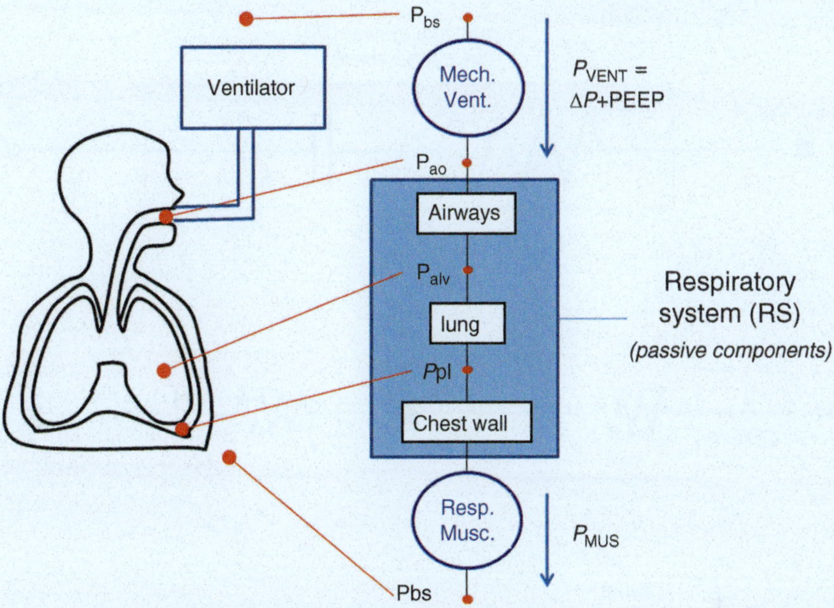

Fig. 14.1 Model of the entire respiratory system (see text for details). Pressures are indicated at specific points, *circles* represent pressure generators, rectangles represent passive components, and *arrows* indicate pressure differences. In this electric- or hydraulic-like representation, the total pressure acting on elements in series is the sum of the pressures acting on the single components, while the flow and volume changes are the same across the system. P_{BS} body surface pressure, P_{AO} airway opening pressure, P_{VENT} sum of the driving pressure necessary to move air into the thorax (ΔP), and the positive end-expiratory pressure (PEEP), P_{ALV} alveolar pressure, P_{PL} pleural pressure P_{MUS} pressure generated by the respiratory muscles

$$\begin{aligned} P_{RS} &= P_{AO} - P_{BS} = \\ &= \left(P_{AO} - P_{PL}\right) + \left(P_{PL} - P_{BS}\right) = \\ &= P_{TP} + P_{CW} \end{aligned} \tag{14.2}$$

Although the significance of Eq. 14.2 is very important, it is often disregarded and is barely considered in the clinical practice when managing ARDS patients. The relevant distending pressure for the lung is P_{TP} [5], but also the chest wall, through the pressure in the pleural space (P_{PL}), plays a significant role in determining lung expansion and stress as well [6, 7]. As shown in Eq. 14.2, if P_{PL} is known, P_{TP} and P_{CW} can be determined. While measuring P_{AO} is relatively simple (all that is required is a lateral pressure tap in a mouthpiece or a section of ventilator tubing, see below), however, measuring P_{PL} in living patients is not. P_{PL} has been estimated in the human physiology laboratory for more than 50 years from measurements of esophageal pressure (P_{ES}) [8, 9]. Most of the existing literature in which P_{ES} is used to estimate P_{PL}, however, reports data obtained with the subject under analysis either in seating or standing position. When the analyzed subject is in supine or prone

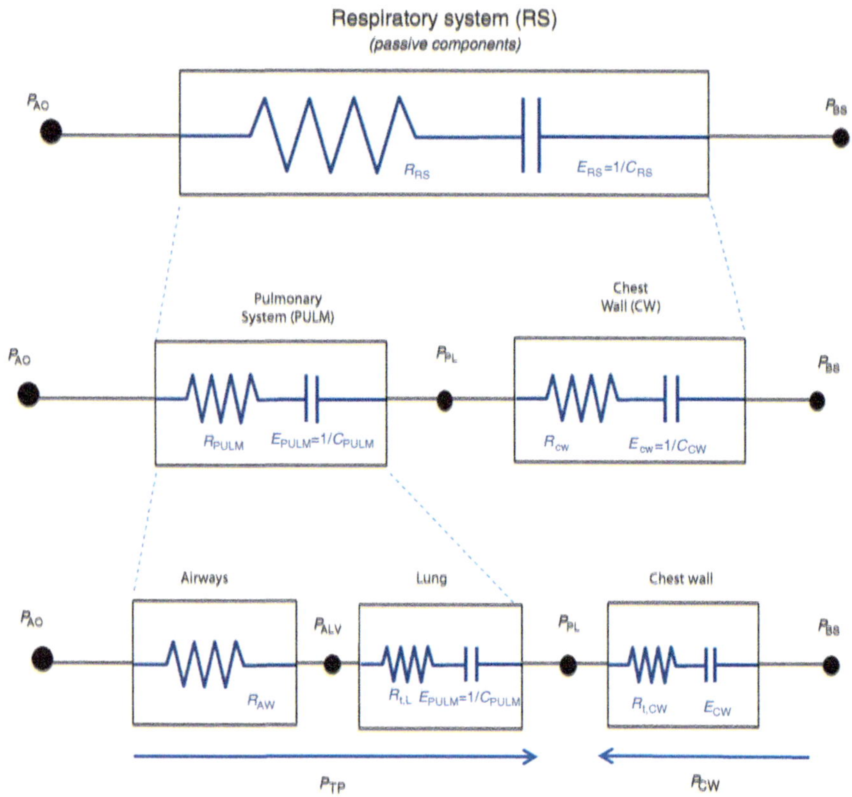

Fig. 14.2 Model of the passive components of the entire respiratory system, divided into the pulmonary system (in turn, composed by airways and lung) and the chest wall. P_{PL} pleural pressure, P_{ALV} alveolar pressure, P_{TP} transpulmonary pressure, P_{CW} thoracic pressure, R_{PULM} pulmonary system resistance, R_{AW} airway resistance, $R_{t,L}$ lung tissue resistance, $R_{t,CW}$ chest wall tissue resistance, E_{PULM} pulmonary system elastance, E_L lung elastance, E_{CW} chest wall elastance, C_{PULM} pulmonary system compliance, C_L lung compliance, and C_{CW} chest wall compliance
See legend of Fig. 14.1 for all the other symbols

position, artifacts caused by mediastinal weight and postural effects have to be considered.

Transpulmonary pressure is the sum of the pressure drop across the airways (P_{AW}, i.e., the pressure difference from airway opening to alveolar space) and lung pressure (P_L, i.e., the lung "transmural" pressure, pressure difference from alveolar space to pleural space):

$$\begin{aligned} P_{RS} &= P_{TP} + P_{CW} \\ &= \left(P_{AO} - P_{ALV}\right) + \left(P_{ALV} - P_{PL}\right) + P_{CW} \\ &= P_{AW} + P_L + P_{CW} \end{aligned} \tag{14.3}$$

Under dynamic conditions, namely, when airflow is present and dV/dt is different than zero, P_{AW} is different than zero. Only under static conditions $P_{AW} = 0$, and therefore $P_{TP} = P_L$.

P_{RS} depends on the mechanical properties of the respiratory system, namely, resistance and elastance, while the "inertance," i.e., the capability to store some energy in the kinetic, form is usually considered negligible, with the exception of the case of high-frequency forced ventilation, where it might play a significant role.

The *elastic behavior* of the respiratory system is everything that makes it spontaneously returning to an equilibrium position. It is described by elastance or its inverse, the compliance, and it depends mostly on the elastic properties of lung and chest wall tissues. Lung tissues consist mainly of *elastin* and *collagen,* structural proteins that have different responses to deformation. The former react to deformation as springs and, up to a certain degree of extension, show a *linear* behavior. The latter are sort of "safety cables," which are entangled in a disordered way in the lung at rest. Collagen fibers do not play any role in the mechanical behavior of the lung at lung volume close to rest, while with increasing lung volume, more and more fibers reach their maximal length, determining a firm increase of lung elastance. The chest wall, namely, all the structures and tissues surrounding the lung and moving with it (rib cage and abdomen), also contributes to the elastance of the respiratory system [4]. The sum of all the elastic forces acting on the respiratory system is expressed by the elastic pressure.

P_{el}, which is proportional to volume V (deviation from the equilibrium position, i.e., deviation from equilibrium volume V_0) by means of elastance E_{RS}.

With *resistance* of the respiratory system (R_{RS}), all those phenomena that oppose to deformation of the respiratory system, thereby dissipating a given amount of energy, are considered. Dissipation means that the energy supplied to the system (work performed by the respiratory muscles) or stored as potential energy (e.g., during mechanical ventilation) is lost as heat. The main source of resistance corresponds to the flow of air through the airways. Due to the viscous effects, most energy provided to the system to ventilate is actually lost as heat in the air. R_{RS}, however, is due not only to the flow resistance of the airways but also contains a significant contribution from the lung ($R_{t,\,L}$) and chest wall ($R_{t,\,CW}$) tissues. When lung and chest wall tissues are stretched, in fact, their constituent fibers, cells, and fluids move against each other and this internal friction produces heat representing another form of dissipation [4].

The sum of all the resistive forces acting on the respiratory system is expressed by the resistive pressure P_{RES}, which is proportional to volumetric flow rate dV/dt (also known as volume flow rate, rate of fluid flow, or volume velocity) by means of resistance R_{RS}.

In summary, the total pressure acting on the respiratory system, P_{RS}, is given by the sum of the elastic pressure (P_{EL}), resistive, (P_{RES}) and inertial (P_{INERT}) components (Fig. 14.3). Being $P_{INERT} \approx 0$, it follows that

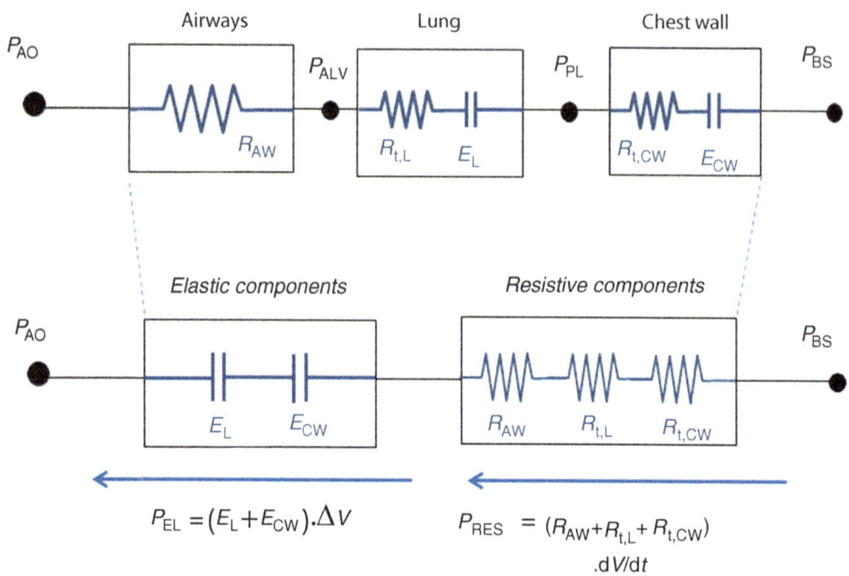

Fig. 14.3 Model of the passive components of the entire respiratory system, divided into the elastic and resistive components. See text for details and legends of Figs. 14.1 and 14.2 for used symbols

$$\begin{aligned} P_{RS} &\cong P_{EL} + P_{RES} \\ &= \frac{1}{C_{RS}} \cdot V + R_{RS} \cdot \frac{\mathrm{d}V}{\mathrm{d}t} \end{aligned} \tag{14.4}$$

Being the pulmonary system and the chest wall mechanically in parallel, total respiratory system elastance and resistance are equal to the sum of pulmonary and chest wall elastances and resistances:

$$\begin{aligned} E_{RS} &= E_L + E_{cw} = \frac{1}{C_{RS}} = \frac{1}{C_L} + \frac{1}{C_{CW}} = \frac{C_L + C_{CW}}{C_L \cdot C_{CW}} \\ R_{RS} &= R_{AW} + R_{t,L} + R_{t,cw} = R_{AW} + R_t \end{aligned} \tag{14.5}$$

Combining Eqs. 14.4 and 14.5, it follows that

$$\begin{aligned} P_{RS} &= P_{el} + P_{res} \\ &= \left(\frac{C_L + C_{CW}}{C_L \cdot C_{CW}} \right) \cdot V + \left(R_{AW} + R_t \right) \cdot \frac{\mathrm{d}V}{\mathrm{d}t} \end{aligned} \tag{14.6}$$

Lung compliance (C_L), defined as the change in lung volume per unit change in P_L, is of particular importance in ARDS and is sometime referred as either "static" or "dynamic," depending on the method of measurement adopted to obtain it (see below). Nevertheless, compliance represents a property that is only static, i.e., it expresses the distensibility of the lung. Lung compliance in ARDS is decreased due to diffused alveolar damage and loss of cellular integrity of the alveoli which are filled with proteinaceous edema fluid that also results in dilution and dysfunction of pulmonary surfactant, leading to alveolar collapse [10], and causes compliance to decrease in inverse proportion to the fraction of lung volume that has been lost by *derecruitment*, i.e., the fraction of the lung to become blocked from receiving ventilation.

Transpulmonary pressure is the relevant distending pressure for the lung [5]. This concept, however, is often disregarded, and the effect of the chest wall in determining lung expansion and stress is barely considered in the clinical practice [6, 7].

Nevertheless, in ARDS patients, it is common that not only the lung but also the chest wall compliance is abnormally low due to the presence of obesity, increased abdominal pressure, chest wall deformities, and resuscitation with large fluid volumes [11, 12, 13].

It must be noted again that only if the pressure in the pleural space (P_{PL}) is estimated by measuring P_{ES}, C_L and C_{CW} can be determined separately. When P_{AO} is measured, the parameters E and R pertain to the entire respiratory system, which includes both the lungs and the chest wall, and therefore it is impossible to identify the separate contribution of the lung and chest wall to the stiffer respiratory system.

Due to several mechanisms, the elastance and compliance of both the lung and the chest wall and, therefore, of the respiratory system are not the same at different lung volumes, in other words the elastic behavior is not linear. The presence and amount of surfactant molecules at the air–liquid interface cause surface tension to vary with lung volume in determining lung hysteresis (i.e., the pressure at a given lung volume is different during inflation compared to deflation) and significant nonlinear mechanical behavior.

14.3 Methods for Assessing Respiratory Mechanics

The methods employed to assess respiratory mechanics in ARDS patients can be classified into two categories: static, or quasi-static, and dynamic.

14.3.1 Static Methods

Static, or quasi-static, methods are based on specific maneuvers that require to discontinue the patient from the normal setting of mechanical ventilation and to provide an estimation of compliance, and eventually resistance. Traditional techniques like the super syringe or the constant flow for *P*–*V* curve assessment and end-inspiratory occlusion can be classified under this category. Because these methods are able to estimate only a single value of compliance and resistance, they need to be repeated periodically in order to have the information regarding variations occurring over time in a given ARDS patient.

In a sedated ventilated patient, the pressure developed by the respiratory muscles (P_{MUS}) is equal to zero, and therefore P_{RS} is only given by the pressure generated by the mechanical ventilator (P_{VENT}) and Eq. 14.1 becomes

$$P_{RS} = P_{AO} - P_{BS} = P_{VENT}$$

Therefore, bringing the respiratory system to a given volume by applying a given pressure, compliance can be determined by measuring the pressure that under static conditions (e.g., by interrupting the flow at end-expiration) equals P_{EL} and by applying Eq. 14.4 in a situation where $P_{RES} = 0$.

The resistance can be determined, in turn, by calculating the pressure (P_{RES}) that has to be added to P_{EL} to reach peak inspiratory pressure just before interrupting the flow.

The measurement of esophageal pressure (P_{ES}), used as an estimate of pleural pressure (P_{PL}), is the only way to distinguish between the pulmonary system (comprising the airways and the lung) and the chest wall. When P_{ES} measurement is available during an end-inspiratory occlusion maneuver, its plateau pressure can be used to evaluate chest wall elastance (E_{CW}) (Fig. 14.4), which can be significantly high in patients with ARDS as a result of intra-abdominal hypertension, pleural effusion, massive ascites, thoracic trauma, and edema of the intrathoracic and intra-abdominal tissues as a result of fluid resuscitation [14. 15, 16, 17].

It must be noted that adjusting the ventilator settings only on the basis of P_{AO} may be incorrect [18], being P_{TP} the real "lung-distending" pressure promoting alveolar recruitment and lung inflation.

Moreover, in patients with ARDS, the reduced chest wall compliance, the presence of edema, or abdominal distension makes Pes very often elevated. Therefore, the calculated P_{TP} can be negative at end-expiration, this indicating closed airways, or flooded or the atelectatic lung, and in this case, PEEP must be increased until P_{TP} becomes positive to keep the airways open.

Super-Syringe Technique

The static reference method is the super-syringe method (Fig. 14.5a) [19]. Fixed increments of gas volume up to a total volume of 1.5–3 liters are applied to the

Fig. 14.4 (**a**) Representative example of airway opening pressure (P_{AO}), flow, and volume tracings obtained during a standard breath (volume-controlled mode with a constant flow) followed by an occlusion maneuver. Rapid interruption of airflow at the airway opening is performed using a mechanical ventilator equipped with facilities for end-inspiratory occlusion. Total respiratory system compliance (C_{RS}) is obtained as the ratio between tidal volume (ΔV) and elastic pressure P_{EL} (difference between plateau pressure Pplat, measured after a few seconds of occlusion, and PEEP). Total respiratory system resistance (R_{RS}) is obtained as the ratio between resistive pressure P_{RES} (difference between peak inspiratory pressure, PIP, and Pplat) and inspiratory flow V'_{INSP}. The patients are sedated and paralyzed (P_{MUS}=0, respiratory muscle generator switched-off in the figure). (**b**) Representative example of airway opening pressure (P_{AO}), esophageal pressure (P_{ES}), and flow and volume tracings obtained during an occlusion maneuver. Chest wall compliance (C_{CW}) is obtained as the ratio between tidal volume (ΔV) and elastic pressure of the chest wall $P_{EL,CW}$ (difference between P_{ES} plateau pressure and P_{ES} at end-expiration. The patients are sedated and paralyzed (P_{MUS}=0, respiratory muscle generator switched-off in the figure)

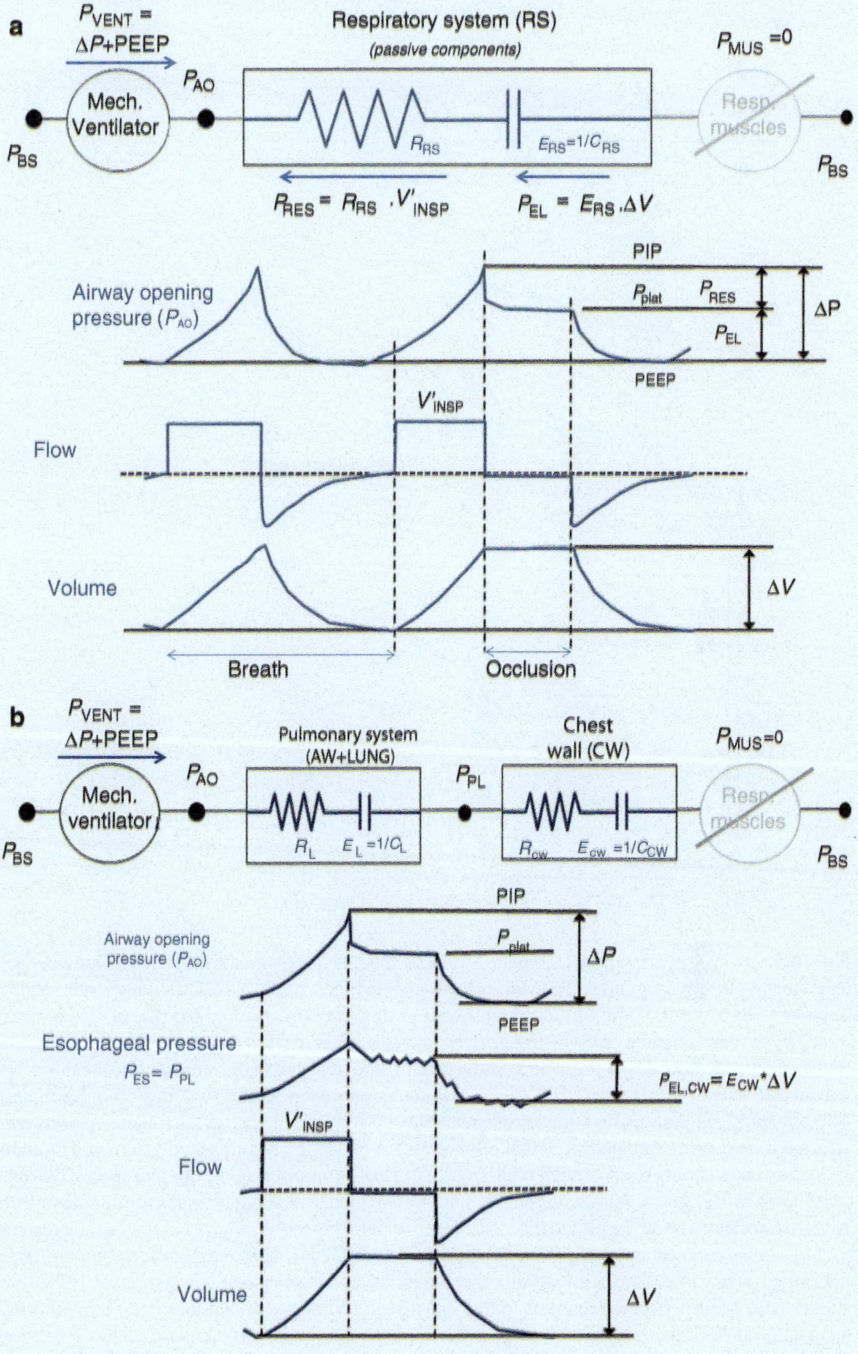
a
PVENT = ΔP+PEEP
Respiratory system (RS)
(passive components)
PMUS =0
PAO
Mech. Ventilator
RRS
ERS=1/CRS
Resp. muscles
PBS
PBS
PRES = RRS .V'INSP
PEL = ERS .ΔV
PIP
Airway opening pressure (PAO)
Pplat
PRES
ΔP
PEL
PEEP
V'INSP
Flow
Volume
ΔV
Breath
Occlusion
b
PVENT = ΔP+PEEP
Pulmonary system (AW+LUNG)
Chest wall (CW)
PMUS=0
PAO
PPL
Mech. ventilator
RL
EL =1/CL
Rcw
Ecw =1/CCW
Resp. muscles
PBS
PBS
PIP
Airway opening pressure (PAO)
Pplat
ΔP
PEEP
Esophageal pressure
PES= PPL
PEL,CW= ECW*ΔV
V'INSP
Flow
Volume
ΔV

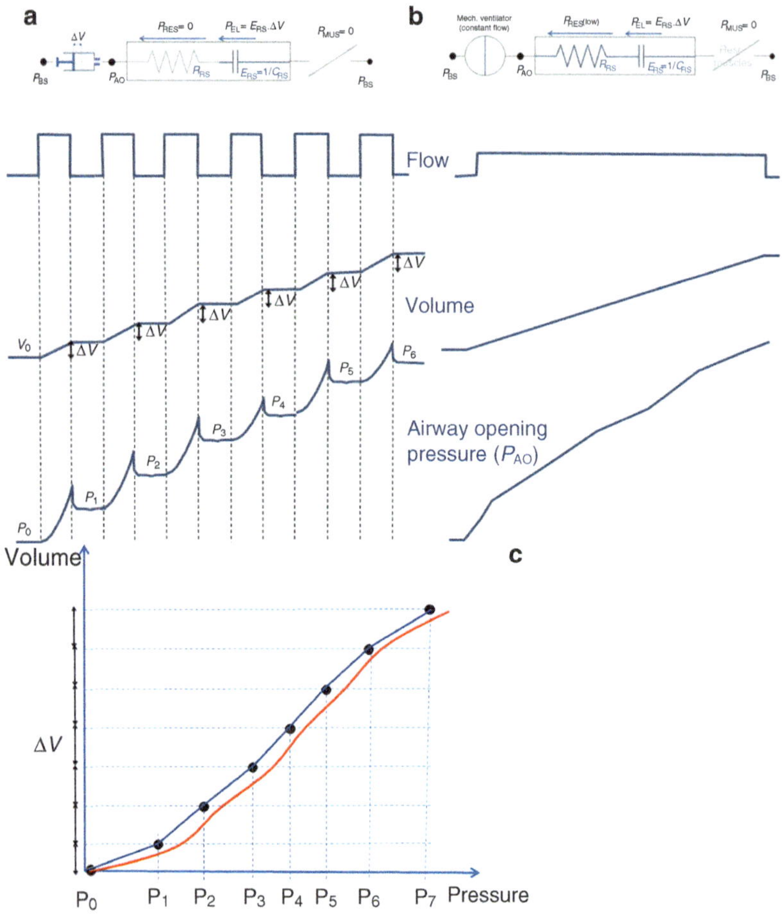

Fig. 14.5 (**a**) The super-syringe technique is a static method consisting of inflating the lungs in volume steps (ΔV in the figure) of 50–100 ml up to 1.5–3 liters, starting from the functional residual capacity (*FRC*). The volume of gas administered (with fractional inspired oxygen of 1.0) is determined by the displacement of the piston. Airway opening pressure (P_{AO}) is measured at the connection of the endotracheal tube by a pressure transducer, with zero referred to the atmospheric pressure. The patients are sedated and paralyzed ($P_{MUS} = 0$, respiratory muscle generator switched-off in the figure). The pressures and the volumes are recorded simultaneously, and the pressure–volume curve is constructed from the different plateau pressures that correspond to the administered volumes. The entire procedure takes about 60 s. A similar maneuver can be performed during deflation in successive steps (not shown in the figure). (**b**) An alternative, simple technique to obtain a pressure volume curve from an ARDS patient without having to disconnect the patient from the ventilator is to inflate the respiratory system by a constant flow delivered by the ventilator [23, 24]. This quasi-static technique can be performed on any intensive care ventilator that is equipped with a constant flow generator. (**c**) Several studies have been performed to compare the quasi-static technique at constant flow with the static technique [25–27]; the results showed that the compliances obtained by the two methods are very similar. An important parameter to be defined is the value of delivered constant flow. High constant flows (between 20 and 60 L/min) reliably estimate only the slope of the P–V curve, while upper and lower inflection points are overestimated because of the resistive effect (Fig. 14.2) [23, 24]. While very low flow allows accurate estimates, long measurement periods are required to inflate the lungs, which may result in a loss of lung volume during the maneuver because of oxygen uptake by the lungs

patient. After each increment, the static airway pressure is measured during a pause of a few seconds when there is no flow, and the pressure is the same in the entire system from the super syringe to the alveoli. The lung is then deflated in a similar way, and the inflation and deflation *P–V* curve is plotted. Oxygen consumption is constant during the whole procedure (i.e., inflation and deflation), which takes 45÷120 seconds. During inflation carbon dioxide removal from the alveoli is null, and its partial pressure in the blood increases. During deflation, carbon dioxide removal is therefore lower than baseline, and this causes expired volume to be less than inspired volume and the *P–V* curve has a marked artifactual hysteresis. In ARDS patients, alveolar recruitment taking place during the stepwise inflation to a high pressure will also cause hysteresis [20, 21].

Multiple Occlusion Technique

The multiple occlusion technique [22, 23] uses a sequence of different-sized volume-controlled inflations with an end-inspiratory pause to allow semi-static pressure measurements. Intrinsic PEEP is determined before each inflation to ensure that the lung volume and the end-expiratory pressure are stable. Pressure and volume are plotted for each end-inspiratory pause to form a static *P–V* curve. If expiratory interruptions are also done, a static expiratory *P–V* curve is obtained. Because the pressure and volume values are obtained during standard, but varying breaths, the artifacts caused by gas exchange do not occur, and no hysteresis is found even in ARDS patients. Although the largest tidal volumes used with this technique may cause recruitment, this is limited because the time at high pressure is very short. The entire set of measurements may take 5÷10 min.

The inspiratory occlusion technique offers the advantage of avoiding disconnection of the patient from the ventilator, and it allows measurements from any level of PEEP. Since the beginning of the 1990s, this technique has been extensively used to determine the lower and upper inflection points on the P–V curve [24, 25] and to quantify the effect of PEEP on alveolar recruitment in patients with ARDS [26]. The sudden change in pressure occurring with interruption of flow is accompanied by rapid damped oscillations and a subsequent further transient change in pressure to a stable plateau. These two phases have been interpreted on the basis of two-compartment models of respiratory mechanics [27, 28].

Low-Flow Inflation Technique

In the low-flow inflation technique [29, 30], a very low constant inspiratory flow is provided to the patient to generate a large total volume (Fig. 14.5b). The low flow causes a minimal but recognizable pressure decrease over the endotracheal tube, which means that the pressure–volume curve obtained under this "quasi-static" (dynamic, in truth) condition is shifted to the right with respect to a "true" static *P–V* curve (Fig. 14.5c). The amount of this shift depends on the resistance offered by the respiratory system, plus the resistance of the endotracheal tube, and the selected flow level. A high flow reduces the time required to obtain the curve, but it increases the shift. The slope of the curve, however, can be considered parallel with the true static *P–V* curve, under the hypothesis that airway resistance is constant throughout the inspiration, which is not true as resistance decreases with the lung volume. A low flow allows to reduce the shift, but the duration of the inspiration becomes long and the gas exchange artifacts above described for the super-syringe technique become significant. Other drawbacks of the low-flow inflation method are that this technique does not allow to obtain the deflation curve, it requires resetting the ventilator, and only volume-controlled ventilation can be used.

14.3.2 Dynamic Methods

Compared to static or quasi-static methods, *dynamic methods* are continuous and can be used as ventilator treatment is applied. Therefore, they are more methods of monitoring rather than of measurement of the mechanical properties of the respiratory system, and their lack of accuracy is counterbalanced to some degree by their capacity to follow trends.

In the past, various methods have been proposed to analyze respiratory mechanics during ongoing mechanical ventilation [31, 32, 33, 34]. The term "dynamic compliance" refers to the calculation of compliance under these conditions and is calculated by dividing the tidal volume by the peak airway pressure (minus PEEP). Dynamic compliance, so calculated, will always be lower than static compliance, as the former includes resistive pressure components, and therefore the term is incorrect. Therefore, methods that consider also the nonlinear mechanical behavior of the respiratory system [35, 36] are preferable.

Among these methods, in the SLICE method [37, 38, 39], the tidal volume of each breath is divided into different volume slices of equal size (Fig. 14.2). Multiple linear regression is then performed for each slice separately, solving the equation of motion (eq. 14.4). Flow-dependent pressure decrease along the artificial airway is also corrected.

A common aspect of all dynamic methods is that a specific model of the respiratory system is considered, and the mechanical properties are estimated in real time by best fitting the model with the data typically available in real time (typically, pressure, and flow) using different algorithms. A wide range of physiologically and clinically relevant models of respiratory mechanics and parameter estimation algorithms and methods have been proposed [4, 40–45], ranging from very simple, like the equations of motion described in the previous section of this chapter, to complex descriptive models. Simpler models are limited in their abilities to describe all respiratory mechanics, while more complex models can suffer from non-identifiability [46].

The dynamic methods are able to analyze the functional mechanics of the respiratory system under its actual ventilatory pattern as chosen by the caregiver. If any of the settings is being varied (e.g., during an incremental PEEP trial [39]), the dynamic analysis may serve to monitor the resulting changes in respiratory mechanics. Although these important advantages are offered by dynamic methods, only static and quasi-static methods are currently used in the clinical practice on ARDS patients. Static measurements are generally considered ideal, and the ventilator settings are based on them. Typically, ventilation is set with an end-inspiratory pause giving quasi-static conditions, so that an adequate plateau pressure indicates the maximal alveolar pressure. Intermittent application of a prolonged hold in expiration gives information about intrinsic PEEP.

Nevertheless, it is still an open question whether static measurements are truly superior to dynamic measurements. In fact, there is a discrepancy between the static methods used for research and the dynamic measurements of respiratory mechanics which are obtained under real clinical condition.

Very probably, the development of robust methods able to reliably minimize the effects of endotracheal tube and airway resistance will determine a wider use of dynamic methods in the future.

14.4 Assessment of "Active" Components

When the patient is spontaneously breathing and his/her respiratory muscles are working, irrespective of the work done by the ventilator, P_{MUS} becomes a significant component of Eq. 14.1. Under this condition, the lung-distending pressure is due to both the action of the ventilator and the patient, and the measurement of P_{ES}, an estimation of P_{PL}, is needed for an accurate estimation of P_{TP}. In presence of spontaneous breathing efforts while receiving mechanical ventilation, direct measurement of effort may help the clinician to better adjust the ventilator settings and/or the sedation level [47].

In the clinical setting, respiratory muscle effort can be assessed by either assessing the work of breathing (WOB) or by the pressure–time product (PTP), which are both useful approaches to estimate the energy dissipated or consumed by the respiratory muscles [48].

The work performed by the respiratory muscles during each inspiration (i.e., from the beginning of inspiratory flow to the end of inspiration) is expressed as the area enclosed between the dynamic esophageal pressure (P_{ES})–volume (V) curve and the static relaxation curve of the chest wall. This is classically referred as the Campbell diagram [49], in which at any time during inspiration, the pressure developed by the inspiratory muscles in expanding the chest wall (P_{MUS}) is determined as the horizontal distance between the current P_{ES}–V point on the diagram and the corresponding point on the chest relaxation curve at the same volume [50]. WOB can be expressed per breathing cycle, per minute (WOB per cycle multiplied by respiratory frequency), or per liter (work per minute divided by minute ventilation).

Respiratory muscle activity can also be assessed using the pressure–time product (PTP) index, which refers to the integral of pressure over time (the cumulative sum of sample-by-sample product of the pressure multiplied by the time difference between two consecutive samples) and not over volume, and, therefore, it can be used whether or not volume is generated. When PTP is calculated using esophageal pressure (PTP_{ES}), it provides an index of the effort done by all of the respiratory muscles. When PTP is calculated using transdiaphragmatic pressure ($P_{DI} = P_{GA} - P_{ES}$, where P_{GA} is gastric pressure, that provides an estimation of abdominal pressure) (PTP_{DI}), it reflects the effort performed by the diaphragm.

WOB is usually highly correlated to oxygen consumption [51]. In conditions like isometric contraction, however, WOB is insensitive to energy expenditure, and PTP_{ES} or PTP_{DI} has to be considered to estimate respiratory muscle oxygen consumption [52].

Although much less accurate than measurements of P_{MUS} or P_{DI}, in the clinical setting, inspiratory effort may be monitored simply by assessing P_{ES} changes during inspiration, in other words not taking into account the static recoil pressure of the relaxed chest wall [53].

14.5 Measurement Issues

14.5.1 Tracheal Pressure

In clinical practice, P_{AO} is measured in the ventilator or at the patient connection. This means that it is affected to a great extent by the endotracheal tube resistance, resulting in a peak inspiratory pressure (PIP) much greater than peak tracheal or peak alveolar pressure [54]. If an end-inspiratory occlusion technique is used, for example, the plateau pressure is the maximum pressure in the airway below the tube. Recording both PIP and plateau pressure gives useful information; for example, increased resistance caused by narrowing of the tube (secretions, kinking) will increase PIP and not affect plateau pressure [55], while the increased resistance is caused by the lungs of the patient below the tube, then both the PIP and the plateau pressure may increase.

By using measurements of flow, P_{AO}, and knowing the resistance of the endotracheal tube, which is obtained from laboratory testing of clean tubes and connectors, tracheal pressure can be calculated continuously. This has been used in commercially available ventilators, and ventilator flow is increased to overcome the endotracheal tube resistance [56]. However, caution should be taken when using a predetermined value of endotracheal tube resistance. Tube resistance is determined on laboratory measurements with clean tubes, which is a rare case in the real intensive care unit environment. Gas humidification and position/angulation of the endotracheal have also significant effects on resistance [57].

Direct tracheal pressure measurements can be made by passing a catheter through the endotracheal tube in order to obtain tracheal pressure values where flow changes caused by the transition from trachea to endotracheal tube are minimized, typically 2 cm above the carina. When using side-hole catheters, the correct position is difficult to be verified. End-hole catheters, on the other hand, are less dependent on position, but measurements are affected by gas kinetic pressure. However, the kinetic energy of gas is so small that this effect on the total measured pressure is negligible.

The pressure catheter can be gas or fluid filled. Fluid-filled catheters, although requiring that the transducer is at the same level as the catheter tip to measure absolute pressure accurately, are less sensitive to secretions and occlusion [55].

Nevertheless, direct tracheal pressure measurements provide correct end-inspiratory and expiratory pressures, including intrinsic PEEP caused by ETT resistance, without stopping ventilation and irrespective of ventilatory mode.

14.5.2 Esophageal Pressure

The most common technique for P_{ES} measurement is to use a catheter with a thin-walled latex balloon sealed at its distal port and filled with air [47, 58]. After anesthetizing the nose and oropharynx, the catheter is inserted through the nostril. The empty balloon catheter is advanced into the stomach, at which time the balloon is inflated. If no diaphragmatic paralysis is present, the presence of an increase in pressure during a spontaneous inspiration generally indicates that the balloon is in the stomach. Afterward, the catheter is slowly withdrawn until a negative pressure deflection replaces the positive deflection, indicating that the balloon is in the lower third of esophagus [59]. The distal part of the catheter is connected to a pressure transducer, which, in turn, can be connected to a dedicated acquisition system, a patient-monitoring system, or an auxiliary pressure port of the ventilator.

There are different types of esophageal catheters available on the market, each one characterized by different length, diameter, and compliance and filling volume of the balloon. These characteristics influence the measurement and must always be taken into account to ensure an accurate estimate of P_{PL}. The filling volume represents a critical issue. Volumes too small determine an underestimation of P_{ES}, while overfilling will stretch the balloon leading to overestimation [60]. New commercially available catheters [61] allow to combine the balloon with a regular nasogastric tube that can be used for enteral feeding, and it is known to not impair the measurement [62].

When inspiratory efforts are made against an occluded airway, the deflections in P_{ES} should match P_{AO}. Thus, a regression of P_{ES} vs. P_{AO} should yield a slope of unity. In practice, slopes that differ from 1.0 by up to 10% are common [63]. In sedated and paralyzed patients, the occlusion test is performed by applying manual compression on the chest during airway occlusion [64]. Factors that should be checked periodically influencing measurement accuracy include the position of the balloon, the amount of air injected into the balloon, the patient's position, and the lung volume. Cardiac artifacts and esophageal contraction due to peristalsis can distort the P_{ES} signal [65].

14.5.3 Abdominal Pressure

A method similar to that for P_{ES} can be used for gastric pressure (P_{GA}) measurements, which will reflect intra-abdominal pressure (P_{AB}). Abdominal pressure can also be measured via a urinary catheter. The bladder is drained of its content after which 50 ± 100 ml of saline is instilled, and the catheter is clamped distal to the pressure measurement position [66]. Measurements of intra-abdominal pressure obtained from a gastric tube and from bladder pressure have been compared, with the two pressures within 2.5 cmH_2O [67].

14.5.4 Lung Volume

Measurements of lung volume variations are usually obtained by integrating the digitized flow signal consisting of a series of data points separated by equal time intervals. A simple method for numerical integration is to calculate the area under the curve defined by the series of measured data. Integration drift represents an important problem. When flow is integrated to yield volume, an upward or downward drift in the volume baseline is invariably seen. This is due to physiological reasons and methodological factors including temperature changes between inspired and expired gas, changes in gas composition between inspiration and expiration, leakages, zero offset in flow calibration, and imperfections in the flowmeter response [68]. It is very difficult, if not impossible, to keep under control all these factors and to avoid drift in volume. Consequently, it is never known how much of the baseline drift in volume is due to drift and how much represents a true change in absolute lung volume.

Monitoring of end-expiratory lung volume (EELV) is essential, however, in the management of patients with ARDS [69]. When dilution techniques are used, mostly for research purposes, the patient breathes in a fixed concentration of helium or methane mixed with oxygen and the concentration in the expired breath can be used to calculate the FRC. An alternative approach is a washout/washin technique using nitrogen or oxygen. By changing the FiO_2 abruptly by 0.1, the FRC could be calculated with acceptable accuracy by using standard gas monitoring equipment [70, 71, 72]. When application of PEEP determines EELV to increase, EELV changes can be combined with compliance values in order to differentiate between recruitment and distention [73]. Knowing compliance, the expected change in EELV for a given change in PEEP is compared to the measured EELV to estimate alveolar recruitment at the bedside [74].

References

1. Acute Respiratory Distress Syndrome Network (2000) Ventilation with lower tidal volume as compared with traditional tidal volumes for acute lung injury and the acute respiratory distress syndrome. N Engl J Med 342:1301–1308
2. Amato MB, Barbas CS, Medeiros DM et al (1998) Effect of protective ventilation strategy on mortality in the acute respiratory distress syndrome. N Engl J Med 338:347–354
3. Amato MBP, Meade MO, Slutsky AS et al (2015) Driving pressure and survival in the acute respiratory distress syndrome. N Engl J Med 372:747–755
4. Bates JHT (2009) Lung mechanics: an inverse modeling approach. Cambridge University Press, New York
5. Mead J, Takishima T, Leith D (1970) Stress distribution in lungs: a model of pulmonary elasticity. J Appl Physiol 28:596–608
6. Loring SH, O'Donnell CR, Behazin N et al (2010) Esophageal pressures in acute lung injury: do they represent artifact or useful information about transpulmonary pressure, chest wall mechanics, and lung stress? J Appl Physiol (1985) 108:515–522
7. Talmor D, Sarge T, Malhotra A et al (2008) Mechanical ventilation guided by esophageal pressure in acute lung injury. N Engl J Med 359:2095–2104
8. Milic-Emili J, Mead J, Turner JM, Glauser EM (1964) Improve technique for estimating pleural pressure from esophageal balloons. J Appl Physiol 19:207–211
9. Mead J, Gaensler EA (1959) Esophageal and pleural pressures in man, upright and supine. J Appl Physiol 14:81–83
10. Cross LJ, Matthay MA (2011) Biomarkers in acute lung injury: insights into the pathogenesis of acute lung injury. Crit Care Clin 27:355–377
11. Hibbert K, Rice M, Malhotra A (2012) Obesity and ARDS. Chest 142:785–790
12. Malbrain MLNG, Chiumello D, Pelosi P et al (2004) Prevalence of intra-abdominal hypertension in critically ill patients: a multicentre epidemiological study. Intensive Care Med 30:822–829
13. Mutoh T, Lamm WJ, Embree LJ, Hildebrandt J, Albert RK (1991) Abdominal distension alters regional pleural pressures and chest wall mechanics in pigs in vivo. J Appl Physiol 70:2611–2618

14. Malbrain ML, Cheatham ML, Kirkpatrick A, Sugrue M, Parr M, De Waele J, Balogh Z, Leppaniemi A, Olvera C et al (2006) Results from the International Conference of Experts on Intra-abdominal Hypertension and Abdominal Compartment Syndrome. I Definitions. Intensive Care Med 32:1722–1732
15. Ranieri VM, Brienza N, Santostasi S, Puntillo F, Mascia L, Vitale N, Giuliani R, Memeo V, Bruno F, Fiore T et al (1997) Impairment of lung and chest wall mechanics in patients with acute respiratory distress syndrome: role of abdominal distension. Am J Respir Crit Care Med 156:1082–1091
16. Kirkpatrick AW, Roberts DJ, De Waele J, Jaeschke R, Malbrain ML, De Keulenaer B, Duchesne J, Bjorck M, Leppaniemi A, Ejike JC et al (2013) Pediatric Guidelines Sub-Committee for the World Society of the Abdominal Compartment Syndrome. Intra-abdominal hypertension and the abdominal compartment syndrome: updated consensus definitions and clinical practice guidelines from the World Society of the Abdominal Compartment Syndrome. Intensive Care Med 39:1190–1206
17. Terragni PP, Filippini C, Slutsky AS, Birocco A, Tenaglia T, Grasso S, Stripoli T, Pasero D, Urbino R, Fanelli V et al (2013) Accuracy of plateau pressure and stress index to identify injurious ventilation in patients with acute respiratory distress syndrome. Anesthesiology 119:880–889
18. Pelosi P, Cereda M, Foti G, Giacomini M, Pesenti A (1995) Alterations of lung and chest wall mechanics in patients with acute lung injury: effects of positive end-expiratory pressure. Am J Respir Crit Care Med 152:531–537
19. Brochard L (1998) Respiratory pressure±volume curves. In: Tobin M (ed) Principles and practice of intensive care monitoring. McGraw Hill, New York, pp 597–616
20. Gattinoni L, Mascheroni D, Basilico E, Foti G, Pesenti A, Avalli L (1987) Volume/pressure curve of total respiratory system in paralysed patients: artefacts and correction factors. Intensive Care Med 13:19–25
21. Chiumello D, Carlesso E, Aliverti A, Dellacà RL, Pedotti A, Pelosi PP, Gattinoni L (2007) Effects of volume shift on the pressure-volume curve of the respiratory system in ALI/ARDS patients. Minerva Anestesiol 73(3):109–118
22. Jonson B, Beydon L, Brauer K, Mansson C, Valind S, Grytzell H (1993) Mechanics of respiratory system in healthy anesthetized humans with emphasis on viscoelastic properties. J Appl Physiol 75:132–140
23. Levy P, Similowski T, Corbeil C et al (1989) A method for studying the static volume±pressure curves of the respiratory system during mechanical ventilation. J Crit Care 4:83–89
24. Roupie E, Dambrosio M, Servillo G et al (1995) Titration of tidal volume and induced hypercapnia in acute respiratory distress syndrome. Am J Respir Crit Care Med 152:121–128
25. Ranieri VM, Mascia LM, Fiore T et al (1995) Cardiorespiratory effects of positive end-expiratory pressure during progressive tidal volume reduction (permissive hypercapnia) in patients with acute respiratory distress syndrome. Anesthesiology 83:710–720
26. Ranieri VM, Giuliani R, Flore T et al (1994) Volume–pressure curve of the respiratory system predicts effects of PEEP in ARDS: 'occlusion' versus 'constant flow' technique. Am J Respir Crit Care Med 149:19–27
27. Bates JH, Baconnier P, Milic-Emili J (1988) A theoretical analysis of interrupter technique for measuring respiratory mechanics. J Appl Physiol 64:2204–2214
28. Bates JH, Rossi A, Milic-Emili J (1985) Analysis of the behavior of the respiratory system with constant inspiratory flow. J Appl Physiol 58:1840–1848
29. Lu Q, Vieira SR, Richecoeur J et al (1999) A simple method for measuring pressure-volume curves during mechanical ventilation. Am J Respir Crit Care Med 159:275–282
30. Servillo G, Svantesson C, Beydon L et al (1997) Pressure-volume curves in acute respiratory failure: automated low flow versus occlusion. Am J Respir Crit Care Med 155:1629–1636
31. Suratt PM, Owens DH, Kilgore WT et al (1980) A pulse method of measuring respiratory system compliance. J Appl Physiol 49:1116–1121
32. Rossi A, Gottfried SB, Higgs BD et al (1985) Respiratory mechanics in mechanically ventilated. patients with respiratory failure. J Appl Physiol 58:1849–1858
33. Wald A, Jason D, Murphy TW et al (1969) A computer system for respiratory parameters. Comput Biomed Res 2:411–429

34. Uhl RR, Lewis FJ (1974) Digital computer calculation of human pulmonary mechanics using a least squares fit technique. Comput Biomed Res 7:489–495
35. Ranieri VM, Zhang H, Mascia L et al (2000) Pressure-time curve predicts minimally injurious ventilatory strategy in an isolated rat lung model. Anesthesiology 93:1320–1328
36. Karason S, Sondergaard S, Lundin S et al (2000) A new method for non-invasive, manoeuvre free determination of "static" pressure-volume curves during dynamic/therapeutic mechanical ventilation. Acta Anaesthesiol Scand 44:578–585
37. Guttmann J, Eberhard L, Fabry B et al (1994) Determination of volume-dependent respiratory system mechanics in mechanically ventilated patients using the new SLICE method. Technol Health Care 2:175–191
38. Mols G, Brandes I, Kessler V et al (1999) Volume dependent compliance in ARDS: Proposal of a new diagnostic concept. Intensive Care Med 25:1084–1091
39. Stahl CA, Möller K, Schumann S, Kuhlen R, Sydow M, Putensen C et al (2006) Dynamic versus static respiratory mechanics in acute lung injury and acute respiratory distress syndrome. Crit Care Med 34:2090–2098
40. Mount LE (1955) The ventilation flow-resistance and compliance of rat lungs. J Physiol 127:157–167
41. van Drunen E, Chiew YS, Chase J, Shaw G, Lambermont B, Janssen N et al (2013) Expiratory model-based method to monitor ARDS disease state. Biomed Eng Online 12:57–71
42. Hickling KG (1998) The pressure–volume curve is greatly modified by recruitment. A mathematical model of ARDS lungs. Am J Respir Crit Care Med 158:194–202
43. Sundaresan A, Yuta T, Hann CE, Geoffrey Chase J, Shaw GM (2009) A minimal model of lung mechanics and model-based markers for optimizing ventilator treatment in ARDS patients. Comput Methods Prog Biomed 95:166–180
44. Salazar E, Knowles JH (1964) An analysis of pressure–volume characteristics of the lungs. J Appl Physiol 19:97–104
45. Schranz C, Docherty PD, Chiew YS, Chase JG, Moller K (2012) Structural identifiability and practical applicability of an alveolar recruitment model for ARDS patients. IEEE Trans Biomed Eng 59:3396–3404
46. Docherty PD, Schranz C, Chiew YS, Möller K, Chase JG (2014) Reformulation of the pressure-dependent recruitment model (PRM) of respiratory mechanics. Biomed Signal Process Control 12:47–53
47. Akoumianaki E, Maggiore SM, Valenza F, Bellani G, Jubran A, Loring SH, Pelosi P, Talmor D, Grasso S, Chiumello D, Guérin C, Patroniti N, Ranieri VM, Gattinoni L, Nava S, Terragni PP, Pesenti A, Tobin M, Mancebo J, Brochard L (2014) PLUG Working Group (Acute Respiratory Failure Section of the European Society of Intensive Care Medicine). The application of esophageal pressure measurement in patients with respiratory failure. Am J Respir Crit Care Med 189(5):520–531
48. Roussos C (1985) Structure and function of the thorax: Energetics. In: Roussos C, Macklem PT (eds) The thorax. Marcel Dekker, New York, pp 437–492
49. Agostoni E, Campbell EJM, Freedman S (1970) Energetics. In: Campbell EJM, Agostoni E, Davis NJ (eds) The respiratory muscles. WB Saunders, Philadelphia, pp 115–137
50. Aliverti A, Carlesso E, Dellacà R, Pelosi P, Chiumello D, Pedotti A, Gattinoni L (2006) Chest wall mechanics during pressure support ventilation. Crit Care 10(2):R54
51. Robertson CH Jr, Foster GH, Johnson RL Jr (1977) The relationship of respiratory failure to the oxygen consumption of, lactate production by, and distribution of blood flow among respiratory muscles during increasing inspiratory resistance. J Clin Invest 59:31–42
52. Tobin MJ, Laghi F, Jubran A (2012) Ventilatory failure, ventilator support, and ventilator weaning. Compr Physiol 2:2871–2921
53. Jubran A, Grant BJ, Laghi F, Parthasarathy S, Tobin MJ (2005) Weaning prediction: esophageal pressure monitoring complements readiness testing. Am J Respir Crit Care Med 171: 1252–1259
54. Conti G, de Blasi RA, Lappa A et al (1994) Evaluation of respiratory system resistance in mechanically ventilated patients: the role of the endotracheal tube. Intensive Care Med 20:421–424

55. Stenqvist O (2003) Practical assessment of respiratory mechanics. Br J Anaesth 91:92–105
56. Guttmann J, Eberhard L, Fabry B, Bertschmann W, Wolff G (1993) Continuous calculation of intratracheal pressure in tracheally intubated patients. Anesthesiology 79:503–513
57. Loring SH, Elliott EA, Drazen JM (1979) Kinetic energy loss and convective acceleration in respiratory resistance measurements. Lung 156:33–42
58. Cherniack RM, Farhi LE, Armstrong BW, Proctor DF (1955) A comparison of esophageal and intrapleural pressure in man. J Appl Physiol 8:203–211
59. Benditt JO (2005) Esophageal and gastric pressure measurements. Respir Care 50:68–75
60. Mojoli F, Chiumello D, Pozzi M et al (2015) Esophageal pressure measurements under different conditions of intrathoracic pressure. An in vitro study of second generation balloon catheters. Minerva Anestesiol 81:855–864
61. Chiumello D, Gallazzi E, Marino A et al (2011) A validation study of a new naso-gastric polyfunctional catheter. Intensive Care Med 37:791–795
62. Niknam J, Chandra A, Adams AB, Nahum A, Ravenscraft SA, Marini JJ (1994) Effect of a nasogastric tube on esophageal pressure measurement in normal adults. Chest 106:137–141
63. Dechman G, Sato J, Bates JHT (1992) Factors affecting the accuracy of esophageal balloon measurement of pleural pressure in dogs. J Appl Physiol 72:383–388
64. D'Angelo E, Robatto FM, Calderini E, Tavola M, Bono D, Torri G, Milic-Emili J (1991) Pulmonary and chest wall mechanics in anesthetized paralyzed humans. J Appl Physiol 70:2602–2610
65. Baydur A, Cha EJ, Sassoon CS (1987) Validation of esophageal balloon technique at different lung volumes and postures. J Appl Physiol 62:315–321
66. Iberti TJ, Kelly KM, Gentili DR, Hirsch S (1987) A simple technique to accurately determine intra-abdominal pressure. Crit Care Med 15:1140–1142
67. Collee GG, Lomax DM, Ferguson C, Hanson GC (1993) Bedside measurement of intraabdominal pressure (IAP) via an indwelling naso-gastric tube: clinical validation of the technique. Intensive Care Med 19(8):478–480
68. Bates JH, Schmalisch G, Filbrun D, Stocks J (2000) Tidal breath analysis for infant pulmonary function testing. Eur Respir J 16:1180–1192
69. Brochard L, Martin GS, Blanch L, Pelosi P, Belda FJ, Jubran A, Gattinoni L, Mancebo J, Ranieri VM, Richard JC, Gommers D, Vieillard-Baron A, Pesenti A, Jaber S, Stenqvist O, Vincent JL (2012) Clinical review: respiratory monitoring in the ICU - a consensus of 16. Crit Care 16(2):219
70. Olegard C, Sondergaard S, Houltz E, Lundin S, Stenqvist O (2005) Estimation of functional residual capacity at the bedside using standard monitoring equipment: a modified nitrogen washout/washin technique requiring a small change of the inspired oxygen fraction. Anesth Analg 101:206–212
71. Chiumello D, Cressoni M, Chierichetti M, Tallarini F, Botticelli M, Berto V, Mietto C, Gattinoni L (2008) Nitrogen washout/washin, helium dilution and computed tomography in the assessment of end expiratory lung volume. Crit Care 12:R150
72. Patroniti N, Saini M, Zanella A, Weismann D, Isgro S, Bellani G, Foti G, Pesenti A (2008) Measurement of end-expiratory lung volume by oxygen washin- washout in controlled and assisted mechanically ventilated patients. Intensive Care Med 34:2235–2240
73. Bikker IG, van Bommel J, Reis Miranda D, Bakker J, Gommers D (2008) End-expiratory lung volume during mechanical ventilation: a comparison with reference values and the effect of positive end-expiratory pressure in intensive care unit patients with different lung conditions. Crit Care 12:R145
74. Bouhemad B, Brisson H, Le-Guen M, Arbelot C, Lu Q, Rouby JJ (2011) Bedside ultrasound assessment of positive end-expiratory pressure-induced lung recruitment. Am J Respir Crit Care Med 183:341–347

15 Noninvasive Ventilatory Support in Acute Respiratory Distress Syndrome

Martin DRES and Laurent Brochard

15.1 Introduction

Invasive mechanical ventilation is the cornerstone of the treatment of acute respiratory failure. Nevertheless, it is now well established that invasive mechanical ventilation can expose patients to several potential complications such as ventilator-induced diaphragm dysfunction [1], ventilator-acquired pneumonia [2], and/or ventilator-induced lung injury (VILI) [3]. These complications, some of them potentially lethal, encouraged clinicians to consider alternatives to invasive mechanical ventilation in patients presenting acute respiratory failure. Noninvasive ventilation (NIV) has become an inescapable strategy in acute hypercapnic respiratory failure related to exacerbation of chronic obstructive pulmonary disease (COPD) and/or cardiogenic pulmonary edema. In these two settings, NIV has been shown to reduce the risk of intubation and mortality [4, 5]. Since more than two decades, the scope of NIV application has largely been expended beyond acute hypercapnic respiratory failure. Currently, NIV is applied in various settings such as immunocompromised patients with acute hypoxemic respiratory failure [6], periprocedural management

M. DRES, MD
Sorbonne Universités, UPMC Univ Paris 06, INSERM, UMRS_1158 Neurophysiologie Respiratoire Expérimentale et Clinique, Paris, France

Keenan Research Centre for Biomedical Science, Li Ka Shing Knowledge Institute, St. Michael's Hospital, 30 Bond St, Toronto, ON M5B 1W8, Canada

Interdepartmental Division of Critical Care Medicine, University of Toronto, Toronto, ON, Canada

L. Brochard, MD (✉)
Keenan Research Centre for Biomedical Science, Li Ka Shing Knowledge Institute, St. Michael's Hospital, 30 Bond St, Toronto, ON M5B 1W8, Canada

Interdepartmental Division of Critical Care Medicine, University of Toronto, Toronto, ON, Canada
e-mail: BrochardL@smh.ca

D. Chiumello (ed.), *Acute Respiratory Distress Syndrome (ARDS)*,
DOI 10.1007/978-3-319-41852-0_15

such as bronchoscopy and bronchoalveolar lavage in hypoxemic patients [7], post-extubation in high-risk patients [8], or in postoperative patients [9] with beneficial results after abdominal surgery [10, 11]. In acute hypoxemic respiratory failure, the benefit of NIV on the reduction of intubation rate and mortality has been suggested in a meta-analysis from five randomized controlled trials [12]. Acute respiratory distress syndrome (ARDS) represents the most severe form of hypoxemic acute respiratory failure [13], and the heterogeneity of circumstances causing this condition makes difficult to perfectly interpret the benefits of NIV in this group of patients. In the present chapter, we will discuss the rationale, benefits, and risks of the use of NIV in acute hypoxemic respiratory failure. We will not strictly focus on ARDS since the criteria for its diagnosis are not always present before intubation, e.g., the need for a positive end-expiratory pressure of 5 cmH_2O or higher, and there are only few studies focusing specifically on NIV in acute hypoxemic respiratory failure fulfilling the most recent ARDS definition [14]. Since the use of high-flow oxygen through nasal cannula (HFNC) has been recently investigated in this setting, we will also review its potential interests. We will discuss the use of NIV and HFNC in a specific group of patients at high risk, namely, immunocompromised patients presenting acute hypoxemic respiratory failure. Last, we will discuss patients with a high drive to breathe where the application of a lung-protective strategy is a necessary treatment, making noninvasive supports mostly contraindicated.

15.2 Standard of Care for Ventilation Strategy of ARDS

ARDS is a life-threatening condition characterized by an acute hypoxemia and respiratory distress and which most often requires mechanical ventilation [13]. A lung-protective ventilation strategy is now proposed as a standard of care for patients presenting ARDS relying on the use of low tidal volume (6 $mL\cdot kg^{-1}$ predicted body weight) and positive end-expiratory pressure and limiting the inspiratory plateau pressure to <28–30 cmH_2O. Probably by optimizing lung-protective ventilation, there is some evidence that the use of neuromuscular-blocking agents at the early phase of ARDS may be beneficial [15]. The cost of such protective strategy may be a complete inactivity of the diaphragm and of the other respiratory muscles that may lead to disuse atrophy and muscle weakness [1]. This can contribute to difficulties in separating patients from the ventilator, prolongation of mechanical ventilation, and poorer prognosis. Hence, there has been a huge interest in the use of noninvasive ventilatory supports such as NIV and HFNC.

15.3 Rationale, Benefits, and Risks of Using NIV in ARDS

Invasive mechanical ventilation increases oxygenation, decreases the work of breathing, helps to reopen or to keep open collapsed alveoli, and improves respiratory mechanics. However, mechanical ventilation per se can aggravate lung injury, a process referred to as ventilator-induced lung injury (VILI) [3]. Moreover, mechanical ventilation can also lead to other complications such as ventilator-induced diaphragm dysfunction [1] and ventilator-acquired pneumonia [2]. In this context, NIV has been used to ensure ventilatory support instead of invasive mechanical ventilation. From a physiological point of view, the application of positive airway pressure can on the one hand reduce the work of breathing [16] and, on the other hand, opens under or non-ventilated alveoli and increases functional residual capacity, thus decreasing right-to-left intrapulmonary shunt and improving lung mechanics. In patients with the mild form of ARDS, NIV has been shown to increase oxygenation, reduce dyspnea, and unload the respiratory muscles [16]. In those patients, continuous positive airway pressure alone improves gas exchange but does not unload the respiratory muscles efficiently, whereas NIV with two levels of pressure proves more efficient, unloading the respiratory muscles and relieving dyspnea, compared to continuous positive airway pressure [16]. Finding the good combination of end-expiratory and inspiratory pressure is not easy, however, since the maximal applied pressure is generally limited to 20 or 25 cmH_2O, because of leaks and discomfort. An individual titration on both oxygenation (PEEP) and comfort and work of breathing (pressure support) is therefore necessary.

15.3.1 What Do the Observational Studies Tell Us?

According to current guidelines [17], the use of NIV is not clearly recommended in acute hypoxemic respiratory failure, but it is interesting to see how NIV is used in real life by physicians. In an observational survey performed in France in 42 intensive care units and published in 2001, Carlucci et al. reported that NIV was employed in 14% of patients with acute hypoxemic respiratory failure [18]. More recently, a cohort study in acute care hospitals in Massachusetts reported that between 2004 and 2007, NIV was used in 37.8% of de novo acute hypoxemic respiratory failure [19]. In an Ontario practice survey, Burns and colleagues reported that 25% of the respondents have used NIV in ARDS/ALI [20]. A population-based study reported that in the USA, the proportion of patients without COPD who received NIV increased from 1.2% in 2000 to 6.0% in 2009 [21]. Interestingly, recent data coming from a longitudinal observational study comparing trends of the use of NIV on a 10-year period, from 2002 to 2010/2011 and performed mostly in France, show slightly different results [22]. In this last study, Demoule et al. described a recent decrease in the use of NIV in de novo acute hypoxemic respiratory failure, from 23% in 2002 to 16% in 2010/2011 [22]. The most recent report is coming from the Large observational study to UNderstand the Global impact of Severe Acute respiratory FailurE (LUNG SAFE) which reported that among 2813 patients with ARDS, 436 (15%) were treated initially with NIV [23].

15.3.2 What Are the Expected Benefits?

The use of NIV to prevent invasive mechanical ventilation is expected to be associated with a decrease in the occurrence of several complications generally attributed to invasive mechanical ventilation. This was shown regarding the risk of nosocomial pneumonia. In 2000, Girou et al. reported in a matched case-control study that the use of NIV was associated with lower rate of ventilator-acquired pneumonia and a reduced ICU mortality as compared to conventional mechanical ventilation [24]. Randomized controlled trials showed reduced mortality with NIV in highly selected populations presenting acute hypoxemic respiratory failure such as patients with immunosuppression [25, 26]. Others have reported similar benefit in non-immunocompromised patients either in very selected population [27] or in heterogeneous groups [28–30]. Hence, it appears that NIV could be beneficial in some patients, but the overall evidence is not entirely consistent. The use of NIV in ARDS is, however, also associated with two potential risks: delaying the time for intubation and possibly favoring lung injury with relative hyperventilation.

15.3.3 NIV Could Delay the Timing of Intubation

By providing high level of inspired oxygen and improving oxygenation, NIV may delay the timing of intubation by masking a progressive worsening. By contrast to hypercapnic acute respiratory failure, where delayed intubation in case of NIV failure does not seem to be associated with worst outcome [28–29, 31], in acute hypoxemic respiratory failure, delayed intubation could be associated with an increase in mortality [32]. Considering that acute hypoxemic acute respiratory failure represents a syndrome of variable etiology and severity, it is not so surprising that the benefit of NIV within this syndrome varies. A recent secondary analysis of a prospective observational cohort study published by Kangelaris et al. analyzed data on 457 patients with ARDS [33]. Among them, 106 (23%) were not intubated at the time of meeting all ARDS criteria. Non-intubated patients had lower morbidity and severity of illness than intubated patients. However, mortality at day 60 was the same (36%) in both groups ($p = 0.91$). Among the 106 non-intubated patients, 36 (34%) required intubation within the subsequent 3 days of follow-up, and this late-intubation subgroup had significantly higher 60-day mortality (56%) when compared with both early intubation group (36%, $p = 0.03$) and patients never requiring intubation (26%; $p = 0.002$). The increased mortality in the late-intubation group persisted at 2-year follow-up. In another prospective cohort, among 170 patients meeting the Berlin definition for ARDS [14], 96 (56%) were initially managed with NIV [34]. Among them, 42 patients (44%) were intubated. NIV failure and mortality were significantly higher in moderate and severe ARDS.

15.3.4 NIV Cannot Counteract an Injurious Breathing Pattern

NIV has been proposed to prevent some of the potential complication of invasive mechanical ventilation such as ventilator-induced lung injury. However, recent data report that NIV cannot prevent its occurrence or can even facilitate it. Alveolar overdistension and alveolar recruitment and derecruitment are thought to be the two main mechanisms of ventilator-induced lung injury (VILI). Carteaux et al. recently assessed expired tidal volume in patients undergoing NIV for acute hypoxemic respiratory failure in a prospective observational study involving 62 patients [35]. They showed first that delivered tidal volumes were higher than expected and could not be controlled by the settings. In particular, the median (interquartile range) tidal volume was 9.8 mL/kg predicted body weight (8.1–11.1 mL/kg predicted body weight), although the targeted tidal volume was 6–8 mL/kg predicted body weight. Therefore, the high tidal volume was primarily driven by a high respiratory drive of the patients, and this could not be controlled by the NIV settings. In this study, high tidal volume was independently associated with NIV failure, which occurred in 51% of the cases. In the subgroup of patients with PaO_2/FiO_2 of less than 200 mmHg, a cumulative tidal volume of 9.5 mL/kg accurately predicted NIV failure with a sensitivity of 82% and a specificity of 87%. These data are remarkable with regard to the potential contributing role of high tidal volume during acute respiratory failure and NIV to a possible lung injury induced by an injurious breathing pattern. The recent FLORALI trial reported a nonsignificantly different 90-day mortality between NIV and spontaneous breathing but a lower mortality with high-flow oxygen therapy [36]. Interestingly, the authors noted that NIV administered to patients with severe lung injury could have increased the incidence of ventilator-induced lung injury by increasing tidal volumes that exceeded 9 mL/kg of predicted body weight. In clinical practice, however, tidal volume is never measured in spontaneously breathing patients, and this injurious breathing pattern may also exist without NIV. It is therefore possible that NIV should be reserved to patients without an excessive drive and able to control tidal volumes around 8 mL/kg PBW.

15.3.5 Clinical Studies Assessing NIV in ARDS

NIV has been chiefly evaluated in two indications in ALI/ARDS: first, as an alternative to invasive mechanical ventilation in patients with acute hypoxemic respiratory failure meeting criteria for intubation, and second, as a mean of avoiding intubation in patients with acute respiratory failure who do not meet criteria for invasive mechanical ventilation.

15.3.5.1 NIV as an Alternative to Invasive Mechanical Ventilation

This indication has been investigated in the seminal study by Antonelli et al. [28]. The authors compared conventional mechanical ventilation and NIV (pressure support plus positive end-expiratory pressure). They reported similar improvement in gas exchange with the two techniques. Notably, only 31% of patients (10/32) treated with NIV required tracheal intubation. Furthermore, authors found that 9 of the 10 patients who were intubated after failing the NIV attempt died in the ICU (90%), whereas only 15 of 32 (47%) who had been intubated without a previous NIV trial died [28]. Complications were decreased in the group using NIV, and mortality tended to be lower with NIV. The study design differs from other NIV studies. The more conventional design has been to randomize patients to NIV or conventional medical therapy as a way to prevent the need for intubation, intubation being an outcome variable. When patients in the control group are intubated per study protocol, it prompts the question of whether intubation was indeed mandatory in all patients in the control group. Furthermore, the study of Antonelli et al. enrolled patients with a variety of diagnoses, making it difficult to apply the study findings to individual patients presenting with acute hypoxemic respiratory failure. Finally, this was a small sample size of patients coming from a single-center study. This kind of protocol has never been replicated. Therefore, the role of NIV with acute hypoxemic respiratory failure as an alternative to intubation remains ambiguous.

15.3.5.2 NIV as a Prophylactic Ventilator Support

This indication has been tested in several studies (Table 15.1). Wysocki et al. randomized 41 patients with acute respiratory failure not related to chronic obstructive pulmonary disease [29]. Patients were randomly assigned to receive conventional therapy (oxygen and medications related to the cause of the respiratory distress (antibiotics, diuretics)) or conventional therapy plus NIV. In this study, respiratory distress was due to pneumonia in 16 patients (39%) but not necessarily associated with ARDS. Seven of these patients were randomly assigned to NIV, none was successful, and all required endotracheal intubation. By contrast, respiratory distress was not due to pneumonia in 25 other patients (61%), and 14 were randomly assigned to receive NIV; 8 were successfully ventilated with NIV ($p = 0.04$). In a larger study, Ferrer et al. randomized 105 patients with severe acute hypoxemic respiratory failure to receive, via oronasal mask, either NIV or high FiO_2 [30]. The main causes were pneumonia and cardiogenic lung edema, but there were 15 patients with ARDS. Overall the study was very positive in favor of NIV, which prevented intubation, reduced the incidence of septic shock, and improved survival compared with high-concentration oxygen therapy. The efficacy of NIV was, however, poor in the ARDS subgroup (intubation rate 86%). This study strictly selected cooperative patients with no other organ dysfunction. Confalonieri et al. randomized 56 patients presenting with acute hypoxemic respiratory failure and community-acquired pneumonia (not ARDS) to receive either NIV or standard treatment [37]. The intubation rate was 21% versus 50% for the NIV group and standard group ($p = 0.03$), respectively. The main limitation of this study was the presence of COPD in many patients, driving the benefits of NIV.

The role of NIV in the treatment of ALI was assessed in critically ill patients with bilateral infiltrates of different origin in a study from the Mayo Clinic [38]. In this observational cohort study, Rana et al. prospectively assessed the outcomes of 54 consecutive patients. They found that 70% of the patients failed NIV. It was of notice that in patients who failed NIV, the observed mortality was higher than APACHE-predicted mortality (68% vs. 39%, $p < 0.01$). Among 113 patients receiving NIV for acute hypoxemic respiratory failure (82 with acute ARDS and 31

Table 15.1 Studies reporting the effect of noninvasive ventilation on acute hypoxemic respiratory failure in immunocompetent patients

First author, year	Patients	Design	Population	Intubation rate	Risk factors for intubation
Wysocki, 1995	41	Monocenter RCT: NIV vs. O_2	ARF not related to AECOPD	NIV: 62% vs. O_2: 70%	Not reported
Antonelli, 1998	64	Monocenter RCT: NIV vs. IMV	ARDS (25%)	10/32 (31%)	Not reported
Confalonieri, 1999	56	Monocenter RCT: NIV vs. O_2	Community acquired pneumonia and ARF	NIV: 21% vs. O_2: 50%	Not reported
Delclaux, 2000	123	Multicenter RCT: CPAP vs. O_2	ALI (1994 definition)	CPAP: 21 (34%) vs. 24 (39%)	High SAPS II Absence of cardiac disease PaO_2/FiO_2 after 1h of NIV
Antonelli, 2001	354	Observational multicenter cohort study	ARDS (25%)	108/354 (30%)	Age > 40 SAPS II > 35 ARDS PaO_2/FiO_2 after 1h
Auriant, 2001	24	Monocenter, RCT: NIV vs. O_2	ARF post lung surgery	NIV: 20% vs. O_2: 50%	Not reported
Ferrer, 2003	105	Multicenter, RCT: NIV vs. O_2	Severe acute hypoxemic respiratory failure, ARDS (14%)	NIV: 25% vs. O_2: 52%	ARDS
Rana, 2006	54	Observational prospective study, NIV first line	ALI, Berlin definition	70%	Metabolic acidosis Severe hypoxemia
Antonelli, 2007	147	Observational first-line NIV	ARDS (1994 definition)	54%	Age>58 Gender male SAPS II>34 pH after 1 h>7.37 PaO_2/FiO_2 after 1 h>175

(continued)

Table 15.1 (continued)

First author, year	Patients	Design	Population	Intubation rate	Risk factors for intubation
Agarwal, 2009	40 (21 ARDS/ALI)	Observational study with NIV in first line	ALI, Berlin definition	47%, 57% in ARDS/ALI and 37% in others	PaO_2/FiO_2 ratio
Zhan, 2012	40	Multicenter RCT: NIV vs. O_2 (Venturi)	ALI, Berlin definition	NIV: 5% vs. O_2: 21%	Not reported
Thille, 2013	113 (87 with ARDS)	Observational with NIV in first line	ALI, Berlin definition	54%	Active cancer Shock Moderate/severe ARDS Low Glasgow coma score
Kangelaris, 2015	457	Observational cohort study	ARDS (Berlin definition)	23% non-intubated	Not reported
Frat, 2015	310	Multicenter RCT: NIV vs. O2 vs. HFNC	ALI/ARDS (Berlin definition)	O_2: 47% vs. HFNC: 38% vs. NIV: 50%	Not reported

ALI acute lung injury, *ARDS* acute respiratory distress syndrome, *ARF* acute respiratory failure, *AECOPD* acute exacerbation of chronic obstructive pulmonary disease, *RCT* randomized controlled trial, *NIV* noninvasive ventilation, *CPAP* continuous positive airway pressure, *IMV* invasive mechanical ventilation, *HFNC* high-flow oxygen through nasal cannula, *SAPS II* simplified acute physiology score without), Thille et al. reported intubation rates significantly different between ARDS and non-ARDS patients (61% vs. 35%, $p = 0.015$) and according to clinical severity of ARDS: 31% in mild, 62% in moderate, and 84% in severe ARDS ($p = 0.0016$) [39].

More recently, Frat et al. randomized 310 patients presenting acute hypoxemic respiratory failure without hypercapnia to receive either high-flow oxygen therapy or standard oxygen therapy delivered through a face mask or NIV [36]. The intubation rate was similar between the three groups (38%, 47%, and 50%, respectively, for the high-flow oxygen group, the standard group, and the NIV group; $p = 0.18$). However, it is important to note that the hazard ratio for death at 90 days was 2.01 (95% confidence interval [CI], 1.01–3.99) with standard oxygen versus high-flow oxygen ($p = 0.046$) and 2.50 (95% CI, 1.31–4.78) with NIV versus high-flow oxygen (p=0.006). Finally, another monocentric study reported intriguing results [40]. In this prospective study, investigators randomized 83 hypoxemic patients after 8 h of NIV to receive NIV provided with a helmet or NIV with a facial mask (as it was previously provided) [40]. The study was stopped earlier for safety since the preestablished criteria for stoppage were met. Hence, the main primary endpoint, the intubation rate, was 61.5% in the face mask group and 18.2% in the helmet group (absolute difference, −43.3%; 95% CI, −62.4% to −24.3%; $p<.001$). The helmet group had a higher PEEP (8 vs. 5 cmH_2O), whereas the pressure support level was higher in the face mask group (11 vs. 8 cmH_2O). With helmet, the assessment of tidal volume is not possible; however, the results could be explained by more protective ventilation provided by the helmet. Since it was a monocentric study, further studies are mandatory to confirm these challenging results.

15.3.6 When NIV Should Not Be Used in Acute Hypoxemic Respiratory Failure

Based on the high intubation rate reported above, it is important to know when NIV should not be applied in patients with acute hypoxemic respiratory failure. Most of the studies that reported the experience of using NIV in acute hypoxemic respiratory failure have proposed predictors of NIV failure. In 2001, Antonelli et al. investigated in a prospective multicenter cohort study factors involved in NIV failure [41]. In a heterogeneous population, the overall efficacy of NIV in avoiding intubation (70%) contrasted with the high rate of failure observed in 86 patients fulfilling the diagnosis of ARDS (51%). The intubation rate was similar among patients with ARDS of pulmonary versus extrapulmonary origin, but sepsis on admission was associated, among other variables, with NIV failure. In a large prospective observational study of NIV in 147 ARDS patients in experienced centers (NIV failure rate around 50%), a high Simplified Acute Physiology Score (SAPS) II and $PaO_2/FiO_2 \leq 175$ mmHg 1 h after initiation of NIV were independently associated with NIV failure [42]. Rana et al. [38] found that NIV success was significantly correlated with low severity scores (Acute Physiology and Chronic Health Evaluation III or Sequential Organ Failure Assessment), with high PaO_2/FiO_2 (147 vs. 112), and with less pronounced acidosis than patients with NIV failure. Last, Thille et al. found that shock, active cancer, low level of consciousness, and mild/severe ARDS were independently associated with NIV failure [39].

15.3.7 Recommendations for clinical practice

The efficiency of NIV in patients with acute hypoxemic respiratory failure due to ALI, ARDS, or severe pulmonary infiltrates, and for whom endotracheal intubation is *not mandatory*, depends on the degree of hypoxia, the presence of comorbidities and complications, and the illness severity scores. It also probably depends on the respiratory drive of the patients. The high rate of NIV failure suggests a cautious approach with these patients, consisting of early NIV trial and no delay of needed intubation. Measurement of tidal volume under NIV may be important, and patients having tidal volume above 8 mL/kg of predicted body weight may be at higher risk of failure and of having an injurious breathing pattern. In those patients, lung-protective ventilation may be considered as a therapy. In addition, when using NIV in a patient with acute hypoxic respiratory failure, in an attempt to avoid intubation, one should always consider the risks of inappropriate intubation delay. Demoule et al. found that the effect of NIV differs between acute hypoxemic respiratory failure (including mainly in this definition, ALI and ARDS) and patients with cardiogenic pulmonary edema or acute exacerbation of COPD, because NIV failure was associated with higher mortality in patients with acute hypoxemic respiratory failure [32]. This finding should therefore raise a note of caution when applying NIV for this indication and make the clinician wonder whether a lung-protective ventilation is not more appropriate. Close monitoring is therefore crucial when using this technique as a first-line therapy in patients with ARDS. Delaying intubation may contribute to mortality [43]. NIV should not be considered primarily as an alternative to invasive ventilation.

15.4 Rationale, Benefits, and Risks of High-Flow Oxygenation Through Nasal Cannula in ARDS

The most conventional form of oxygen delivery relies on face masks, nasal cannula, or nasal prongs. However, some drawbacks limit their use in case of severe hypoxemia if oxygen flow higher than 15 L/min is needed and in case of high patients' inspiratory flow that may induce a certain amount of oxygen dilution. An alternative to conventional oxygen therapy has received growing attention: heated, humidified high-flow nasal cannula oxygen (HFNC) is a technique that can deliver heated and humidified oxygen, with a controlled FiO_2, at a maximum flow of 60 L/min of gas via nasal prongs or cannula. Many data with this technique have been published in the neonatal field where it is increasingly used [44]. Since a decade, the use of HFNC has been considered for patients with acute hypoxemic respiratory failure. The high flow rates used generate low levels of positive pressure in the upper airways [45, 46]. The high flow rates may also decrease physiological dead space by flushing the expired carbon dioxide from the upper airway [47, 48], a process that potentially explains the observed decrease in the respiratory rate and the work of breathing [49]. In patients with acute respiratory failure of various origins, HFNC has been shown to result in better comfort and oxygenation than standard oxygen therapy delivered through a face mask [50–52]. HFNC has gained increasing clinical and scientific interest [36, 50–53]. The larger study on the use of HFNC in patients with acute hypoxemic respiratory failure was conducted by Frat and coworkers in 2015 [36]. In this randomized controlled trial, investigators aimed at determining whether HFNC administered through a large-bore close-fitting nasal cannula or NIV could reduce the intubation rate and improve outcomes in acute hypoxemic patients compared with standard oxygen administration [36]. In this trial, patients had mild or moderate ARDS (PaO_2/FiO_2 ratio around 155 mmHg) mainly due to pneumonia. The primary outcome, the rate of endotracheal intubation, was lower among patients treated with high-flow oxygen than among those who received standard oxygen therapy or NIV, but the rates did not differ significantly (38% vs. 47% and 50%, respectively) ($p = 0.18$). However, in a post hoc adjusted analysis that included the 238 patients with severe initial hypoxemia ($PaO_2/FiO_2 \leq 200$ mmHg), the intubation rate was significantly lower among patients who received high-flow oxygen than among patients in the other two groups ($p = 0.009$). Furthermore, the hazard ratio for death at 90 days after randomization was 2.01 in the standard oxygen group versus the high-flow oxygen group ($p = 0.046$) and 2.5 in the NIV group versus the high-flow oxygen group ($p = 0.006$). One explanation proposed by the authors was that NIV and spontaneous breathing could have provided tidal volume greater than 9 mL/kg of predicted body weight. Hence, the degree of lung injury might have been increased in this group, contributing to a higher mortality than that observed in the high-flow oxygen group.

15.5 Noninvasive Ventilator Support in Immunocompromised Patients with ARDS

Acute respiratory failure remains the most common and severe life-threatening complication in immunocompromised patients [54, 55]. Many immunocompromised patients with acute respiratory failure require ventilatory support within a few hours after admission to the ICU. Avoiding invasive mechanical ventilation significantly decreases the risk of death. Thus, choosing the optimal device for delivering oxygen is of the utmost importance. In a large multicenter study of 1,004 patients with solid or hematologic malignancies and ARDS meeting the new operational Berlin definition, Azoulay et al. reported that NIV was used initially in one-third of the patients. They frequently failed, with the highest failure rates occurring in the most severe ARDS category [55]. Nevertheless, a favorable impact of NIV has been described in retrospective studies [56–58] and in a few randomized controlled trials including a relatively small number of patients [25, 26, 59] (Table 15.2). Hence, the efficacy of NIV in this population appears to be promising. More recently, the use

Table 15.2 Studies exploring the effect of noninvasive ventilation on acute hypoxemic respiratory failure in immunocompromised patients

First author, year	Patients	Design	Population description	Intubation rate	Risk factors for intubation
Hilbert, 2000	52	Monocenter RCT: NIV vs. O_2	Immunocompromised patients with ARF	46% vs. 77% ($p = 0.03$)	Not reported
Antonelli, 2000	40	Monocenter RCT: NIV vs. O_2	Immunocompromised patients with ARF	20% vs. 70% ($p = 0.002$)	Not reported
Adda, 2008	99	Retrospective cohort study, NIV in first line	Immunocompromised patients with ARF (32% ARDS)	54%	Respiratory rate under NIV Need for vasopressor Need for RRT ARDS
Squadrone, 2010	40	Monocenter RCT, CPAP vs. O_2	Hematologic malignancy	40% vs. 10% ($p< 0.001$)	Not reported
Wermke, 2012	86	Monocenter RCT, NIV vs. 0_2	Allogenic hematopoietic stem cell transplant	14% vs. 25% ($p = 0.3$)	Not reported
Lemiale, 2015	374	Multicenter RCT: NIV vs. O_2	Immunocompromised patients with ARF	44.8% vs. 38.2% ($p = 0.2$)	Not reported

ARDS acute respiratory distress syndrome, *ARF* acute respiratory failure, *RCT* randomized controlled trial, *NIV* noninvasive ventilation, *CPAP* continuous positive airway pressure, *RRT* renal replacement therapy of HFNC has also been investigated in immunocompromised patients. Below, we will discuss the advantages and limits of using NIV and HFNC in immunocompromised patients.

15.5.1 NIV in Immunocompromised Patients

The first study that assessed NIV in immunocompromised patients was published by Hilbert et al. in 2001 [25]. In this single-center randomized controlled trial, 52 immunosuppressed patients (not only patients with hematologic malignancies but several modalities of immunosuppression) were enrolled if they had pulmonary infiltrates, fever, and hypoxemic acute respiratory failure, defined by the presence of dyspnea at rest, respiratory rate greater than 30 breaths per minute, and a PaO_2/FiO_2 ratio of less than 200 mmHg while breathing oxygen. These patients were randomly allocated to receive either standard oxygen treatment via face mask or intermittent NIV. Compared to standard oxygen therapy, the group treated with NIV had lower rates of endotracheal intubation (12/26 patients vs. 20/26, $p = 0.03$), and in-hospital mortality (50% vs. 81%, $p = 0.02$). The main limits of this study were that the patients were recruited at a single center and that the mortality rate among patients managed with invasive mechanical ventilation was considerably higher than current rates (90%). Antonelli et al. reported the efficacy of NIV in reducing the need of endotracheal intubation and invasive mechanical ventilation in immunocompromised patients after solid organ transplantation with hypoxemic respiratory failure [28]. Forty patients with a PaO_2/FiO_2 ratio of less than 200 mmHg while breathing oxygen and active use of accessory respiratory muscles were randomized to receive either NIV or treatment with supplemental oxygen via Venturi mask. The group treated with NIV demonstrated significantly lower rates of endotracheal intubation (20% vs. 70%, $p = 0.002$) and ICU mortality (20% vs. 50%, $p = 0.05$). However, no significant difference was found in the in-hospital mortality rate. A more recent randomized controlled trial investigated the potential role of early use of continuous positive airway pressure (CPAP) in patients with hematologic malignancies delivered before ICU admission [59]. Forty patients of the ward with bilateral infiltrates, respiratory rate greater than 25 breaths/minute, and an oxygen saturation of less than 90% while breathing on room air were randomized to receive oxygen (FiO_2 = 50%) either by face mask or helmet CPAP at 10 cmH_2O. Overall, significantly fewer patients treated with CPAP required ICU admission and NIV or invasive mechanical ventilation (4 vs. 16 patients; $p = 0.0002$). This was associated with an improved survival. However, these very encouraging results have not been confirmed in subsequent observational [60] and randomized clinical studies [61]. To assess the potential benefit of early NIV in reducing the mortality rate among immunocompromised patients who developed acute hypoxemic respiratory failure, Lemiale underwent a randomized controlled trial [6]. In 28 intensive care units from France and Belgium, 374 immunocompromised patients with PaO_2 less than 60 mmHg on room air, or respiratory rate greater than 30/min, or signs of respiratory distress, were randomized to receive NIV or conventional oxygen therapy. Of note, patients were stratified according to the cause of immune deficiency in two groups, one with hematologic malignancy or solid cancer and one with solid organ transplant or long-term/high-dose immunosuppressive treatment. No difference was found between groups with regard to the primary endpoint, the mortality rate at 28 days after randomization (NIV 24.1% vs. oxygen 27.3%; 95% CI: −12.1 to 5.6; $p = 0.47$). Also the analysis of the two prespecified subgroups did not result in any significant difference. Nevertheless, it must be outlined that this trial was underpowered since the authors anticipated a mortality of 35% in the oxygen-treated group, whereas the observed mortality rate was 27.3%. As a result, the possibility of drawing definitive conclusions and a clinically meaningful effect based on the study findings is limited. A recent post hoc analysis, restricted to the subgroup of immunosuppressed patients of the FLORALI trial, in a population of patients with acute hypoxemic respiratory failure suggested no benefit of NIV neither for intubation nor for survival [62]. In contrast to what it was expected, NIV may not be the panacea for the main reason than discussed in non-immunosuppressed patients. The possible role of injurious breathing pattern, potentially aggravated by NIV, may hence provide another explanation for the lack of efficacy of NIV in immunocompromised patients.

15.5.2 High-Flow Nasal Cannula in Immunocompromised Patients with Acute Hypoxemic Respiratory Failure

A multicenter parallel randomized controlled trial in four intensive care units assessing the role of HFNC versus Venturi mask oxygen in immunocompromised patients with acute hypoxemic respiratory failure has been conducted [53]. Patients were randomized to only 2 h of HFNC or Venturi mask oxygen [53]. The primary endpoint was a need for invasive mechanical ventilation or NIV during the 2-h oxygen therapy period. They found no significant difference between the two groups (15% with HFNC and 8% with the Venturi mask, $p = 0.36$). None of the secondary endpoints, which included comfort, dyspnea, and thirst, differed significantly between the two groups. The authors concluded that in immunocompromised patients with hypoxemic acute respiratory failure, a 2-h trial with HFNC did not improve mechanical ventilatory assistance or patient comfort compared with oxygen delivered via a simple Venturi mask. However, this study was underpowered given the low event rate and use of a one-sided hypothesis only. Furthermore, this trial focused only upon the initial 2 h after ICU admission, and thus the role of HFNC for longer periods of time remains to be assessed.

Conclusion

The benefits of NIV on the outcome of acute hypercapnic respiratory failure are well demonstrated. By contrast, there is less evidence in the setting of acute hypoxemic respiratory failure. This is in part due to the fact that acute hypoxemic respiratory group is gathering very different diagnoses leading to a heterogeneous group. As first-line approach, NIV should not be considered as a ventilatory support therapy among the most severe patients with ARDS though the meaning of "severe" is subjective. Indeed, some patients with a high drive and spontaneous large tidal volumes may benefit from a lung protection best offered by intubation and sedation. NIV can be beneficial in other patients. Nevertheless, if NIV is initiated in such patients, a close monitoring is mandatory. Clinicians need also to be aware of the potential deleterious effects of delaying intubation. This highlights the potential interest of high-flow oxygenation through nasal cannula. A first step has been reached with the FLORALI study. Future studies will have to determine the respective indications of HFNC, NIV, and lung-protective ventilation in ARDS.

References

1. Petrof BJ, Jaber S, Matecki S (2010) Ventilator-induced diaphragmatic dysfunction. Curr Opin Crit Care 16:19–25
2. Klompas M (2013) Complications of mechanical ventilation–the CDC's new surveillance paradigm. N Engl J Med 368:1472–1475
3. Slutsky AS, Ranieri VM (2014) Ventilator-induced lung injury. N Engl J Med 370:980
4. Masip J, Roque M, Sánchez B, Fernández R, Subirana M, Expósito JA (2005) Noninvasive ventilation in acute cardiogenic pulmonary edema: systematic review and meta-analysis. JAMA 294:3124–3130
5. Keenan SP, Sinuff T, Cook DJ, Hill NS (2003) Which patients with acute exacerbation of chronic obstructive pulmonary disease benefit from noninvasive positive-pressure ventilation? A systematic review of the literature. Ann Intern Med 138:861–870
6. Lemiale V, Mokart D, Resche-Rigon M et al (2015) Effect of noninvasive ventilation vs oxygen therapy on mortality among immunocompromised patients with acute respiratory failure: a randomized clinical trial. JAMA 314:1–9
7. Cracco C, Fartoukh M, Prodanovic H et al (2013) Safety of performing fiberoptic bronchoscopy in critically ill hypoxemic patients with acute respiratory failure. Intensive Care Med 39:45–52
8. Girault C, Bubenheim M, Abroug F et al (2011) Noninvasive ventilation and weaning in patients with chronic hypercapnic respiratory failure: a randomized multicenter trial. Am J Respir Crit Care Med 184:672–679
9. Lorut C, Lefebvre A, Planquette B et al (2014) Early postoperative prophylactic noninvasive ventilation after major lung resection in COPD patients: a randomized controlled trial. Intensive Care Med 40:220–227
10. Squadrone V, Coha M, Cerutti E et al (2005) Continuous positive airway pressure for treatment of postoperative hypoxemia: a randomized controlled trial. Jama 293:589–595
11. Jaber S, Lescot T, Futier E et al (2016) Effect of noninvasive ventilation on tracheal reintubation among patients with hypoxemic respiratory failure following abdominal surgery: a randomized clinical trial. JAMA 315:1345–1353
12. Hess DR (2004) The evidence for noninvasive positive-pressure ventilation in the care of patients in acute respiratory failure: a systematic review of the literature. Respir Care 49:810–829
13. Ware LB, Matthay MA (2000) The acute respiratory distress syndrome. N Engl J Med 342:1334–1349
14. Definition Task Force ARDS, Ranieri VM, Rubenfeld GD, Thompson BT, Ferguson ND, Caldwell E, Fan E, Camporota L, Slutsky AS (2012) Acute respiratory distress syndrome: the Berlin Definition. JAMA 307:2526–2533
15. Rittayamai N, Brochard L (2015) Recent advances in mechanical ventilation in patients with acute respiratory distress syndrome. Eur Respir Rev Off J Eur Respir Soc 24:132–140

16. L'Her E, Deye N, Lellouche F, Taille S, Demoule A, Fraticelli A, Mancebo J, Brochard L (2005) Physiologic effects of noninvasive ventilation during acute lung injury. Am J Respir Crit Care Med 172:1112–1118
17. Evans TW (2001) International Consensus Conferences in Intensive Care Medicine: non-invasive positive pressure ventilation in acute respiratory failure. Organised jointly by the American Thoracic Society, the European Respiratory Society, the European Society of Intensive Care Medicine, and the Société de Réanimation de Langue Française, and approved by the ATS Board of Directors, December 2000. Intensive Care Med 27:166–178
18. Carlucci A, Richard JC, Wysocki M, Lepage E, Brochard L, SRLF Collaborative Group on Mechanical Ventilation (2001) Noninvasive versus conventional mechanical ventilation. An epidemiologic survey. Am J Respir Crit Care Med 163:874–880
19. Ozsancak Ugurlu A, Sidhom SS, Khodabandeh A et al (2014) Use and outcomes of noninvasive positive pressure ventilation in acute care hospitals in Massachusetts. Chest 145:964–971
20. Burns KEA, Sinuff T, Adhikari NKJ, Meade MO, Heels-Ansdell D, Martin CM, Cook DJ (2005) Bilevel noninvasive positive pressure ventilation for acute respiratory failure: survey of Ontario practice. Crit Care Med 33:1477–1483
21. Walkey AJ, Wiener RS (2013) Use of noninvasive ventilation in patients with acute respiratory failure, 2000-2009: a population-based study. Ann Am Thorac Soc 10:10–17
22. Demoule A, Chevret S, Carlucci A et al (2015) Changing use of noninvasive ventilation in critically ill patients: trends over 15 years in francophone countries. Intensive Care Med. doi:10.1007/s00134-015-4087-4
23. Bellani G, Laffey JG, Pham T et al (2016) Epidemiology, patterns of care, and mortality for patients with acute respiratory distress syndrome in intensive care units in 50 countries. JAMA 315:788–800
24. Girou E, Schortgen F, Delclaux C, Brun-Buisson C, Blot F, Lefort Y, Lemaire F, Brochard L (2000) Association of noninvasive ventilation with nosocomial infections and survival in critically ill patients. JAMA 284:2361–2367
25. Hilbert G, Gruson D, Vargas F, Valentino R, Gbikpi-Benissan G, Dupon M, Reiffers J, Cardinaud JP (2001) Noninvasive ventilation in immunosuppressed patients with pulmonary infiltrates, fever, and acute respiratory failure. N Engl J Med 344:481–487
26. Antonelli M, Conti G, Bufi M, Costa MG, Lappa A, Rocco M, Gasparetto A, Meduri GU (2000) Noninvasive ventilation for treatment of acute respiratory failure in patients undergoing solid organ transplantation: a randomized trial. JAMA 283:235–241
27. Auriant I, Jallot A, Hervé P, Cerrina J, Le Roy LF, Fournier JL, Lescot B, Parquin F (2001) Noninvasive ventilation reduces mortality in acute respiratory failure following lung resection. Am J Respir Crit Care Med 164:1231–1235
28. Antonelli M, Conti G, Rocco M, Bufi M, De Blasi RA, Vivino G, Gasparetto A, Meduri GU (1998) A comparison of noninvasive positive-pressure ventilation and conventional mechanical ventilation in patients with acute respiratory failure. N Engl J Med 339:429–435
29. Wysocki M, Tric L, Wolff MA, Millet H, Herman B (1995) Noninvasive pressure support ventilation in patients with acute respiratory failure. A randomized comparison with conventional therapy. Chest 107:761–768
30. Ferrer M, Esquinas A, Leon M, Gonzalez G, Alarcon A, Torres A (2003) Noninvasive ventilation in severe hypoxemic respiratory failure: a randomized clinical trial. Am J Respir Crit Care Med 168:1438–1444
31. Squadrone E, Frigerio P, Fogliati C, Gregoretti C, Conti G, Antonelli M, Costa R, Baiardi P, Navalesi P (2004) Noninvasive vs invasive ventilation in COPD patients with severe acute respiratory failure deemed to require ventilatory assistance. Intensive Care Med 30:1303–1310
32. Demoule A, Girou E, Richard JC, Taille S, Brochard L (2006) Benefits and risks of success or failure of noninvasive ventilation. Intensive Care Med 32:1756–1765
33. Kangelaris KN, Ware LB, Wang CY, Janz DR, Zhuo H, Matthay MA, Calfee CS (2016) Timing of intubation and clinical outcomes in adults with acute respiratory distress syndrome. Crit Care Med 44:120–129

34. Chawla R, Mansuriya J, Modi N, Pandey A, Juneja D, Chawla A, Kansal S (2016) Acute respiratory distress syndrome: Predictors of noninvasive ventilation failure and intensive care unit mortality in clinical practice. J Crit Care 31:26–30
35. Carteaux G, Millán-Guilarte T, De Prost N, Razazi K, Abid S, Thille AW, Schortgen F, Brochard L, Brun-Buisson C, Mekontso Dessap A (2016) Failure of noninvasive ventilation for De Novo acute hypoxemic respiratory failure: role of tidal volume. Crit Care Med 44:282–290
36. Frat J-P, Thille AW, Mercat A et al (2015) High-flow oxygen through nasal cannula in acute hypoxemic respiratory failure. N Engl J Med 372:2185–2196
37. Confalonieri M, Potena A, Carbone G, Porta RD, Tolley EA, Umberto Meduri G (1999) Acute respiratory failure in patients with severe community-acquired pneumonia. A prospective randomized evaluation of noninvasive ventilation. Am J Respir Crit Care Med 160:1585–1591
38. Rana S, Jenad H, Gay PC, Buck CF, Hubmayr RD, Gajic O (2006) Failure of non-invasive ventilation in patients with acute lung injury: observational cohort study. Crit Care Lond Engl 10:R79
39. Thille AW, Contou D, Fragnoli C, Córdoba-Izquierdo A, Boissier F, Brun-Buisson C (2013) Non-invasive ventilation for acute hypoxemic respiratory failure: intubation rate and risk factors. Crit Care Lond Engl 17:R269
40. Patel BK, Wolfe KS, Pohlman AS, Hall JB, Kress JP (2016) Effect of noninvasive ventilation delivered by helmet vs face mask on the rate of endotracheal intubation in patients with acute respiratory distress syndrome: a randomized clinical trial. JAMA. doi:10.1001/jama.2016.6338
41. Antonelli M, Conti G, Moro ML et al (2001) Predictors of failure of noninvasive positive pressure ventilation in patients with acute hypoxemic respiratory failure: a multi-center study. Intensive Care Med 27:1718–1728
42. Antonelli M, Conti G, Esquinas A et al (2007) A multiple-center survey on the use in clinical practice of noninvasive ventilation as a first-line intervention for acute respiratory distress syndrome. Crit Care Med 35:18–25
43. Carrillo A, Gonzalez-Diaz G, Ferrer M, Martinez-Quintana ME, Lopez-Martinez A, Llamas N, Alcazar M, Torres A (2012) Non-invasive ventilation in community-acquired pneumonia and severe acute respiratory failure. Intensive Care Med 38:458–466
44. Dani C, Pratesi S, Migliori C, Bertini G (2009) High flow nasal cannula therapy as respiratory support in the preterm infant. Pediatr Pulmonol 44:629–634
45. Parke R, McGuinness S, Eccleston M (2009) Nasal high-flow therapy delivers low level positive airway pressure. Br J Anaesth 103:886–890
46. Parke RL, Eccleston ML, McGuinness SP (2011) The effects of flow on airway pressure during nasal high-flow oxygen therapy. Respir Care 56:1151–1155
47. Ricard J-D (2012) High flow nasal oxygen in acute respiratory failure. Minerva Anestesiol 78:836–841
48. Roca O, Riera J, Torres F, Masclans JR (2010) High-flow oxygen therapy in acute respiratory failure. Respir Care 55:408–413
49. Pham TMT, O'Malley L, Mayfield S, Martin S, Schibler A (2015) The effect of high flow nasal cannula therapy on the work of breathing in infants with bronchiolitis. Pediatr Pulmonol 50:713–720
50. Lenglet H, Sztrymf B, Leroy C, Brun P, Dreyfuss D, Ricard J-D (2012) Humidified high flow nasal oxygen during respiratory failure in the emergency department: feasibility and efficacy. Respir Care 57:1873–1878
51. Spoletini G, Alotaibi M, Blasi F, Hill NS (2015) Heated humidified high-flow nasal oxygen in adults: mechanisms of action and clinical implications. Chest 148:253–261
52. Sztrymf B, Messika J, Bertrand F, Hurel D, Leon R, Dreyfuss D, Ricard J-D (2011) Beneficial effects of humidified high flow nasal oxygen in critical care patients: a prospective pilot study. Intensive Care Med 37:1780–1786
53. Lemiale V, Mokart D, Mayaux J, Lambert J, Rabbat A, Demoule A, Azoulay E (2015) The effects of a 2-h trial of high-flow oxygen by nasal cannula versus Venturi mask in immunocompromised patients with hypoxemic acute respiratory failure: a multicenter randomized trial. Crit Care Lond Engl 19:380

54. Azevedo LCP, Caruso P, Silva UVA et al (2014) Outcomes for patients with cancer admitted to the ICU requiring ventilatory support: results from a prospective multicenter study. Chest 146:257–266
55. Azoulay E, Lemiale V, Mokart D et al (2014) Acute respiratory distress syndrome in patients with malignancies. Intensive Care Med 40:1106–1114
56. Depuydt PO, Benoit DD, Vandewoude KH, Decruyenaere JM, Colardyn FA (2004) Outcome in noninvasively and invasively ventilated hematologic patients with acute respiratory failure. Chest 126:1299–1306
57. Adda M, Coquet I, Darmon M, Thiery G, Schlemmer B, Azoulay E (2008) Predictors of noninvasive ventilation failure in patients with hematologic malignancy and acute respiratory failure. Crit Care Med 36:2766–2772
58. Azoulay E, Alberti C, Bornstain C, Leleu G, Moreau D, Recher C, Chevret S, Le Gall JR, Brochard L, Schlemmer B (2001) Improved survival in cancer patients requiring mechanical ventilatory support: impact of noninvasive mechanical ventilatory support. Crit Care Med 29:519–525
59. Squadrone V, Massaia M, Bruno B et al (2010) Early CPAP prevents evolution of acute lung injury in patients with hematologic malignancy. Intensive Care Med 36:1666–1674
60. Azoulay E, Thiéry G, Chevret S et al (2004) The prognosis of acute respiratory failure in critically ill cancer patients. Medicine (Baltimore) 83:360–370
61. Wermke M, Schiemanck S, Höffken G, Ehninger G, Bornhäuser M, Illmer T (2012) Respiratory failure in patients undergoing allogeneic hematopoietic SCT–a randomized trial on early noninvasive ventilation based on standard care hematology wards. Bone Marrow Transplant 47:574–580
62. Frat JP, Ragot S, Girault C, Perbet S, Prat G, Boulain T et al (2016) Impact of non-invasive oxygenation strategies in immunocompromised patients with severe acute respiratory failure: post hoc analysis of a randomized trial. Lancet Resp Med 4(8):646–652

Interaction Between the Heart and Lungs

16

Fabio Guarracino and Rubia Baldassarri

16.1 Introduction

The main reason for the heart and lungs to interact physiologically is that they share the same space within the chest (Fig. 16.1), and their physiologies are both submitted to and driven by the interaction among different pressures (viz. airways, intrathoracic and intracardiac pressures).

The heart and lung (H-L) interaction can be defined as the effects of airway pressure and volume on venous return, ventricular function and arterial outflow [1]. Such effects are summarised in Fig. 16.2.

H-L interactions are different in healthy and diseased conditions and between spontaneous and positive pressure ventilation.

Under normal conditions and in spontaneous ventilation, the H-L interaction is subtle. In the presence of cardiac and respiratory disease states, or when the compensatory reserve is limited, such as in critically ill patients, and under positive pressure ventilation (either invasive either non-invasive), H-L interactions are elicited, and the cardiovascular function can be affected by respiratory changes.

As ARDS (Acute Respiratory Distress Syndrome) pathology involves both alveoli and pulmonary capillaries, as reported long ago [2], it represents a typical predisposing situation for the H-L interaction to influence the circulation.

F. Guarracino (✉), R. Baldassarri
Department of Anaesthesia and Critical Care Medicine, Azienda Ospedaliero Universitaria Pisana, Via Paradisa, 2, Pisa 56123, Italy
e-mail: fabiodoc64@hotmail.com

D. Chiumello (ed.), *Acute Respiratory Distress Syndrome (ARDS)*,
DOI 10.1007/978-3-319-41852-0_16

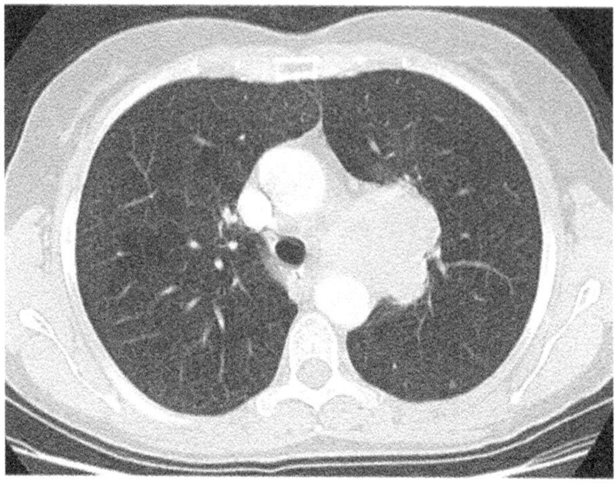

Fig. 16.1 A CT scan of human chest showing the close spatial relationship between the heart and the lungs

Fig. 16.2 Effects of increase in airway pressure and volume on the heart

Effects of increase in airway pressure and volume	
Right ventricle	**Left ventricle**
Decreased preload Increased afterload Reduced contractility Compression of heart in cardiac fossa	Decreased preload Decreased compliance Variable effects on (autonomous nervous system control of) contractility Decreased afterload compression of heart in cardiac fossa

16.2 H-L Interactions: The Impact of Cardiorespiratory System Characteristics

The description of the anatomy and function of the heart and lungs is basic knowledge that is beyond the scope of this chapter. Therefore, only some key aspects of the cardiorespiratory system relevant to the H-L interaction issue of the ARDS patient will be addressed here.

The human heart shows the interesting combination of physiologically consisting of a double pump system where the two pumps, the left and right ventricles, work in series, with each pump ejecting the blood received from the other pump, and anatomically consisting of two pumps sharing the interventricular septum and the pericardium, thus being anatomically in parallel (Fig. 16.3). One more important aspect to underline in this contest is the anatomic and functional presence of the pulmonary circulation between the two pumps within the chest. This peculiar anatomic and functional condition of two pumps structurally made in parallel and mechanically working in series, with the pulmonary circulation being the circuit connecting the right ventricular ejection to the left ventricle, represents the main reason for the H-L interactions to occur and to have consequences in diseased states,

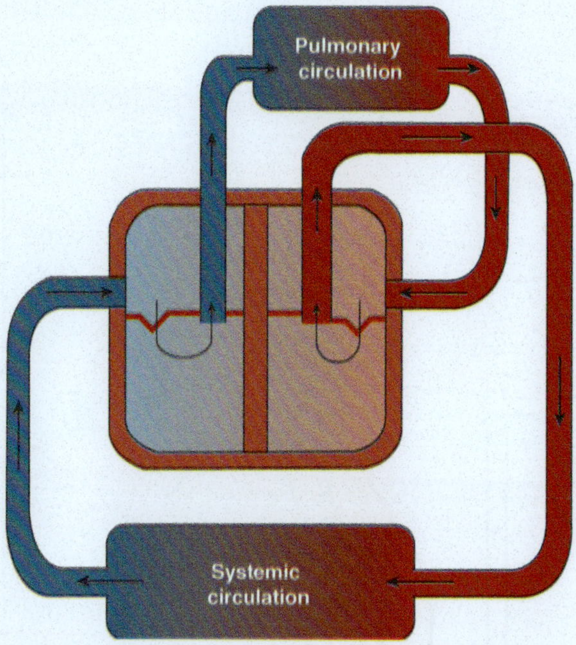

Fig. 16.3 Pulmonary and systemic circulation (to modify) (Modified with permission from F. Guarracino "Ecocardiografia in Area critica" 2013 Elsevier, Milan)

and it is pivotal to understanding the ventricular interdependence. In fact, any acute and relevant change of the anatomy and/or the function of one pump or of the pulmonary circulation will cause the H-L interactions to be clinically significant.

In the setting of ARDS, it is the relationship between the right ventricle (RV) and the pulmonary circulation that plays a major role, in a setting where the physiological interplay of the pump and vascular elastances is pivotal in determining the right ventriculo-arterial coupling.

It is wise to distinguish H-L interactions under spontaneous ventilation from those observed under positive pressure ventilation.

16.3 H-L Interactions in Spontaneous Ventilation

Heart-lung interactions occur at every breath. Under normal conditions, the changes in pressure and volume within the lungs (Fig. 16.4) will have no relevant haemodynamic effect. However, if a respiratory or cardiac disease is present, either acute or chronic, then the normal respiratory physiology is altered, and this may have circulatory consequences.

In the setting of acute dyspnoea, such as in asthma, or in the acute exacerbation of a chronic respiratory disease, the increased swing in pleural pressure leads to an increasingly negative intrathoracic pressure during inspiration [3], which increases the venous return. This increased venous return increases the right ventricular

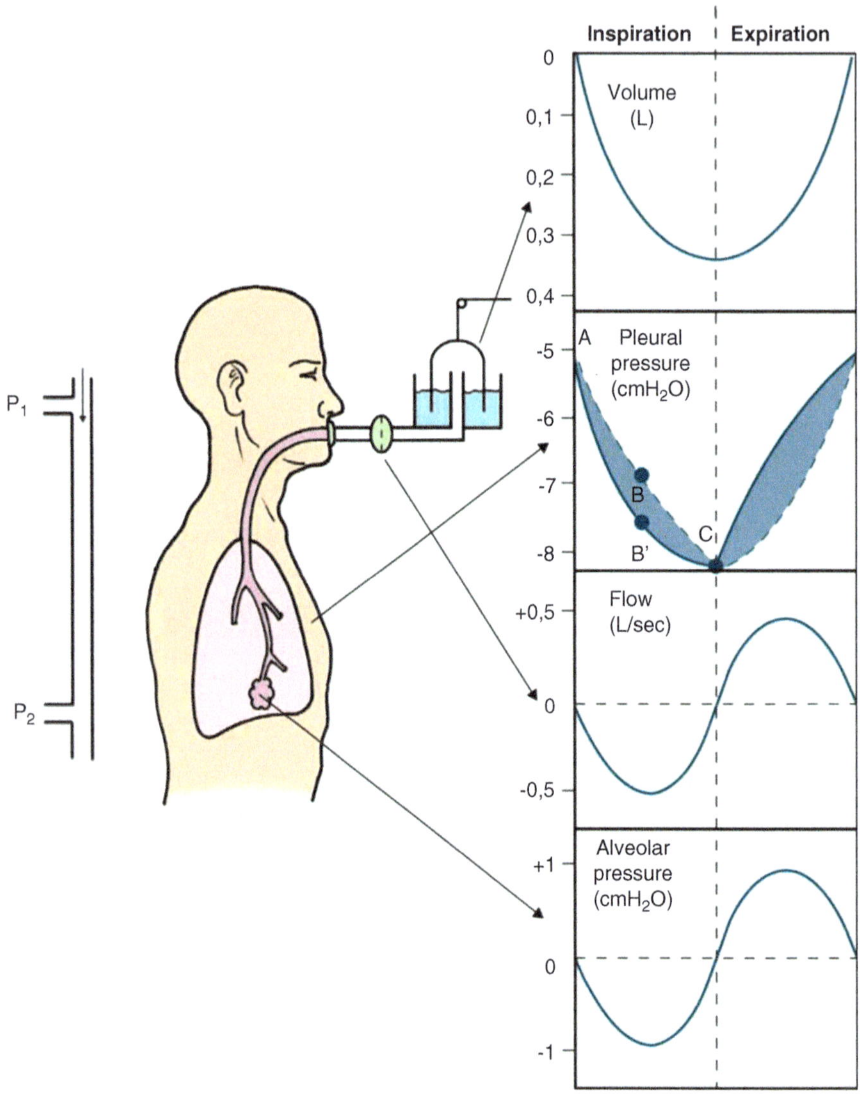

Fig. 16.4 Changes of airways pressure, flow and volume and of pleural pressure during spontaneous ventilation (Modified with permission from F. Guarracino "Ecocardiografia in Area critica" 2013 Elsevier, Milan)

volume, causing the intraventricular septum to move into the left ventricle. This leads to a decreased left ventricular diastolic compliance and a decrease in left ventricular filling volume during the inspiratory phase. As a consequence, the stroke volume and pulse pressure are reduced, and the features of pulsus paradoxus appear.

Therefore, during dyspnoea under spontaneous ventilation, the greater the pleural pressure, the greater the pulsus paradoxus.

This increased negative shift in intrathoracic pressure is not only responsible for the pulsus paradoxus but also causes acute changes in the cardiac transmural pressure, with increased myocardial oxygen consumption, reduced cardiac output and reduced flow to the respiratory muscles. The consequences of this H-L interaction will be haemodynamic impairment and further deterioration of the respiratory state.

An acute hypoxaemia from any respiratory cause will lead to pulmonary vasoconstriction and an increased RV afterload. The consequence will be an increased RV afterload and an RV/pulmonary circulation uncoupling.

Acute changes in the pulmonary circulation, such as in pulmonary embolism or in pulmonary oedema, will also affect H-L interactions and cause RV/pulmonary circulation uncoupling through an increased afterload to the RV [4]. The effect will be a reduced systemic flow and, again, an acute increase in the myocardial transmural pressure via the increased negativisation of inspiratory pleural pressure.

In some of the described acute disease states, the treatment includes positive pressure ventilation, which contributes to further elicit the H-L interactions.

16.4 H-L Interactions in Positive Pressure Ventilation

When a patient is under positive pressure ventilation (PPV), the interaction between the lungs and the heart is elicited, and haemodynamic effects can be observed [1, 5].

The effects of airway pressure and volume can be addressed separately.

The inspiratory positive pressure is transmitted to the right atrium (RA) and vena cava and below the diaphragm to the abdominal district. A direct compression of the great veins in the cardiac fossa and of the RA wall by the lungs must also be taken into account. This process causes a reduction in the venous return to the right heart [6] due to an increase in the difference between the transpulmonary pressure (TP) and filling pressure, which represents the gradient for the venous return. Such a reduction in the RV preload causes a reduction in the RV stroke volume and then a reduction in the cardiac output.

A specific aspect related to the effects of ventilatory pressure in the setting of mechanical ventilation in ARDS patients regards the decreased lung compliance that such a disease carries [7, 8]. In fact, a reduction in lung compliance leads to a reduced transmission of inspiratory positive pressure, with potentially fewer haemodynamic effects. However, if a patient with ARDS is kept at a constant tidal volume (TV), then his/her airway pressure will be increased regardless if compared to baseline healthy conditions; thus, both the intrathoracic pressure and the right heart pressure will increase and cause a reduction in the venous return. Therefore, despite a reduction in lung compliance in ARDS, the haemodynamic consequences of H-L interactions under mechanical positive pressure ventilation cannot be excluded.

The inspired volume mechanically delivered to the lungs has effects on both the alveolar and extra-alveolar capillaries. The alveolar capillaries are directly compressed, reducing the available pulmonary vascular bed; the extra-alveolar capillaries are simultaneously stretched with an opposite effect on their cross section. Taken

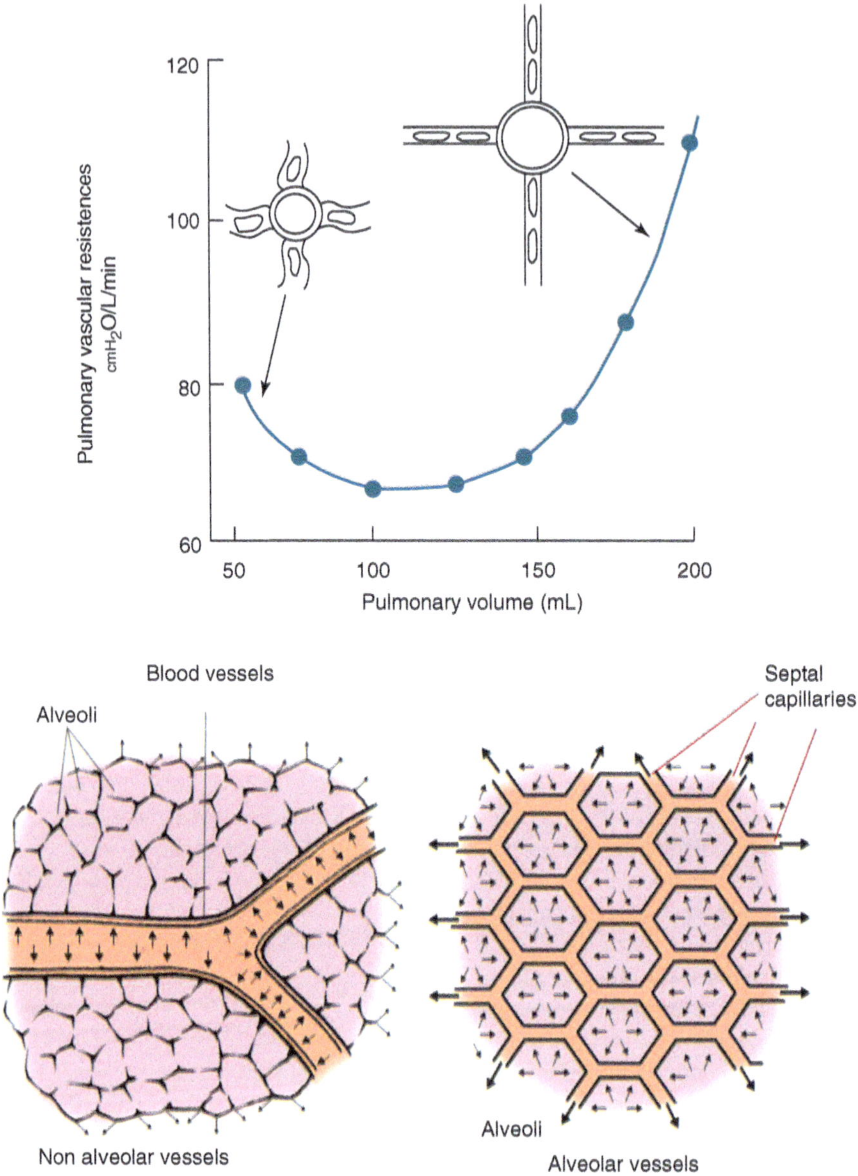

Fig. 16.5 Effect of pulmonary volumes on pulmonary vascular resistances. At low pulmonary volumes the effect is exerted on non-alveolar capillaries; high pulmonary volumes stretch the alveolar capillaries (Modified with permission from F. Guarracino "Ecocardiografia in Area critica" 2013 Elsevier, Milan)

all together, the net effect of the tidal volume on pulmonary circulation consists of an increase in the pulmonary vascular resistances (PVR) followed by an increase in the afterload to the RV (Fig. 16.5). Such an effect can add to the pressure-related preload effect, worsening the reduction in the RV stroke volume.

Again, a specific aspect regarding ARDS should be underlined: because the right ventricle acts as a "passive conduit" in normal conditions [5], *ACP* may be induced by adding the effects of PPV to the pulmonary vascular dysfunction occurring in ARDS, which leads to an abrupt increase in pulmonary artery pressure.

The H-L interaction under PPV leads to a fluctuating systolic arterial pressure waveform or stroke volume measure on the monitor screens whose variation represents a dynamic parameter to assess whether the patient is a fluid responder.

Interestingly, if a volume-related increase in the RV afterload predominates over the reduction in venous return, then the RV end-diastolic volume may increase with rising airway pressures, and an acute cor pulmonale (ACP) may develop [5]. This condition is not rare, being reported in up to 25% of patients with ARDS on mechanical ventilation [5]. If ACP occurs, then besides the RV dilatation and the reduction in cardiac output, other pathophysiological aspects characterising the acute ventricular interdependence deserve careful attention by the physician. In particular, it should be considered that in ACP, the RV undergoes a reduction of subendocardial flow, with myocardial ischaemia further contributing to impaired systolic function, hypotension and low systemic flow state and that the RV dilatation strongly affects the left ventricle (LV) filling. In fact, the pressure overload and dilated RV show a septal geometry ranging from flattened to leftward shifted, with the LV becoming acutely hypodiastolic [11].

In this scenario, tricuspid regurgitation may appear secondary to RV remodelling. IT adds prognostic information and affects the haemodynamic monitoring (cardiac output measured by PAC will no longer be reliable), impacting patient care.

16.5 H-L Interaction May Be Affected by Underlying Conditions

Pre-existing respiratory disease amplifies the normal effects of breathing, and cardiovascular disease jeopardises the response to these stresses. Pulsus paradoxus and Kussmaul's sign are common signs of the mechanical effects of respiration upon the circulation [10].

Chronic lung disease is often complicated with hyperinflation and/or pulmonary hypertension (PH). In the context of airway obstruction, alveolar pressure increases and can exert a compressive effect on the surrounding alveolar vasculature. Therefore, marked hyperinflation increases pulmonary vascular resistances. This scenario is especially relevant during the extremes of hyperinflation, as observed in patients with acute exacerbations of asthma or chronic respiratory disease. Pulsus paradoxus may be found in asthmatic patients representing a typical picture of H-L interaction under spontaneous ventilation.

Hypoxic pulmonary vasoconstriction commonly accompanies exacerbations: if PH is already present, this can impose a dangerous further overload to the RV ejection under mechanical ventilation. An ACP can then more easily occur in a chronic respiratory patient under PPV, independent of the cause leading to the respiratory failure being exacerbation or ARDS.

Underlying cardiac conditions, such as coronary artery disease (CAD) and cardiomyopathies, or the adequacy of the circulating volume will also affect the haemodynamic consequences of H-L interaction under PPV.

A CAD involving the RV may increase the risk of RV subendocardial ischaemia if ACP occurs. A baseline RV dysfunction will influence the haemodynamic significance of any added vascular load imposed by the airway pressure on pulmonary resistance.

On the other hand, a patient with reduced LV function may take advantage of the reduction in transmural pressure induced by PEEP application, and this effect may predominate the reduced preload to the RV [1]. Finally, one more example from the real world consists of the hypotensive effect of PPV, for instance, when increasing PEEP, in patients with hypovolaemia.

16.6 Clinical Implications of H-L Interaction in the ARDS Patient

While the protective ventilation regimen applied in ARDS makes standard dynamic indices of fluid responsiveness based on H-L interaction unreliable, the pathophysiology of the haemodynamic effects of H-L interaction represents a strong rationale for managing mechanical ventilation in the light of RV physiology and for addressing weaning failure from a different pathophysiological approach.

Therefore, the main clinical implication with regard to ARDS management consists of preventing or improving ACP by adhering to lung-protective strategies during mechanical ventilation [5, 9, 11–13] and in addressing the cardiac issue at the time of difficult weaning.

The management of mechanical ventilation to prevent effects on the RV requires an echocardiographic approach. Echocardiography is currently considered the gold standard in this setting [5].

The comprehensive description of the ultrasound assessment of the heart under mechanical ventilation goes beyond the aim of this chapter. However we suggest that any ARDS patient under PPV should be evaluated by echocardiography on a daily basis, and reassessed any time the clinical situation shows changes in the haemodynamic profile or the clinician suspects that a RV dysfunction is developing. The echo approach should aim at evaluating the RV anatomy and function, addressing the RV/LV ratio, and detecting and assessing the tricuspid valve.

The RV assessment allows one to balance lung recruitment and lung overdistention [5]. A strategy based on the use of echocardiography in combination with a protective ventilatory approach allows one to pursue the following: “what is good for the lung is good for the right ventricle” [5].

Positive pressure ventilation can also have beneficial effects on haemodynamics in ARDS patients if appropriately managed. The use of PEEP to treat hypoxaemia may reduce pulmonary vascular resistance through lung recruitment and aeration of hypoxic alveoli, which contribute to blunt hypoxic pulmonary vasoconstriction. Applying the least amount of PEEP necessary to achieve an adequate PaO_2/FiO_2

ratio should lead to the least detrimental haemodynamic effects. This application can be achieved by titrating PEEP under echocardiography monitoring of the RV response [12, 13].

Conclusions

The heart and lung physiologically interact both in spontaneous and mechanical ventilation. Under mechanical ventilation, the H-L interactions are elicited, and the positive pressure and the tidal volume applied to the lungs cause haemodynamic changes. Such changes are observed as variation in the stroke volume and pulse pressure peripherally, with the meaning ranging between slight haemodynamic change and severe circulatory alteration. This result will depend both on the presence of pre-existing respiratory and cardiac conditions and the severity of RV involvement by the respiratory stressor. In ARDS pathology, factors leading to capillary damage and increased PVR contribute to a major impact of PPV on the RV and can increase the risk of ACP. Echocardiography plays a pivotal role in elucidating the cardiac function during mechanical ventilation and in promptly detecting signs of RV dysfunction. By doing so, the echo assessment is helpful in titrating both the ventilatory and haemodynamic treatments in critically ill patient with ARDS.

References

1. Pinsky MR (2007) Heart–lung interactions. Curr Opin Crit Care 13:528–531
2. Zapol WM, Kobayashi K, Snider MT, Greene R, Laver MB (1977) Vascular obstruction causes pulmonary hypertension in severe acute respiratory failure. Chest 71(Suppl 2):306–307
3. Pinsky MR (2012) Heart lung interactions during mechanical ventilation. Curr Opin Crit Care 18:256–260
4. Price LC, Wort SJ, Finney SJ, Marino PS, Brett SJ (2010) Pulmonary vascular and right ventricular dysfunction in adult critical care: current and emerging options for management: a systematic literature review. Crit Care 14(5):R169
5. Repessé X, Charron C, Vieillard-Baron A (2015) Acute Cor Pulmonale in ARDS rationale for protecting the right ventricle. Chest 147(1):259–265
6. Smeding L, Lust E, Plötz FB, ABJ G (2010) Clinical implications of heart-lung interactions during mechanical ventilation: an update. Neth J Med 68(2):56–61
7. Romand JA, Shi W, Pinsky MR (1995) Cardiopulmonary effects of positive pressure ventilation during acute lung injury. Chest 108:1041–1048
8. Scharf SM, Ingram RH Jr (1977) Effects of decreasing lung compliance with oleic acid on the cardiovascular response to PEEP. Am J Phys 233:H635–H641
9. Pinsky MR, Desmet JM, Vincent JL (1992) Effect of positive endexpiratory pressure on right ventricular function in humans. Am Rev Respir Dis 146(3):681–687
10. Vieillard-Baron A, Prin S, Chergui K, Dubourg O, Jardin F (2002) Echo-Doppler demonstration of acute cor pulmonale at the bedside in the medical intensive care unit. Am J Respir Crit Care Med 166:1310–1319
11. Forfia PR, Vaidya A, Wiegers SE (2013) Pulmonary heart disease: the heart-lung interaction and its impact on patient phenotypes. Pulm Circ 3:5–19
12. Jardin F, Vieillard-Baron A (2007) Is there a safe plateau pressure in ARDS? The right heart only knows. Intensive Care Med 33(3):444–447
13. Jardin F (2005) Acute leftward septal shift by lung recruitment maneuver. Intensive Care Med 31:1148–1149

Stem Cells and Their Immunomodulatory Potential for the Treatment of ARDS

17

Claudia C. dos Santos

17.1 Introduction

Despite significant advances in supportive ICU care, acute respiratory distress syndrome (ARDS) remains a leading cause of death and disability worldwide [1–4]. Many potential therapies have been found ineffective, including corticosteroids and immunomodulation agents. Reasons behind the failed trials in ARDS have been discussed [5–8]. From the preclinical research perspective, the largely disappointing results from clinical trials can be explained in part by our incomplete understanding of the molecular responses to injury and the mechanisms that promote repair [9–13]. Dysregulated inflammation, inappropriate accumulation and activity of leukocytes, and disruption of the alveolar-capillary barrier remain central to the pathophysiology of ARDS. A therapeutic approach that can successfully target injurious inflammation and restore alveolar-capillary barrier function, while maintaining host defense and augmenting tissue repair, would be an ideal strategy for the treatment of ARDS. Rapid and exciting progresses in the field of cell immunotherapy have recently emerged as a disruptive strategy that can modulate the immune system and overcome the immunological derailment characterizing the pathophysiology of ARDS. This chapter focuses on summarizing current knowledge on the immunomodulatory actions of mesenchymal stromal cell (MSC) as novel immunotherapeutics for the treatment of ARDS and the translation of new knowledge to clinical trials.

C.C. dos Santos, MSc, MD, FRCPC
The Keenan Centre for Biomedical Research, The Li Ka Shing Knowledge Institute and the Interdepartmental Division of Critical Care, University of Toronto, Toronto, ON, Canada

St. Michael's Hospital, 30 Bond Street, Bond Wing, Room 4-008, Toronto, ON, Canada
e-mail: claudia.santos@utoronto.ca; dossantosc@smh.ca

D. Chiumello (ed.), *Acute Respiratory Distress Syndrome (ARDS)*,
DOI 10.1007/978-3-319-41852-0_17

17.2 Mesenchymal Stem/Stromal Cell (MSCs)

Although mesenchymal stem/stromal cells can be derived from a variety of different tissue sources, bone marrow-derived mesenchymal stem/stromal cells (BM-MSCs) have been the most extensively studied in the field of acute lung injury (ALI, the pro-clinical correlate of human ARDS) and will be the main focus of this review. Some controversy remains regarding how to name these pluripotent cells [14], stem vs. stromal, and minimal criteria to define them have been established [15]. First, MSC should be adherent to plastic in standard culture conditions. Second, they should express CD105, CD73, and CD90 and lack expression of CD45, CD34, CD14 or CD11b, CD79alpha or CD19, and HLA-DR surface molecules. Finally, they should differentiate to osteoblasts, adipocytes, and chondroblasts in vitro [15]. MSCs possess various favorable biological characteristics underscoring their clinical utility, including their convenient isolation, their rapid expansion in culture, and high clonogenicity while preserving their genetic stability and minimal immunogenicity making them a viable option for allogenic transplantation. The latter has recently come into question as MSCs may be immune evasive rather than immune privileged [16].

MSCs also preferentially home to the wounded or damaged tissue sites [17]. Traffic of MSCs to areas of tissue injury appears to be driven by different interactions between chemokines released from the injured tissue and chemokine receptors expressed on MSCs. For example, stromal cell-derived factor 1/CXCR4 pathway can mediate traffic of MSCs to ischemic or hypoxic tissues [18–20], while CD44 expressed on MSCs may interact with hyaluronic acid where interstitial matrices are exposed following injury [21–23]. Following intravenous administration, MSCs become entrapped in the capillary beds; this occurs primarily in the lung and liver [24]. In the context of ARDS, the relative biological significance of MSC entrapment is unclear since MSCs from bone marrow, adipose, and other tissues stay in the lungs for only about 24–48 h prior to being cleared [25, 26]. The overall opinion is that these cells may exert their beneficial effect through mechanisms that may not require cell-cell contact, and although cell engraftment with differentiation, transdifferentiation, or cell fusion may contribute to reconstitution of normal organ function, these are of uncertain therapeutic significance [27–29]. In contrast to the engraftment hypothesis, several alternative mechanistic explanations have been proposed for how these cells exert their therapeutic effects including:

(i) Their potential for enhancing tissue-endogenous stem/progenitor cell activity
(ii) Regulation of genes that modulate the response to injury and repair
(iii) Transfer of cellular and genomic contents such as mitochondria and microRNAs
(iv) Secretion of paracrine factors that target key aspects of the pathophysiology of injury and repair in ARDS

17.3 Performance of MSCs in Preclinical Models of ALI and Translation to Clinical Trials

The growing interest in the therapeutic potential of these cells for the treatment of ARDS rests solidly on their robust and reproducible performance in preclinical models of organ injury including lung bleomycin [30], intratracheal [31–33] or intraperitoneal [34, 35] endotoxin, cecal ligation and puncture [36], pseudomonal abdominal sepsis [37], and *E. coli* pneumonia [38]. In most, if not all models, stem cell administration reduces the odds of death [39, 40]. This is true for overall mortality, as well as mortality at predefined time intervals [39]. MSC administration reduces death even when the initiation of MSC therapy is delayed to 6 h post induction of ALI (or sepsis). In terms of secondary outcomes, MSCs may exert their beneficial effect by reducing inflammation while enhancing bacterial clearance [41], augmenting lung repair [42], and restoring alveolar-capillary barrier function [43, 44]. The dramatic results in preclinical models of ALI has propelled rapid translation to the clinic, with a recent phase I trial completed [45, 46], a phase 2 trial in progress (NCT02097641), and another phase 1/2 randomized, double-blind, placebo-controlled trial (NCT01902082) on the way. The latter targets not only safety but also efficacy outcomes, using allogeneic adipose-derived MSCs. In both studies, cells will be administered intravenously, inclusion criteria are similar, and MSC therapeutic doses vary from 1 to 10 × 10^6 cells/kg. In parallel, the Canadian Critical Care Trials Group has also initiated the first human trial using stem cell as immunotherapy for the treatment of sepsis (Cellular Immunotherapy for Septic Shock, CISS Trial, NCT02421484).

As we transition from preclinical to clinical studies, many questions remain about how we will translate knowledge acquired on the bench or in animal models to the clinic. We will highlight some of these questions throughout the review, but the issue of potency deserves brief attention. The International Society for Cellular Therapy (ISCT) released in 2015 their perspective on immune functional assays for MSC potency [47]. The proposal springs from a broad consensus in the community that, despite different tissue sourcing and culture expansion protocols, human MSCs likely share fundamental mechanisms of action. Identification of functional markers of potency and harmonization of standard operating procedures to measure biological properties of stem cells intended for therapy is a primary goal of future studies. The preferred analytic methods proposed by the ISCT focus on (a) gene, (b) protein (secretome), and (c) cell marker expression that reflect current knowledge in the field. While safety and tolerability of human MSCs remain the main primary study end points, future studies will aim to address secondary efficacy end points by assessing respiratory, systemic, and biological markers of function. Here, we will briefly discuss the state of knowledge of the immunoregulatory properties of these cells and their potential for future therapeutics in ARDS.

17.3.1 Enhancing Tissue-Endogenous Stem/Progenitor Cell Activity

The adult lung is a tissue with relatively slow cellular turnover. The turnover of airway epithelial cells is less than 1% per day during steady-state conditions, in contrast to the regenerative capacity of a continuously renewing tissue, such as bone marrow, which has the ability to generate approximately 10^9 hematopoietic cells per day [48]. Repair in the lung in turn depends on the regenerative capacity of over 40 different types of cells for tissue regeneration or replacement. Following severe injury, self-renewing potential of stromal and other progenitor cells of the lung increases significantly [49]. Initially, it was thought that MSCs participated directly in the repair process by incorporating into regenerated tissues and replacing cells [50, 51]. It has been difficult to resolve the fate of grafted MSCs because of the short half-life of engrafted MSCs, lack of sensitive means for isolation and detection, and low targeting efficiency [17]. Cumulative evidence suggests exogenous MSCs are unlikely to replace/regenerate lung tissue. Differentiation and/or transdifferentiation of specific progenitor cells along the trachea, bronchioles, or alveoli depends on distinct progenitor populations (and specific signals) that contribute to lung maintenance and repair [52]. Recent evidence suggests exogenously administered MSCs may enhance resident stem cell "niches," that in turn repopulate the lung and repair damaged tissue.

The ability of MSCs to stimulate endogenous progenitor cells was first demonstrated in experiments where human MSCs were injected directly into the hippocampus of immune-deficient rats [53] where they enhanced the proliferation of the endogenous neural stem cells increasing their migration and differentiation into neural cells. Similar findings were documented in a model of intracerebral hemorrhage, where the number of endogenous progenitor cells was increased in MSC-treated animals compared to controls [54]. More recently, in a model of excisional wound repair that mimics wound reepithelialization and granulation tissue formation, labeled human MSCs and species-specific markers demonstrated that exogenous MSCs initiate the formation of a niche in the injured environment and promote recruitment of endogenous stem/progenitor cells to the site of injury [55]. Critical signals such as Wnt, vascular endothelial growth factor (VEGF), and platelet-derived growth factor receptor-α (PDGFRA) within these "niches" of repair suggest that the role of MSCs is largely limited to signaling that initiates the recruitment and direction of endogenous (progenitor) cells to sites of injury to promote repair [56].

Although it is now evident that the lung harbors a diverse population of progenitor cells [57, 58], direct evidence demonstrating the role of exogenous stem cells in enhancing the recruitment and repair activity of endogenous progenitors after lung injury is scant. Gotts et al. recently reviewed the various lines of evidence in support for an endogenous cell-based pathway for recovery in the lung [44], highlighting the diversity of lung epithelial/endothelial progenitor cell populations and their regulation [44]. In a murine model of cigarette smoke-induced COPD, MSCs transplantation can relieve lung injury by promoting proliferation of endogenous lung stem cells [59] although there is immense controversy about how to demonstrate the presence and activity of true lung progenitors [44, 60]. Bronchoalveolar stem cells increase after MSC treatment in a mouse model of bronchopulmonary dysplasia [61, 62]. A recent report suggests that MSCs may also promote repair through activation of endogenous distal lung airway progenitor cell populations in mouse models [61]. Further indirect evidence in support for exogenous stem cells as coordinators of an endogenous progenitor cell response comes from pneumonectomy experiments that demonstrate VEGF signaling in lung endothelium promotes matrix metalloproteinase 14 expression, which in turn releases EGF receptor ligands that drive epithelial progenitor proliferation and alveologenesis. Moreover, there are MSCs that reside in the lung. Resident lung MSCs niches can be found along the proximal-distal axis of the airway tree. Lung MSCs secrete FGF-10, a critical factor necessary for directing lung differentiation [63]. How these resident MSCs respond to exogenous MSC administration and their contribution to lung repair remains to be elucidated.

17.3.2 Secretion of Paracrine Factors

Diffusion of autocrine and paracrine signaling molecules enables cells to communicate in the absence of physical contact. MSCs possess strong immunoregulatory properties, affecting both innate and adaptive immune systems [14]. Specific factors secreted by stem cells have various functional properties such as being antiapoptotic, immunomodulatory, and angiogenic, playing a role in cell mobilization, evoking responses from resident cells in the extracellular environment, and facilitating collateral remodeling [64]. The activity of various immune cells, including T cells, B cells, neutrophils, NK cells, and dendritic cells, is modulated in the presence of MSCs. For example, MSCs suppress T-cell activation and proliferation, inhibit monocyte differentiation, and block proliferation of B cells [65–68]. Interestingly, the immunosuppressive ability of MSCs may be dose dependent, where a low dose (below a threshold which is yet to be determined) elicits pronounced lymphocyte expansion [69], while a sufficient MSC "dose" suppresses T-lymphocyte proliferation, resulting in anergy of activated T lymphocytes [68, 70]. MSCs also inhibit B-lymphocyte proliferation in vitro by arresting the G0/G1 phase of the cell cycle rather than inducing apoptosis [67, 71], thus reducing antibody production [72]. Of note, in the absence of an inflammatory stimulus, naıve MSCs are unable to influence B-lymphocyte proliferation [73] underscoring the importance of the "inflammatory milieu" in guiding MSC responses: a phenomenon which is actively being exploited to engineer MSCs with specific biotherapeutic properties.

The immunosuppressive properties of MSCs are thought to depend on secretion of various soluble factors, including cytokines, indoleamine 2,3- dioxygenase (IDO), nitric oxide (NO), prostaglandin E2 (PGE2), and tumor necrosis factor-α-induced protein 6 (TSG-6) [52]. Although most studies rely on in vitro data to define specific mechanisms of action, in vivo, the interaction between endogenous and exogenous MSCs may lead to a complex interplay between specific factors: (i) multiple paracrine factors are involved in MSC-mediated modulation of the immune response, (ii) various factors share redundant functions, and (iii) many factors affect multiple processes (perhaps even simultaneously). For example, IL-1 receptor antagonist mediates both the anti-inflammatory and anti-fibrotic effects of MSCs after lung injury [74]. A further layer of complexity is provided by the existence of resident MSCs [75, 76]. The ability of tissue-resident MSCs to physiologically modulate the immune system (or be modulated by exogenous MSC administration) is unknown [52].

In specific reference to models of ALI, MSC regulation of angiopoietin1 (ANGPT1) has been identified as a critical event to promote survival of endothelial cells, protect against vascular inflammation and leakage, and reduce loss of barrier function [32]. MSCs engineered to produce ANGPT1 significantly reduced ALI in preclinical models indicating that the beneficial effects of MSCs can be further enhanced by gene therapy approaches [33]. Another mediator that has gained much attention in lung research is keratinocyte growth factor (KGF). In an ex vivo human lung injury model, KGF was shown to be essential for the beneficial effect of human MSCs on alveolar epithelial fluid transport [77]. In addition, hepatocyte growth factor (HGF) has been implicated in ameliorating lung injury in models of both emphysema and pulmonary fibrosis [77–79]. In vitro data suggests HGF acts on endothelial cells, restoring integrity and permeability [80]. Recently, it has been suggested that the therapeutic effects of MSCs can be reproduced, at least in part, by components of MSC secretome including KGF [77, 81] and ANGPT1 [32]. An intriguing property of MSCs is their ability to enhance bacterial phagocytosis and killing [36, 82, 83]. Bonfield et al. reported that systemic administration of MSCs significantly reduced weight loss, chronic infection, circulating neutrophils relative to macrophages, and lung pathologies in a murine cystic fibrosis infection and inflammation model [84]. In our own work, we demonstrated that treatment with MSCs significantly enhances gene expression pathways related to antigen presentation and bacterial killing [36, 85]. How MSCs enhance antibacterial clearance is an active area of research. Stimulated MSCs, in vitro and in vivo, synthesize antimicrobial peptide LL-37 and β-defensins. Increased β-defensin 2 levels and antibacterial effects of MSCs are abolished by specific antagonist or by siRNA-mediated knockdown of TLR4, but not TLR2, and restored by β-defensin 2 supplementation [86]. This discovery suggests that MSCs are a potential therapeutic agent for acute and systemic infections; this will be tested in further trials looking at the role of stem cell therapy for the treatment of sepsis.

Moreover, MSCs have been implicated in "educating" professional phagocytes such as macrophages. Recent studies have suggested an emerging role for macrophages in the reduction of inflammation and promotion of tissue repair [87, 88]. Coculture or stimulation of immune cells with MSCs alters the expression of a number of pattern recognition receptors, which appear to play a role in their immunoregulatory actions [83, 89]. Human MSCs cocultured with macrophages induce macrophage M1/M2 phenotype transformation. The M2 macrophages have high phagocytosis capacity [90], increased migratory and proliferative capacity to produce extracellular matrix (ECM) components, angiogenic and chemotactic factors, increased levels of IL-10, decreased TNF-α and IL-12, and low co-stimulatory molecule CD86 and HLA class II [91]. In addition to the pathogen defense, M2 macrophages clear apoptotic cells, can mitigate inflammatory response, and promote wound healing. Also, M2 macrophages have complex roles outside the context of inflammation, such as organ morphogenesis, tissue turnover, and endocrine signaling. This effect of MSC is at least partially mediated by soluble mechanisms and PGE-2 has been indicated to be one of the factors involved [90, 91]. The current classification of macrophage immune activation is challenging because two very distinct aspects are considered: the in vitro effects of selected immune-related ligands on the phenotype of macrophages and the in vivo. The biological relevance of MSCs in the reciprocal regulation of M1/M2 macrophages is evidenced in studies where after injection of MSCs into myocardium and adjacent macrophages adopted an M2 phenotype characterized by strong expression of arginase-1 [92]. Inhibiting M2 macrophages abrogated myocardial repair and regeneration post-injury [87, 93].

The cellular and inflammatory microenvironment determines MSC phenotype and their effects on the immune system. MSCs may be induced to adopt either pro- or an anti-inflammatory phenotype (reviewed in detail in [94]). MSCs with a predominantly pro-inflammatory signature are associated with early stage infection and inflammation. For example, stimulation of Toll-like receptor 4 (TLR4) with LPS or TLR2 (peptidoglycan) results in a pro-inflammatory, "MSC1" phenotype (analogous to the M1 macrophage), whereas priming of TLR3 with poly I:C or ds DNA results in a MSC2 phenotype with secretion of immunosuppressive mediators [95]. It has been recently suggested that in vitro MSC expansion media can affect this phenotype, with platelet lysate-supplemented media favoring a pro-inflammatory MSC phenotype [96], highlighting the fundamental importance of the culture expansion conditions for the success of future trials.

In addition to targeting inflammation, MSC administration may enhance active biochemical and metabolic repair. Specifically, MSCs secrete lipoxins, derived by the sequential actions of lipoxygenases and other enzymes to produce bioactive trihydroxytetraenes, structures that are found in all eicosanoids of this class, e.g., lipoxin A4 (LXA4). LXA4 is a specialized proresolving lipid mediator that dampens excessive inflammation, promotes resolution, and protects from leukocyte-mediated tissue damage. Although the mechanisms of action are not fully understood, previous studies suggested that aspirin-triggered 15-epi-LXA4 induces apoptosis in neutrophils in situ and facilitates resolution of myeloperoxidase-sustained neutrophil-dependent pulmonary inflammation [42]. Coculture of human MSCs with alveolar epithelial type II cells in the presence of cytomix significantly increased the production of LXA4. In vivo, blocking the LXA4 receptor with WRW4, a LXA4 receptor antagonist, in a murine model of LPS-induced lung injury significantly reversed the protective effect of MSCs on both survival and the accumulation of pulmonary edema [42].

17.3.3 Regulation of Genes That Modulate the Response to Injury and Repair

Studies looking at changes in gene expression in recipients following MSC administration point to the role of MSCs in "reprogramming" the inflammatory response network [97]. MSC administration results in a coordinated modulation of the host transcriptional response characterized by an overall downregulation of inflammation and inflammation-related genes and a shift toward upregulation of genes involved in reducing inflammation, phagocytosis, and bacterial killing. MSC administration results in transcriptional reprogramming of multiple genes involved in the host response to injury and repair. As well, MSC administration alters the expression of genes responsible for the pro-inflammatory M1 macrophage phenotype together with an increase in anti-inflammatory M2 macrophage determinants. Our own group employed a genome-wide expression microarray approach to perform an "unsupervised" network analysis in major organs commonly affected by sepsis following MSC administration. In addition to the expected changes in pathways associated with inflammation and tissue repair, we found that treatment with MSCs returned transcriptional pathways responsible for maintaining mitochondrial function and consequently cellular bioenergetics to control levels. This finding is consistent with the possibility of mitochondrial transfer between MSCs and cells of the host organs as proposed by Islam et al. [31]. Moreover, reduction in innate immune pro-inflammatory transcription responses was also observed concurrently with upregulation of genes tasked with maintaining microvasculature integrity [98]. This data indicates that the paradigm that a single MSC-derived paracrine mediator is responsible for the global pleotropic effect of MSCs on transcriptional and network reprogramming is absurd. A much more plausible explanation is that MSC-conferred protection from acute injury involves a range of complementary activities, resulting in mitigation of the innate and acquired immune and inflammatory responses while also affecting complex networks of host cell-cell, cell-matrix, metabolism and bioenergy substrate utilization, and functional pathways. The dramatic effect of stem cells on gene transcription suggests MSCs may generate a coordinated genetic response by regulating gene expression at a higher gene organizational level that depends on complex network of transcription factors and histone modifiers, in concert with specific transcriptional co-activators and co-repressors that activate or repress MSCs [99, 100].

Regulation of gene expression at the epigenetic level occurs via modifications of chromatin architecture by facilitating the opening of DNA (euchromatin) to permit transcription or the condensing of DNA (heterochromatin) to repress transcription [101]. Accordingly, the architecture of chromatin is essential for the regulation of various chromatin-based cellular processes and is dynamically modulated through the orchestration of multiple mechanisms including histone modification, DNA methylation, chromatin remodeling, and noncoding RNA. At present, a large number of studies are focusing on identifying extrinsic regulators and their intrinsic target transcription factors that regulate MSC properties and functions. So far we know that a variety of histone-modifying enzymes are involved in the dynamic regulation of MSC trilineage differentiation [100]. In addition, epigenetic changes seem to play a critical role in the ability of MSCs to cross oligolineage boundaries and differentiate into different cell types, such as neurons, cardiomyocytes, hepatocytes, and endothelial cells, under appropriate culture conditions, indicating that these cells are extremely plastic. Importantly, various chemical genetic approaches, specific combination of small cell-permeable biological active compounds that are involved in the regulation of chromatin structure and function, and interfere with specific cell signaling pathways, may be used for reprogramming MSCs [102]. For example, histone modifiers alter the differentiation of MSCs into neuronal [103,

104] or cardiomyocyte [102, 105] cells. Moreover, the epigenetic-modifying drug such as BIX-01294 (a histone G9a methyltransferase inhibitor) can enhance endothelial differentiation of adipose tissue-derived MSCs through upregulation of several endothelial markers and factors associated with blood vessel formation [106]. The relative biological significance of the role of epigenetic regulation to the therapeutic potential of MSCs comes from the diabetes and the senescence literature. MSCs are responsive to metabolic cues including circulating glucose levels. Long-term exposure of undifferentiated human adipose tissue stromal cells to high glucose upregulates a subset of inflammation response genes by altering their promoter histone methylation patterns in a manner consistent with transcriptional derepression [107]. Genetic alteration studies demonstrate that DNA methyltransferases are responsible for maintaining methylation, and their loss results in significant myeloid skewing and self-renewal defects (reviewed in detail in [108]). Evidence that MSCs can be primed to express epigenetic "marks" provides an argument for priming cells in an effort to engineer MSCs that can impart specific biological properties to recipients [109, 110].

17.3.4 Transfer of Cellular and Genomic Contents such as Mitochondria and MicroRNAs

Recently, a novel mechanism for cellular communication involving long-distance intercellular connections called tunneling nanotubes (TNTs) has come to light [111]. TNTs are actin-based cytoplasmic extensions that not only facilitate direct communication between distant cells and intercellular trafficking [112] but also are associated with the transfer of biomolecular cargos such as organelles, Golgi vesicles, plasma membrane components, and even pathogens [113–115]. BM-derived MSCs have been shown to have the ability to transfer mitochondria to other cell types via these TNTs, thus restoring aerobic respiratory function in cells with defective mitochondria [116]. Mitochondrial transfer is thought to augment macrophage function by improving mitochondrial bioenergetics. As reported for alveolar epithelial cells, recovery of the energetic function of macrophages is characterized by an increased ability to generate ATP under conditions in which the cells exhibit mitochondrial uncoupling or an enhanced proton leak and involves protection of the macrophage by reducing mitochondrial ROS generation [117, 118]. In a mouse model of ALI, intratracheal delivery of BM-derived MSCs resulted in mitochondrial transfer from MSCs to alveolar epithelial cells via Connexin-43- containing gap junctions [31]. Following lung injury, human mitochondrial DNA was detected in mouse lungs, and human MSCs and their exosomes were shown to prevent accumulation of inflammatory (Ly6Chigh) monocytes and reduce the production of inflammatory and pro-fibrotic cytokines [119]. Importantly, MSCs carrying defective mitochondria did not ameliorate lung injury, and increased mouse survival was only evident following administration of wild-type MSCs. More recent studies demonstrate that mitochondrial Rho GTPase 1 (MIRO1), a Rho GTPase, functions as a calcium-sensitive adaptor protein that drives mitochondria along microtubules [120].

Cells can also communicate with each other by secreting small vesicles into the extracellular milieu, known as extracellular vesicles (EVs) [121, 122]. EVs are submicron vesicles, which, based on their size, origin, morphology, and mode of release, can be categorized into exosomes (40–200 nm), microvesicles (50–1000 nm), apoptotic bodies (50–5000 nm), or Golgi vesicles [123]. EVs are secreted by a multitude of cell and can be isolated via several conventional as well as high-throughput technologies. Importantly, these vesicles carry a repertoire of mRNAs, miRNAs, DNA, proteins, and lipids that can be transferred to neighboring cells, modifying their phenotype as well as the microenvironment [123–125]. The molecular signatures of EVs are selective to each cell/tissue type, which makes them ideal source for clinical applications [126]. Various studies have shown stem cell-EVs traffic stem cell-associated transcription factors associated with self-renewal of stem cells such as Nanog, Oct-4, HoxB4, and Rex-1 [127] key factors in the maintenance of pluripotency. They have also been shown to express MSC markers such as CD105 [128], prominin-1/CD133 [129–131], and KIT [132]. More direct effectors of the stem cell phenotype such as WNT [133], β-catenin [134], and Hedgehog [135] have also been identified on stem cell-EVs. Moreover, key biological features of stem cells, such as self-renewal, differentiation, and maturation, could be mimicked by stem cell-associated EVs [136–138].

Targeting of proteins into shedding vesicles appears to be entirely selective [139]. Specific proteins may be included or excluded from membrane EVs, leading to the expression of proteins arrays that differ from those present on the surface of the cells from which they originated. The most comprehensive proteomic characterization of MSCs and exosomes to date detected 580 membrane-associated proteins including those required to meet the minimal criteria for MSC classification (CD73, CD90, CD105) across various MSC samples [139]. Precondition alters the proteins in exosomes [140, 141]. Exposure to ischemic tissue conditions enhanced the proangiogenic properties of exosomes, facilitating localized tissue healing. A total of 1927 proteins were identified in MSC-derived exosomes from three different donors following exposure to ischemic conditions, of which 457 were not expressed under baseline conditions, suggesting MSCs can be made to generate "tailored" exosomes [142].

Exosomes derived from MSCs may have the capability to mediate much of the functionality traditionally associated with canonical secretory proteins such as growth factors of the MSC secretome [143–147]. Exosomes, in particular, are small lipid-bound, cellularly secreted vesicles [148] that mediate some of the tissue healing properties of MSCs [149]. In addition, EVs from lung cells have been shown to induce bone marrow cells to express mRNAs coding for lung-specific proteins such as Clara cell protein, aquaporin-5, and surfactants. Furthermore, this phenomenon is enhanced significantly during lung injury [150]. Of importance to the management of ARDS, KGF mRNA is present in microvesicles, suggesting that the reparative function might stem from boosting certain growth factors in the recipient. Administration of MVs derived from human MSCs can improve survival in part through KGF secretion and decreased the influx of inflammatory cells, cytokines, protein, and bacteria in mice injured with bacterial pneumonia. In primary cultures of human monocytes or alveolar type 2 cells, the uptake of MVs may be mediated by CD44 receptors. MVs enhance monocyte phagocytosis of bacteria while decreasing inflammatory cytokine secretion and increased intracellular ATP levels in injured alveolar epithelial type 2 cells. Prestimulation of MSCs with TLR3 agonist further enhances the therapeutic effects of the released MVs [151].

Of specific interest is the transfer of microRNAs in exosomal vesicles. Until recently it was thought that stem cells can rejuvenate damaged cells by mitochondrial transfer, but recently it has been shown that mitochondrial transfer by MSCs may not be an altruistic event but rather may serve to enhance the survival of MSCs. By unloading partially depolarized mitochondria, MSCs can obviate death. MSCs manage intracellular oxidative stress by targeting depolarized mitochondria to the plasma membrane via arrestin, a domain-containing protein 1 (ARRDC1)- mediated microvesicles. Vesicles containing these depolarized mitochondria are in turn engulfed by macrophages. Elimination of depolarized mitochondria is a priority for MSCs that experience high mitochondrial ROS generation when cultured under stressful conditions (such as in the presence of atmospheric oxygen tension) [152]. In parallel, however, MSCs also shed microRNA-containing exosomes that inhibit macrophage activation by suppressing TLR signaling, thereby desensitizing macrophages to the ingested mitochondria [119]. Exosomes modulate TLR signaling and cytokine secretion in macrophages, in part, by transfer of regulatory microRNAs. A microRNA contained within MSC-derived exosomes is miR-451, known to suppress TNF, and macrophage migration inhibitory factor [153, 154]. Based on this new evidence, it seems that transfer of mitochondria that have escaped mitophagy may be pro-inflammatory and pro-injurious [155, 156]. Therefore, silencing TLR responses in macrophages is likely necessary to induce tolerance to transferred mitochondria. Circumstances would have it that the immunomodulatory activities of MSC-derived exosomes may have evolved, in part, as a mechanism by which MSCs survive oxidative stress and serendipitously confer on cells the ability to suppress inflammation, in lung injury models [119].

17.4 Summary and Future Directions

Although this is an exciting time for immunotherapy for ARDS, the issue of safety remains a lingering concern in the field. A recent meta-analysis has comprehensively summarized the safety of systemic MSC administration in humans. Lalu et al. were unable to detect associations between MSC treatment and the development of acute infusional toxicity, organ system complications, infection, death, or malignancy. Importantly, this group also showed that there was no evidence of increased susceptibility to infection with MSC administration. Although MSC immunomodulatory effects may be beneficial in pro-inflammatory diseases, these same effects may leave a patient susceptible to infection. Development of novel stem cell or stem cell-like products with wide pleotropic effects that target competing pathological processes in ARDS offers a unique opportunity for advancement in the field. Many questions remain including identifying specific mechanisms of action, potency, dose, frequency, and markers of biological efficacy and response to therapy. As we move toward large-scale multicenter randomized clinical trials, it will be important to define specific mechanisms of action, the potential for engineering performance enhanced cell-products, and the development of cell-free adjuncts that may perhaps replace cell therapy.

References

1. Bellani G et al (2016) Epidemiology, patterns of care, and mortality for patients with acute respiratory distress syndrome in intensive care units in 50 countries. JAMA 315:788–800
2. Clark BJ, Moss M (2016) The acute respiratory distress syndrome: dialing in the evidence? JAMA 315:759–761
3. Herridge MS et al (2003) One-year outcomes in survivors of the acute respiratory distress syndrome. N Engl J Med 348:683–693
4. Herridge MS et al (2011) Functional disability 5 years after acute respiratory distress syndrome. N Engl J Med 364:1293–1304
5. Annane D (2009) Improving clinical trials in the critically ill: unique challenge–sepsis. Crit Care Med 37:S117–S128
6. Angus DC, Mira JP, Vincent JL (2010) Improving clinical trials in the critically ill. Crit Care Med 38:527–532
7. Zeni F, Freeman B, Natanson C (1997) Anti-inflammatory therapies to treat sepsis and septic shock: a reassessment. Crit Care Med 25:1095–1100
8. Eichacker PQ et al (2002) Risk and the efficacy of antiinflammatory agents: retrospective and confirmatory studies of sepsis. Am J Respir Crit Care Med 166:1197–1205
9. Marshall JC (2003) Such stuff as dreams are made on: mediator-directed therapy in sepsis. Nat Rev Drug Discov 2:391–405
10. Hotchkiss RS, Coopersmith CM, McDunn JE, Ferguson TA (2009) The sepsis seesaw: tilting toward immunosuppression. Nat Med 15:496–497
11. Mongardon N, Dyson A, Singer M (2009) Is MOF an outcome parameter or a transient, adaptive state in critical illness? Curr Opin Crit Care 15:431–436
12. Dyson A, Singer M (2009) Animal models of sepsis: why does preclinical efficacy fail to translate to the clinical setting? Crit Care Med 37:S30–S37
13. Monneret G, Venet F (2010) Immunomodulatory cell therapy in sepsis: have we learnt lessons from the past? Expert Rev Anti Infect Ther 8:1109–1112
14. Keating A (2012) Mesenchymal stromal cells: new directions. Cell Stem Cell 10:709–716
15. Dominici M et al (2006) Minimal criteria for defining multipotent mesenchymal stromal cells. The International Society for Cellular Therapy position statement. Cytotherapy 8:315–317
16. Ankrum JA, Ong JF, Karp JM (2014) Mesenchymal stem cells: immune evasive, not immune privileged. Nat Biotechnol 32:252–260
17. Karp JM, Leng Teo GS (2009) Mesenchymal stem cell homing: the devil is in the details. Cell Stem Cell 4:206–216
18. Honczarenko M et al (2006) Human bone marrow stromal cells express a distinct set of biologically functional chemokine receptors. Stem Cells 24:1030–1041
19. Hung SC et al (2007) Short-term exposure of multipotent stromal cells to low oxygen increases their expression of CX3CR1 and CXCR4 and their engraftment in vivo. PLoS One 2:e416
20. Togel F, Isaac J, Hu Z, Weiss K, Westenfelder C (2005) Renal SDF-1 signals mobilization and homing of CXCR4-positive cells to the kidney after ischemic injury. Kidney Int 67:1772–1784
21. Zhu H et al (2006) The role of the hyaluronan receptor CD44 in mesenchymal stem cell migration in the extracellular matrix. Stem Cells 24:928–935
22. Goransson V et al (2004) Renal hyaluronan accumulation and hyaluronan synthase expression after ischaemia-reperfusion injury in the rat. Nephrol Dial Transplant 19:823–830

23. Herrera MB et al (2007) Exogenous mesenchymal stem cells localize to the kidney by means of CD44 following acute tubular injury. Kidney Int 72:430–441
24. Gao J, Dennis JE, Muzic RF, Lundberg M, Caplan AI (2001) The dynamic in vivo distribution of bone marrow-derived mesenchymal stem cells after infusion. Cells Tissues Organs 169:12–20
25. Weiss DJ, Bates JHT, Gilbert T, Liles WC, Lutzko C, Rajagopal J, Prockop DJ (2013) Vermont stem cell conference report: stem cells and cell therapies in lung biology and diseases. Ann Am Thorac Soc 10:25–44
26. Matthay MA et al (2013) Cell therapy for lung diseases. Report from an NIH-NHLBI workshop, November 13-14, 2012. Am J Respir Crit Care Med 188:370–375
27. Bianco P et al (2013) The meaning, the sense and the significance: translating the science of mesenchymal stem cells into medicine. Nat Med 19:35–42
28. Prockop DJ, Oh JY (2012) Medical therapies with adult stem/progenitor cells (MSCs): a backward journey from dramatic results in vivo to the cellular and molecular explanations. J Cell Biochem 113:1460–1469
29. Prockop DJ, Oh JY (2012) Mesenchymal stem/stromal cells (MSCs): role as guardians of inflammation. Mol Ther 20:14–20
30. Ortiz LA et al (2003) Mesenchymal stem cell engraftment in lung is enhanced in response to bleomycin exposure and ameliorates its fibrotic effects. Proc Natl Acad Sci U S A 100:8407–8411
31. Islam MN et al (2012) Mitochondrial transfer from bone-marrow-derived stromal cells to pulmonary alveoli protects against acute lung injury. Nat Med 18:759–765
32. Mei SH et al (2007) Prevention of LPS-induced acute lung injury in mice by mesenchymal stem cells overexpressing angiopoietin 1. PLoS Med 4:e269
33. McCarter SD et al (2007) Cell-based angiopoietin-1 gene therapy for acute lung injury. Am J Respir Crit Care Med 175:1014–1026
34. Xu J et al (2007) Prevention of endotoxin-induced systemic response by bone marrow-derived mesenchymal stem cells in mice. Am J Physiol Lung Cell Mol Physiol 293:L131–L141
35. Rojas M, Woods CR, Mora AL, Xu J, Brigham KL (2005) Endotoxin-induced lung injury in mice: structural, functional, and biochemical responses. Am J Physiol Lung Cell Mol Physiol 288:L333–L341
36. Mei SH et al (2010) Mesenchymal stem cells reduce inflammation while enhancing bacterial clearance and improving survival in sepsis. Am J Respir Crit Care Med 182:1047–1057
37. Krasnodembskaya A et al (2012) Human mesenchymal stem cells reduce mortality and bacteremia in gram-negative sepsis in mice in part by enhancing the phagocytic activity of blood monocytes. Am J Physiol Lung Cell Mol Physiol 302:L1003–L1013
38. Lee JW et al (2013) Therapeutic effects of human mesenchymal stem cells in ex vivo human lungs injured with live bacteria. Am J Respir Crit Care Med 187:751–760
39. McIntyre LA et al (2016) Efficacy of mesenchymal stromal cell therapy for acute lung injury in preclinical animal models: a systematic review. PLoS One 11:e0147170
40. Lalu MM et al (2014) Efficacy and safety of mesenchymal stromal cells in preclinical models of acute lung injury: a systematic review protocol. Syst Rev 3:48
41. Devaney J et al (2015) Human mesenchymal stromal cells decrease the severity of acute lung injury induced by *E. coli* in the rat. Thorax 70:625–635
42. El Kebir D et al (2009) 15-epi-lipoxin A4 inhibits myeloperoxidase signaling and enhances resolution of acute lung injury. Am J Respir Crit Care Med 180:311–319
43. Gupta N et al (2007) Intrapulmonary delivery of bone marrow-derived mesenchymal stem cells improves survival and attenuates endotoxin-induced acute lung injury in mice. J Immunol 179:1855–1863
44. Gotts JE, Matthay MA (2014) Endogenous and exogenous cell-based pathways for recovery from acute respiratory distress syndrome. Clin Chest Med 35:797–809
45. Liu KD et al (2014) Design and implementation of the START (STem cells for ARDS Treatment) trial, a phase 1/2 trial of human mesenchymal stem/stromal cells for the treatment of moderate-severe acute respiratory distress syndrome. Ann Intensive Care 4:22

46. Wilson JG et al (2015) Mesenchymal stem (stromal) cells for treatment of ARDS: a phase 1 clinical trial. Lancet Respir Med 3:24–32
47. Galipeau J et al (2016) International Society for Cellular Therapy perspective on immune functional assays for mesenchymal stromal cells as potency release criterion for advanced phase clinical trials. Cytotherapy 18:151–159
48. Klimczak A, Kozlowska U (2016) Mesencheymal stromal cells and tissue-specific progenitor cells: their role in tissue homeostasis. Stem Cells Int 2016:1–12
49. Bertoncello I, McQualter JL (2013) Lung stem cells: do they exist? Respirology 18:587–595
50. Wu Y, Chen L, Scott PG, Tredget EE (2007) Mesenchymal stem cells enhance wound healing through differentiation and angiogenesis. Stem Cells 25:2648–2659
51. Prockop DJ, Gregory CA, Spees JL (2003) One strategy for cell and gene therapy: harnessing the power of adult stem cells to repair tissues. Proc Natl Acad Sci U S A 100(Suppl 1):11917–11923
52. Savukinas UB, Enes SR, Sjoland AA, Westergren-Thorsson G (2016) The bystander effect: MSC-mediated lung repair. Stem Cells 4(6):1437–1444
53. Munoz JR, Stoutenger BR, Robinson AP, Spees JL, Prockop DJ (2005) Human stem/progenitor cells from bone marrow promote neurogenesis of endogenous neural stem cells in the hippocampus of mice. Proc Natl Acad Sci U S A 102:18171–18176
54. Fatar M et al (2008) Lipoaspirate-derived adult mesenchymal stem cells improve functional outcome during intracerebral hemorrhage by proliferation of endogenous progenitor cells stem cells in intracerebral hemorrhages. Neurosci Lett 443:174–178
55. Shin L, Peterson DA (2013) Human mesenchymal stem cell grafts enhance normal and impaired wound healing by recruiting existing endogenous tissue stem/progenitor cells. Stem Cells Transl Med 2:33–42
56. Burdon TJ, Paul A, Noiseux N, Prakash S, Shum-Tim D (2011) Bone marrow stem cell derived paracrine factors for regenerative medicine: current perspectives and therapeutic potential. Bone Marrow Res 2011:207326
57. Kumar ME et al (2014) Mesenchymal cells. Defining a mesenchymal progenitor niche at single-cell resolution. Science 346:1258810
58. Hogan BL et al (2014) Repair and regeneration of the respiratory system: complexity, plasticity, and mechanisms of lung stem cell function. Cell Stem Cell 15:123–138
59. Liu HM, Ma LJ, Wu JZ, Li YG (2015) MSCs relieve lung injury of COPD mice through promoting proliferation of endogenous lung stem cells. J Huazhong Univ Sci Technolog Med Sci 35:828–833
60. Weiss DJ (2014) Concise review: current status of stem cells and regenerative medicine in lung biology and diseases. Stem Cells 32:16–25
61. Tropea KA et al (2012) Bronchioalveolar stem cells increase after mesenchymal stromal cell treatment in a mouse model of bronchopulmonary dysplasia. Am J Physiol Lung Cell Mol Physiol 302:L829–L837
62. Rock JR et al (2011) Multiple stromal populations contribute to pulmonary fibrosis without evidence for epithelial to mesenchymal transition. Proc Natl Acad Sci U S A 108:E1475–E1483
63. Leeman KT, Fillmore CM, Kim CF (2014) Lung stem and progenitor cells in tissue homeostasis and disease. Curr Top Dev Biol 107:207–233
64. Kinnaird T et al (2004) Local delivery of marrow-derived stromal cells augments collateral perfusion through paracrine mechanisms. Circulation 109:1543–1549
65. Nauta AJ, Fibbe WE (2007) Immunomodulatory properties of mesenchymal stromal cells. Blood 110:3499–3506
66. Beyth S et al (2005) Human mesenchymal stem cells alter antigen-presenting cell maturation and induce T-cell unresponsiveness. Blood 105:2214–2219
67. Corcione A et al (2006) Human mesenchymal stem cells modulate B-cell functions. Blood 107:367–372
68. Glennie S, Soeiro I, Dyson PJ, Lam EW, Dazzi F (2005) Bone marrow mesenchymal stem cells induce division arrest anergy of activated T cells. Blood 105:2821–2827

69. Le Blanc K, Tammik L, Sundberg B, Haynesworth SE, Ringden O (2003) Mesenchymal stem cells inhibit and stimulate mixed lymphocyte cultures and mitogenic responses independently of the major histocompatibility complex. Scand J Immunol 57:11–20
70. Benvenuto F et al (2007) Human mesenchymal stem cells promote survival of T cells in a quiescent state. Stem Cells 25:1753–1760
71. Rafei M et al (2008) Mesenchymal stromal cell-derived CCL2 suppresses plasma cell immunoglobulin production via STAT3 inactivation and PAX5 induction. Blood 112:4991–4998
72. Comoli P et al (2008) Human mesenchymal stem cells inhibit antibody production induced in vitro by allostimulation. Nephrol Dial Transplant 23:1196–1202
73. Krampera M et al (2006) Role for interferon-gamma in the immunomodulatory activity of human bone marrow mesenchymal stem cells. Stem Cells 24:386–398
74. Ortiz LA et al (2007) Interleukin 1 receptor antagonist mediates the antiinflammatory and antifibrotic effect of mesenchymal stem cells during lung injury. Proc Natl Acad Sci U S A 104:11002–11007
75. Lama VN et al (2007) Evidence for tissue-resident mesenchymal stem cells in human adult lung from studies of transplanted allografts. J Clin Invest 117:989–996
76. Rolandsson S et al (2014) Primary mesenchymal stem cells in human transplanted lungs are CD90/CD105 perivascularly located tissue-resident cells. BMJ Open Respir Res 1:e000027
77. Lee JW, Fang X, Gupta N, Serikov V, Matthay MA (2009) Allogeneic human mesenchymal stem cells for treatment of *E. coli* endotoxin-induced acute lung injury in the ex vivo perfused human lung. Proc Natl Acad Sci U S A 106:16357–16362
78. Lan YW et al (2015) Hypoxia-preconditioned mesenchymal stem cells attenuate bleomycin-induced pulmonary fibrosis. Stem cell Res Ther 6:97
79. Katsha AM et al (2011) Paracrine factors of multipotent stromal cells ameliorate lung injury in an elastase-induced emphysema model. Mol Ther 19:196–203
80. Chen QH, Liu AR, Qiu HB, Yang Y (2015) Interaction between mesenchymal stem cells and endothelial cells restores endothelial permeability via paracrine hepatocyte growth factor in vitro. Stem cell Res Ther 6:44
81. Atabai K et al (2002) Keratinocyte growth factor can enhance alveolar epithelial repair by nonmitogenic mechanisms. Am J Physiol Lung Cell Mol Physiol 283:L163–L169
82. Gonzalez-Rey E et al (2009) Human adult stem cells derived from adipose tissue protect against experimental colitis and sepsis. Gut 58:929–939
83. Nemeth K et al (2009) Bone marrow stromal cells attenuate sepsis via prostaglandin E(2)-dependent reprogramming of host macrophages to increase their interleukin-10 production. Nat Med 15:42–49
84. Sutton MT et al (2016) Antimicrobial properties of mesenchymal stem cells: therapeutic potential for cystic fibrosis infection, and treatment. Stem Cells Int 2016:5303048
85. Amatullah H, Shan Y, Beauchamp BL, Gali PL, Gupta S (2016) Canadian critical care translational biology group (CCCTBG). DJ-1/PARK7 impairs bacterial clearance in sepsis. Am J Respir Crit Care Med. [Epub ahead of print]
86. Sung DK et al (2016) Antibacterial effect of mesenchymal stem cells against Escherichia coli is mediated by secretion of beta- defensin- 2 via toll- like receptor 4 signalling. Cell Microbiol 18:424–436
87. Godwin JW, Pinto AR, Rosenthal NA (2013) Macrophages are required for adult salamander limb regeneration. Proc Natl Acad Sci U S A 110:9415–9420
88. Pinto AR et al (2012) An abundant tissue macrophage population in the adult murine heart with a distinct alternatively-activated macrophage profile. PLoS One 7:e36814
89. Tomchuck SL et al (2008) Toll-like receptors on human mesenchymal stem cells drive their migration and immunomodulating responses. Stem Cells 26:99–107
90. Maggini J et al (2010) Mouse bone marrow-derived mesenchymal stromal cells turn activated macrophages into a regulatory-like profile. PLoS One 5:e9252
91. Kim J, Hematti P (2009) Mesenchymal stem cell-educated macrophages: a novel type of alternatively activated macrophages. Exp Hematol 37:1445–1453
92. Cho DI et al (2014) Mesenchymal stem cells reciprocally regulate the M1/M2 balance in mouse bone marrow-derived macrophages. Exp Mol Med 46:e70

93. Aurora AB et al (2014) Macrophages are required for neonatal heart regeneration. J Clin Invest 124:1382–1392
94. Bernardo ME, Fibbe WE (2013) Mesenchymal stromal cells: sensors and switchers of inflammation. Cell Stem Cell 13:392–402
95. Waterman RS, Tomchuck SL, Henkle SL, Betancourt AM (2010) A new mesenchymal stem cell (MSC) paradigm: polarization into a pro-inflammatory MSC1 or an Immunosuppressive MSC2 phenotype. PLoS One 5:e10088
96. Le Blanc K, Davies LC (2015) Mesenchymal stromal cells and the innate immune response. Immunol Lett 168:140–146
97. Zhao YD et al (2014) Endothelial FoxM1 mediates bone marrow progenitor cell-induced vascular repair and resolution of inflammation following inflammatory lung injury. Stem Cells 32:1855–1864
98. dos Santos CC et al (2012) Network analysis of transcriptional responses induced by mesenchymal stem cell treatment of experimental sepsis. Am J Pathol 181:1681–1692
99. Mohammadzadeh A et al (2014) Immunomodulatory effects of adipose-derived mesenchymal stem cells on the gene expression of major transcription factors of T cell subsets. Int Immunopharmacol 20:316–321
100. Huang B, Li G, Jiang XH (2015) Fate determination in mesenchymal stem cells: a perspective from histone-modifying enzymes. Stem Cell Res Ther 6:35
101. Elgin SC (1996) Heterochromatin and gene regulation in Drosophila. Curr Opin Genet Dev 6:193–202
102. Zhang Z, Maiman DJ, Kurpad SN, Crowe MJ, Alexanian AR (2011) Feline bone marrow-derived mesenchymal stem cells express several pluripotent and neural markers and easily turn into neural-like cells by manipulation with chromatin modifying agents and neural inducing factors. Cell Reprogram 13:385–390
103. Yu YL et al (2011) EZH2 regulates neuronal differentiation of mesenchymal stem cells through PIP5K1C-dependent calcium signaling. J Biol Chem 286:9657–9667
104. Jeong SG, Ohn T, Kim SH, Cho GW (2013) Valproic acid promotes neuronal differentiation by induction of neuroprogenitors in human bone-marrow mesenchymal stromal cells. Neurosci Lett 554:22–27
105. Li L, Zhu J, Tian J, Liu X, Feng C (2010) A role for Gcn5 in cardiomyocyte differentiation of rat mesenchymal stem cells. Mol Cell Biochem 345:309–316
106. Culmes M et al (2013) Endothelial differentiation of adipose-derived mesenchymal stem cells is improved by epigenetic modifying drug BIX-01294. Eur J Cell Biol 92:70–79
107. Ronningen T, Shah A, Reiner AH, Collas P, Moskaug JO (2015) Epigenetic priming of inflammatory response genes by high glucose in adipose progenitor cells. Biochem Biophys Res Commun 467:979–986
108. Choudry FA, Frontini M (2016) Epigenetic control of haematopoietic stem cell aging and its clinical implications. Stem Cells Int 2016:5797521
109. Alexanian AR, Liu QS, Zhang Z (2013) Enhancing the efficiency of direct reprogramming of human mesenchymal stem cells into mature neuronal-like cells with the combination of small molecule modulators of chromatin modifying enzymes. SMAD signaling and cyclic adenosine monophosphate levels. Int J Biochem Cell Biol 45:1633–1638
110. Ankrum JA, Dastidar RG, Ong JF, Levy O, Karp JM (2014) Performance-enhanced mesenchymal stem cells via intracellular delivery of steroids. Sci Rep 4:4645
111. Rustom A, Saffrich R, Markovic I, Walther P, Gerdes HH (2004) Nanotubular highways for intercellular organelle transport. Science 303:1007–1010
112. Marzo L, Gousset K, Zurzolo C (2012) Multifaceted roles of tunneling nanotubes in intercellular communication. Front Physiol 3:72
113. Gerdes HH, Bukoreshtliev NV, Barroso JF (2007) Tunneling nanotubes: a new route for the exchange of components between animal cells. FEBS Lett 581:2194–2201
114. Lou E et al (2012) Tunneling nanotubes provide a unique conduit for intercellular transfer of cellular contents in human malignant pleural mesothelioma. PLoS One 7:e33093

115. Abounit S, Zurzolo C (2012) Wiring through tunneling nanotubes–from electrical signals to organelle transfer. J Cell Sci 125:1089–1098
116. Spees JL, Olson SD, Whitney MJ, Prockop DJ (2006) Mitochondrial transfer between cells can rescue aerobic respiration. Proc Natl Acad Sci U S A 103:1283–1288
117. King MP, Attardi G (1988) Injection of mitochondria into human cells leads to a rapid replacement of the endogenous mitochondrial DNA. Cell 52:811–819
118. King MP, Attardi G (1989) Human cells lacking mtDNA: repopulation with exogenous mitochondria by complementation. Science 246:500–503
119. Phinney DG et al (2015) Mesenchymal stem cells use extracellular vesicles to outsource mitophagy and shuttle microRNAs. Nat Commun 6:8472
120. Ahmad T et al (2014) Miro1 regulates intercellular mitochondrial transport & enhances mesenchymal stem cell rescue efficacy. EMBO J 33:994–1010
121. Valadi H et al (2007) Exosome-mediated transfer of mRNAs and microRNAs is a novel mechanism of genetic exchange between cells. Nat Cell Biol 9:654–659
122. Turturici G, Tinnirello R, Sconzo G, Geraci F (2014) Extracellular membrane vesicles as a mechanism of cell-to-cell communication: advantages and disadvantages. Am J Physiol Cell Physiol 306:C621–C633
123. Tetta C, Bruno S, Fonsato V, Deregibus MC, Camussi G (2011) The role of microvesicles in tissue repair. Organogenesis 7:105–115
124. Camussi G et al (2011) Exosome/microvesicle-mediated epigenetic reprogramming of cells. Am J Cancer Res 1:98–110
125. Gatti S et al (2011) Microvesicles derived from human adult mesenchymal stem cells protect against ischaemia-reperfusion-induced acute and chronic kidney injury. Nephrol Dial Transplant 26:1474–1483
126. Nawaz M et al (2016) Extracellular vesicles: evolving factors in stem cell biology. Stem Cells Int 2016:1073140
127. Ratajczak J et al (2006) Embryonic stem cell-derived microvesicles reprogram hematopoietic progenitors: evidence for horizontal transfer of mRNA and protein delivery. Leukemia 20:847–856
128. Grange C et al (2011) Microvesicles released from human renal cancer stem cells stimulate angiogenesis and formation of lung premetastatic niche. Cancer Res 71:5346–5356
129. Bauer N et al (2011) Haematopoietic stem cell differentiation promotes the release of prominin-1/CD133-containing membrane vesicles–a role of the endocytic-exocytic pathway. EMBO Mol Med 3:398–409
130. Rappa G et al (2013) Wnt interaction and extracellular release of prominin-1/CD133 in human malignant melanoma cells. Exp Cell Res 319:810–819
131. Huttner HB et al (2008) The stem cell marker prominin-1/CD133 on membrane particles in human cerebrospinal fluid offers novel approaches for studying central nervous system disease. Stem Cells 26:698–705
132. Xiao H et al (2014) Mast cell exosomes promote lung adenocarcinoma cell proliferation – role of KIT-stem cell factor signaling. Cell Commun Signal 12:64
133. Gross JC, Chaudhary V, Bartscherer K, Boutros M (2012) Active Wnt proteins are secreted on exosomes. Nat Cell Biol 14:1036–1045
134. Chairoungdua A, Smith DL, Pochard P, Hull M, Caplan MJ (2010) Exosome release of beta-catenin: a novel mechanism that antagonizes Wnt signaling. J Cell Biol 190:1079–1091
135. Gradilla AC et al (2014) Exosomes as Hedgehog carriers in cytoneme-mediated transport and secretion. Nat Commun 5:5649
136. Nair R et al (2014) Extracellular vesicles derived from preosteoblasts influence embryonic stem cell differentiation. Stem Cells Dev 23:1625–1635
137. McIver SC et al (2014) The exosome complex establishes a barricade to erythroid maturation. Blood 124:2285–2297
138. Forterre A et al (2014) Myotube-derived exosomal miRNAs downregulate Sirtuin1 in myoblasts during muscle cell differentiation. Cell Cycle 13:78–89
139. Anderson JD et al (2016) Comprehensive proteomic analysis of mesenchymal stem cell exosomes reveals modulation of angiogenesis via NFkB signaling. Stem Cells 34(3):601–613

140. Rosova I, Dao M, Capoccia B, Link D, Nolta JA (2008) Hypoxic preconditioning results in increased motility and improved therapeutic potential of human mesenchymal stem cells. Stem Cells 26:2173–2182
141. Beegle J et al (2015) Hypoxic preconditioning of mesenchymal stromal cells induces metabolic changes, enhances survival, and promotes cell retention in vivo. Stem Cells 33:1818–1828
142. Hultin-Rosenberg L, Forshed J, Branca RM, Lehtio J, Johansson HJ (2013) Defining, comparing, and improving iTRAQ quantification in mass spectrometry proteomics data. Mol Cell Proteomics 12:2021–2031
143. Zhang HC et al (2012) Microvesicles derived from human umbilical cord mesenchymal stem cells stimulated by hypoxia promote angiogenesis both in vitro and in vivo. Stem Cells Dev 21:3289–3297
144. Li T et al (2013) Exosomes derived from human umbilical cord mesenchymal stem cells alleviate liver fibrosis. Stem Cells Dev 22:845–854
145. Katsuda T et al (2013) Human adipose tissue-derived mesenchymal stem cells secrete functional neprilysin-bound exosomes. Sci Rep 3:1197
146. Bruno S et al (2009) Mesenchymal stem cell-derived microvesicles protect against acute tubular injury. J Am Soc Nephrol 20:1053–1067
147. Xin H et al (2013) MiR-133b promotes neural plasticity and functional recovery after treatment of stroke with multipotent mesenchymal stromal cells in rats via transfer of exosome-enriched extracellular particles. Stem Cells 31:2737–2746
148. E.L. Andaloussi S, Mager I, Breakefield XO, Wood MJ (2013) Extracellular vesicles: biology and emerging therapeutic opportunities. Nat Rev Drug Discov 12:347–357
149. Zhu YG et al (2014) Human mesenchymal stem cell microvesicles for treatment of *Escherichia coli* endotoxin-induced acute lung injury in mice. Stem Cells 32:116–125
150. Aliotta JM et al (2007) Alteration of marrow cell gene expression, protein production, and engraftment into lung by lung-derived microvesicles: a novel mechanism for phenotype modulation. Stem Cells 25:2245–2256
151. Monsel A et al (2015) Therapeutic efects of human mesenchymal stem cell-derived microvesicles in severe pneumonia in mice. Am J Respir Crit Care Med 192:324–336
152. Boregowda SV et al (2012) Atmospheric oxygen inhibits growth and differentiation of marrow-derived mouse mesenchymal stem cells via a p53-dependent mechanism: implications for long-term culture expansion. Stem Cells 30:975–987
153. Zhang Z et al (2012) MicroRNA-451 regulates p38 MAPK signaling by targeting of Ywhaz and suppresses the mesangial hypertrophy in early diabetic nephropathy. FEBS Lett 586:20–26
154. Bandres E et al (2009) microRNA-451 regulates macrophage migration inhibitory factor production and proliferation of gastrointestinal cancer cells. Clin Cancer Res 15:2281–2290
155. Oka T et al (2012) Mitochondrial DNA that escapes from autophagy causes inflammation and heart failure. Nature 485:251–255
156. Ishikawa K et al (2010) The innate immune system in host mice targets cells with allogenic mitochondrial DNA. J Exp Med 207:2297–2305

18 Sedation

Giovanni Mistraletti, Paolo Formenti, and Giovanni Sabbatini

18.1 Introduction

The severity of the acute respiratory failure, the necessity of lifesaving invasive procedures, and the harsh intensive care unit (ICU) environment make sedation necessary in ARDS patients [1]. Such patients may experience a dangerous condition, both physical and psychological, and need the most appropriate and individualized neurological treatment. Among many other vital organ failures, the early and long-term consequences of ARDS may lead to severe brain dysfunction [2].

Pain, agitation, delirium, anxiety, and alteration of consciousness are common conditions in ARDS patients [3]. They are frequently triggered by treatable causes, like hypoxemia, hypercarbia, acidosis, hypoglycemia, hypo- or hypernatremia, sepsis, hypovolemia, and alcohol or drug withdrawal, or by lifesaving medical treatments comprehending mechanical ventilation, invasive procedures, forced body postures, and uninterrupted noise and light stimulation, together with their consequences like sleep deprivation or the impossibility of communicating with the staff [4]. International guidelines recommend to face and treat first all organic and metabolic causes of distress and to minimize environment-linked stressors [5, 6]. As a second step, they suggest the administration of analgesic, sedative, and antipsychotic drugs to ensure comfort, at all stages of the illness. Adequate levels of sedation, therefore, represent a primary target for managing ARDS patients. However, since neuroactive therapy is related to several important side effects like hemodynamic instability and cardiac dysrhythmias [7], sepsis [8], ileus, delirium [9], and lengthening of respiratory weaning [10], it is important to titrate it to the lowest effective amount [11].

G. Mistraletti, MD (✉) • P. Formenti, MD • G. Sabbatini, MD
Università degli Studi di Milano, Dipartimento di Fisiopatologia medico-chirurgica e dei trapianti, A.S.S.T. dei Santi Paolo e Carlo, Ospedale San Paolo – Polo Universitario, Via A. Di Rudinì, 8, 20142 Milan, Italy
e-mail: giovanni.mistraletti@unimi.it

D. Chiumello (ed.), *Acute Respiratory Distress Syndrome (ARDS)*,
DOI 10.1007/978-3-319-41852-0_18

Several authors have pointed out the need for light sedation [12, 13], due both to the detrimental effects of neuroactive therapy itself and to the clinical and economical costs associated with deeper-than-needed sedation levels [1, 14, 15]. Daily interruption of intravenous short-term sedative administration [16] in association with a spontaneous breathing trial [17] may decrease the mechanical ventilation length and reduce both complications and prevalence of delirium. Analgesia-based sedation could be another effective way to manage ARDS patients, relying on the opiates' ability to maintain adaptation to mechanical ventilation while preserving patients' consciousness [18]. However, the use of short-half-life analgesics (remifentanil) is only indicated for short-stay patients, while there is no difference among opiates for patients requiring mechanical ventilation longer than 3 days [19, 20]. In 2010, Strom et al. demonstrated that a protocol based only on morphine 5 mg boluses allows minimal sedation and provides better outcomes, rather than adding propofol to achieve deeper sedation levels [21].

The conscious sedation target is an innovation of the utmost relevance in the field of ICU care. Nonetheless, some intensivists tend to consider it unfeasible, considering the potential higher risk of ventilation-related lung damage, the risk of self-removal of invasive devices [22], and the possible stress/discomfort for patients [23]. From an ICU staff perspective, it also raises the issue of an increased workload. These beliefs, however, are at least partially unfounded [24]. Intensivists have to face the side effects of both pharmacological and physical "restraint" methods, continuously pursuing the best approach for patient security and healing.

Despite guideline suggestions and the fact that between 60 and 80% of ICUs use a specific score to evaluate the level of sedation [25], many physicians routinely maintain [26] a deeper than desired level of sedation [27], probably causing avoidable side effects. Pragmatically, it is important to underline the concept that it does not exist in one-and-only sedative treatment which can be always adequate; at the same time, a disproportionate fear to use sedative drugs is inappropriate. Even if the clinical course of each ARDS patient is different from the others, it is useful to distinguish at least two different scenarios, leading to the neuroactive drug prescription (Fig. 18.1) in ARDS patients. In the acute phase, intubation and placing of vascular catheters and other maneuvers devoted to clinical stabilization require a deep sedation target, similar to general anesthesia. On the other hand, in the subsequent phase, it is important to change the target toward a lighter sedation, by using the lowest amount of neuroactive drugs in order to only obtain a patient adaptation to critical illness. This second phase has to begin as soon as possible, frequently after the second/third ICU day. Other practices such as adjustment of the mechanical ventilation settings, of the drug therapies, and of the environment to the specific necessities of each specific patient can help in reducing discomfort.

18.2 The Key Importance of Continuous Neurological Assessment with Validated Tools

International guidelines clearly recommend systematic assessment of pain, agitation/sedation, and delirium in all ICU patients, with validated tools [4–6]. They provide repeatable and comparable measurements, able to adequately titrate the

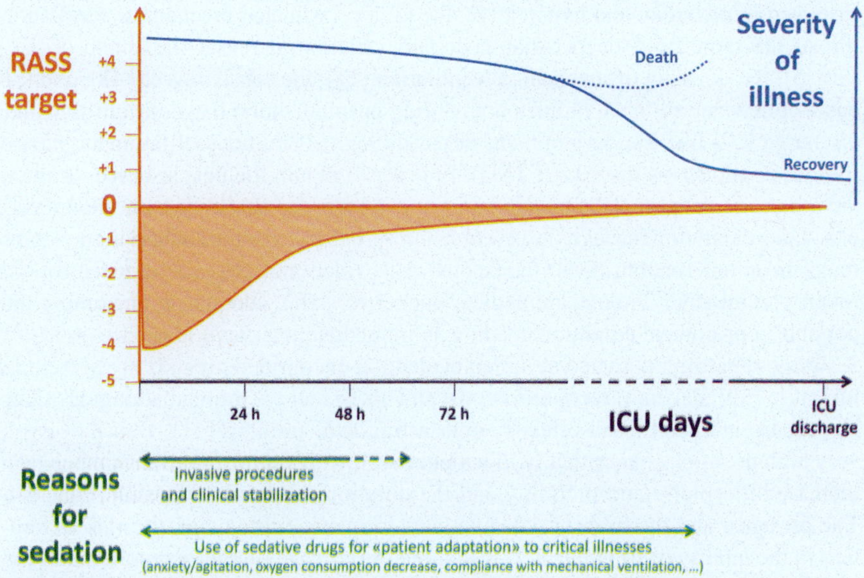

Fig. 18.1 The target level of sedation is different from the first period, devoted to clinical stabilization and protective ventilation, to the second one, when patients need to receive lighter sedation, intended to join and maintain a calm, conscious, and cooperative neurological state

analgesic, sedative, and antipsychotic therapy. The goal is to control the stress response and the neurological symptoms together keeping ARDS patients awake, cooperative, and well adapted to the necessary invasive procedures as soon as possible [28]. An excessive use of neuroactive drugs [26] correlates with longer mechanical ventilation and ICU stay, as well as with an increased risk of serious neurological consequences in both the short- and long-term [10, 29].

Among the validated tools, the scales with the highest psychometric properties [30] are the Verbal Numeric Rating (VNR), the Behavioral Pain Scale (BPS) [31], or the Critical-Care Pain Observation Tool (CPOT) [32] for the pain assessment, the Richmond Agitation-Sedation Scale (RASS) [33] and the Sedation-Agitation Scale (SAS) [34] for the agitation/sedation assessment, and the Confusion Assessment Method for the Intensive Care Unit (CAM-ICU) [35] and the Intensive Care Delirium Screening Checklist (ICDSC) [36] for the delirium assessment.

Pain assessment has become culturally essential for intensivists, both nurses and physicians. Proper identification of pain symptoms in critically ill patients represents a challenge because of complexity in communication with patients needing endotracheal respiratory prostheses, because of altered state of consciousness or because of neuroactive drugs use. To address these issues, specific behavioral scales were designed and validated both in unconscious/sedated [37] and in conscious/awake patients [38] and established as a valid, reliable, and simple tool to be used in clinical practice.

Regarding sedative drugs, their under- or overuse may compromise clinical stability. Life-threatening side effects of untreated agitation and stress response are evident: self-removal of life-sustaining devices, tachypnea, tachycardia, hypertension, sustained hypoxemia, and hypercarbia due to uncoordinated mechanical ventilation [6]. At the same time, deeper-than-necessary sedation increases the length of ICU stay [5], the duration of mechanical ventilation [21], the sepsis severity [8], and the onset of new neurological failures both during hospitalization like delirium and after discharge [29] like the development of psychological reactions of traumatic nature (posttraumatic stress disorder, PTSD). In order to obtain the best sedative titration, the use of validated tools is mandatory. For example, the RASS describes ten levels of sedation/agitation through observation and verbal and physical stimulation. Scores range from −5 (unconscious, unresponsive to voice and physical stimuli) to + 4 (overtly combative, violent, immediate danger to staff), adequately describing the possible neurological condition needing an immediate intervention.

While regarding pain and agitation evaluation encouraging results are present in literature [39], delirium recognition [40] and assessment is more challenging, since its success is linked to an effective and lasting staff training [41]. Delirium has a very high prevalence in critically ill patients [42], with a direct relationship between increased morbidity and mortality and the duration (in days) of delirium [43, 44]. The presence and duration of delirium also correlates with a significant deterioration in the quality of life after ICU discharge [45]. Large literature recommends the use of validated tools [46], like the Confusion Assessment Method for the ICU (CAM-ICU) and the Intensive Care Delirium Screening Checklist (ICDSC). The CAM-ICU has excellent sensitivity and specificity and is based on only four items (acute modification of consciousness, inattention, disorganized thinking, altered level of consciousness). This allows a shorter training to teach ICU staff members a validated way to evaluate delirium.

All these measurements have to be reported in the clinical chart at least once per shift, together with an evaluation of adequacy of sedative treatment. The neurological monitoring plays a key role in ARDS patients, and it is quick to perform. A complete example of evaluations recommended by international guidelines is reported in Fig. 18.2. Physicians have to state the desired sedation target for that specific patient at that specific moment of clinical course; nurses, on their part, report the actual neurological state, describing pain, anxiety, agitation, sleep, need for physical restraints, and delirium, together with a comprehensive evaluation of sedative therapy, in order to get the most adequate treatment titration.

18.3 Sedation Assessment

The appropriate target level of sedation primarily depends on a patient's acute disease process and on the therapeutic and supportive interventions required. After the first few days of ICU stay, characterized by clinical stabilization and invasive procedures, the sedation target is a calm patient, awake during the day and asleep at night. The use of deep levels of sedation to facilitate mechanical ventilation or painful procedures should be minimized with ventilation setting optimization and adequate analgesia, rather than deepening unconsciousness [12, 47].

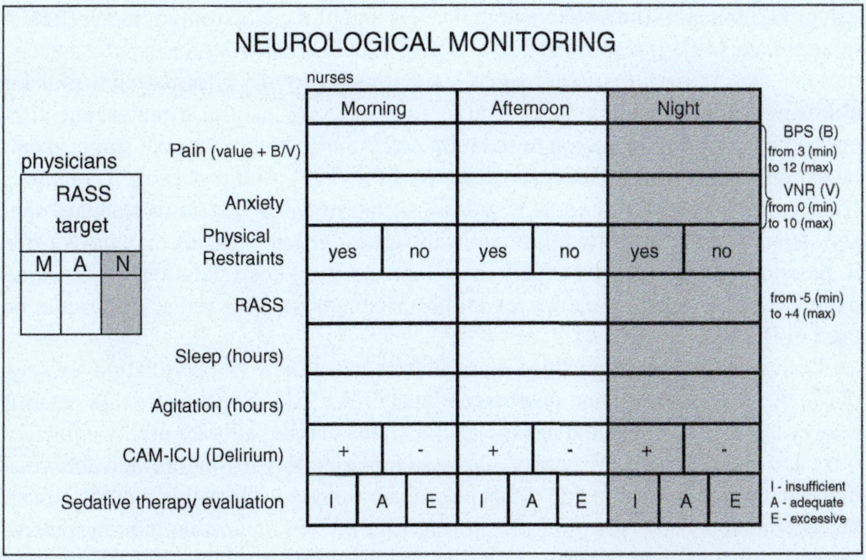

Fig. 18.2 An example of very simple neurological monitoring card, used in a general ICU of the University Hospital (A.O. San Paolo, Milano), to be added within a dedicated spot in nursing sheets. For each shift – morning, afternoon, and night – physicians have to state the target level of sedation, while nurses have to monitor and record, through appropriate validated tools, neurological parameters, and also to evaluate the adequacy of sedative therapy as prescribed by physicians

The appropriate balance of sedation and analgesia is difficult to be achieved and maintained. Without a rational agreement upon "target levels" of sedation, different members of the healthcare team will have disparate treatment goals, increasing the chance for iatrogenic complications and potentially delaying recovery [48].

The target level of sedation should be discussed and defined at the beginning of each staff shift and reevaluated regularly as the clinical condition of the patient changes. The pharmacological treatment should be planned with the appropriate flexibility to allow titration to the desired endpoint, anticipating fluctuations in sedation requirements throughout the day. Frequent monitoring with validated tools improves communication among clinicians and plays an important role in detecting and treating pain, agitation, and delirium while avoiding excessive or prolonged sedation [25].

18.3.1 Sedation Assessment with Objective Methods

Within several objective methods to sedation assessment proposed, none of them have fully yielded satisfying results. For example, bispectral index (BIS) monitor is a four-channel electroencephalographic (EEG) monitor which generates a single number that correlates with depth of consciousness during general anesthesia. The poor correlation between BIS and validated ICU sedation scales is related with BIS values variability at the awake/agitated levels and of the electromyography (EMG) interference [49]. Based on the analysis of EEG signal irregularity, the entropy monitor also utilizes the EMG signal, which may provide information useful for assessing whether a patient is responding to an external, painful stimulus, but without adding useful information to sedation assessment. In this context, some advantages could be offered by the responsiveness index [50]. Auditory evoked potentials (AEP) are electrophysiological responses of the nervous system to standard sensory stimulation transmitted through headphones. These methods may have a role in monitoring sedation levels only in patients needing deep sedation, or receiving neuromuscular blocking agents, as in this circumstance sedation scales cannot be used [49].

Monitoring blood drug values is useful only when there is a correlation between plasmatic concentration and pharmacological effect [51]. However, ARDS patients may be affected by renal and hepatic dysfunctions that impair their ability to metabolize and excrete drugs. Moreover, hypoxia, inflammatory mediators, and abnormal diets are common, too, and all affect enzymatic function. Thus, this method cannot be recommended for sedation monitoring [52, 53]. Spontaneous, non-propulsive lower esophageal contractility (LOC) is definitely stress related and increases in frequency as the dose of anesthetic is reduced. Deepening of anesthesia resulted in progressive suppression of LOC. However, LOC has great inter-variability and is affected by drugs such as atropine. The electromyogram responsiveness is not sufficiently sensitive to monitor sedation in ICU patients [51].

Actigraphy provides a continuous measure of body movements and was initially developed to measure sleep-wake cycles. This small electronic device containing an accelerometer continuously senses and records minimal movements, summarizing such data in numerical form. Wrist actigraphy provides useful nonspecific observations in ICU patients. Even if it does not discriminate the lack (or the excess) of analgesics and sedatives from other acute neurological dysfunctions, preliminary observations suggest that the measurement of body movements could provide a timely indication of acute changes in neurological status generating motor agitation or hypoactive behavior [54]. This objective method is relatively new in this context. It presents interesting properties, worthy of future investigation [55].

18.3.2 Sedation Assessment with Subjective Methods

Individual assessments of sedation, performed at the bedside by nurses or physicians, can be hampered by a lack of objectivity. Guidelines recommend establishing a sedation target and regularly redefining it for each patient, using a validated sedation assessment scale. The use of such a scale is a key component of sedation algorithms [1, 4–6]. It helps in managing agitation and establishing a target level of sedation for medication titration, in order to promptly detect oversedation when the target level is exceeded. All sedation algorithms recommend to use a sedation scale, such as Ramsay Sedation Scale (RSS), Richmond Agitation-Sedation Scale (RASS), and Riker Sedation-Agitation Scale (SAS) [56].

The use of a scale to assess level of consciousness dates to the introduction of a six-point scale by Ramsay et al. (RSS) more than 40 years ago [57]. Nowadays, it continues to be a widely used scale for monitoring sedation in daily practice [58]. Some experts consider that it is more a scale of consciousness than a tool for the measurement of sedation. RSS has been extensively tested but it has never been validated. Moreover, it does not grade agitation. Consequently, this scale is excessively subjective and has poor validity. Many other scales have been proposed [59]; some of them are not validated. They are not recommended for clinical use.

The ideal scoring system should be easy, reliable, sensitive, and with minimal interobserver variability. Moreover, it should give no or minimal additional discomfort to the patient. Even though a complex scoring system is not suitable for the ICU, oversimplification brings risk of neglecting important information. Most of the proposed tools are a compromise between accuracy and time required for evaluation of sedation [60].

Recently developed scales often combine the sedation/arousal domain with an assessment of agitation, like the SAS, the RASS, the Motor Activity Assessment Scale (MAAS), the Observer's Assessment of Alertness and Sedation (OAAS), the Nursing Instrument for the Communication of Sedation (NICS) [61], and the Bloomsbury Sedation Score (Fig. 18.3).

Unlike other validated instruments, the RASS separates verbal from physical stimulation so that the patient's level of arousal may be graded according to the potency of the stimulus. Interestingly, RASS is validated also to assess patients' sedation over time, both in spontaneously breathing/mechanically ventilated and in sedated/nonsedated critically ill patients.

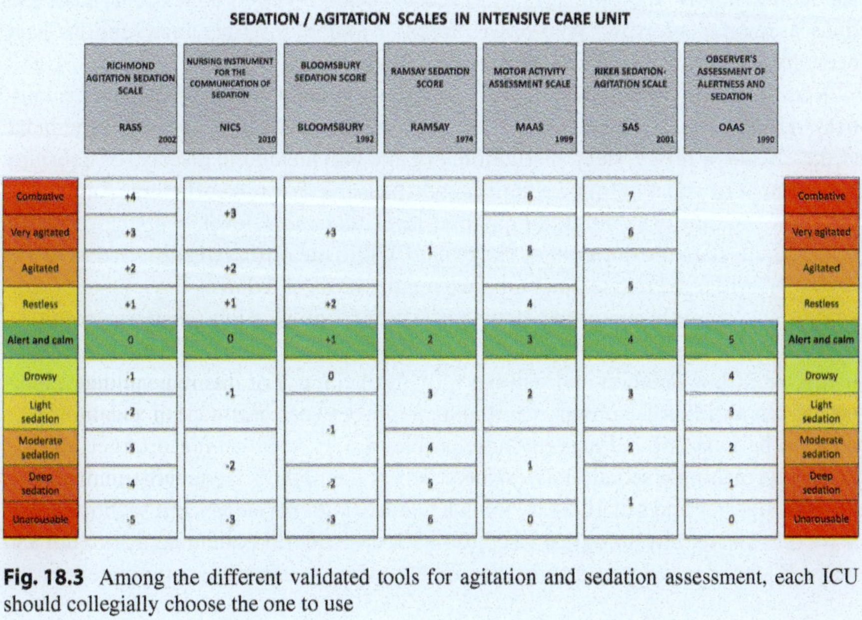

Fig. 18.3 Among the different validated tools for agitation and sedation assessment, each ICU should collegially choose the one to use

Other multiple-item sedation scales are described in literature. The Adaptation to the Intensive Care Environment scale (ATICE) consists of five items [62]: awareness and comprehension combined in a "Conscious" domain; calmness, ventilator synchrony, and facial relaxation are combined in a "Tolerance" domain. As for ATICE, the Minnesota Sedation Assessment Tool (MSAT) evaluates the level of consciousness of patients receiving invasive mechanical ventilation. It measures arousability, spontaneous muscle activity, and global sedation quality. The Vancouver Interaction and Calmness Scale (VICS) consists of two five-item subscales quantifying separately calmness and interaction with operators. These more complex scoring systems are usually adopted in clinical trials to evaluate a new drug or a new objective tool for sedation assessment, whereas in daily practice, easily applied scores are usually preferred.

18.3.3 Choosing and Implementing an Evaluation Scale

Desirable features of sedation evaluation instruments should include rigorous multidisciplinary development; ease of administration, recall, and interpretation; well-designed discrete criteria for each level; sufficient sedation levels for effective drug titration; assessment of agitation; and demonstration of inter-rater reliability and validity in relevant patient populations [48]. Each ICU has to choose the best tools for its patient population and to plan specific intervention to introduce it in daily care [63].

Teaching protocols used for implementation of sedation scales have shown good results among ICU caregivers. Different methods have been used to implement evaluation tools in clinical practice. Typically, they are based on introductory in-service for nurses and operators followed by graded, staged educational interventions at regular intervals. Web-based, freely available teaching interventions have been also proposed (www.icudelirium.org, www.sedaicu.it).

Some emerging problems remain, particularly about the fluctuation of consciousness. ARDS patients are prone to sudden changes in their state of consciousness due to the effects of drugs, sleep disruption, organic and metabolic disease, or delirium. Assessment of sedation once a shift is indispensable but not sufficient. Among the different possibilities (minimal/maximal level, prevalent level, worst level), it is important to state the duration of each value within the observed shift. Sedation and agitation need to be reassessed both on a regular basis and during any clinical modification, to promptly capture all the modifications requiring intervention. Moreover, it is relatively common for patients to manifest sudden aggressive behavior when recovering from sedation and without fully awakening. For this reason, it is important to boost interdisciplinary communication between nurses and physicians in order to be aware of and prevent these problems.

Lastly, making a sedation assessment during the night is frequently challenging. Most analgesics and sedatives are known to make patients sleepy, but without reaching a restorative, physiological sleep [64]. If a critically ill patient appears calm and keeps his/her eyes closed during the night, he/she should not be stimulated just to make a sedation assessment. He/she could be observed during unavoidable procedures happening in the ICU during the night, in order to discriminate normal sleep (with arousals due to noise or light) from sedation or coma.

18.4 Clinical Practice Flowcharts for Pain, Agitation, and Delirium Management

Recognition that heavy sedation may increase mortality and morbidity has led to a new approach that maximizes the comfort of the patients while they remain awake, interactive, and oriented. This new approach relies on strategies such as daily interruptions of sedation, analgesia-based sedation, enteral sedation, avoidance of paralytic agents, early mobilization, and use of validated tools for sedation assessment [1]. In recent years, many guidelines have been proposed [4–6], representing a guide to symptom-oriented prevention, diagnosis, and treatment of delirium, anxiety, stress, and protocol-based analgesia, sedation, and sleep management. They comprehensively describe all attentions to be paid to perform the best neurological treatment. Nevertheless, even in guidelines with a high-quality rating, numerous recommendations have moderate or low levels of evidence [65].

Overall, the principal recommendation regarding analgesia is to evaluate pain and maintain its level ≤ 4/10, by beginning early than late the treatment of pain, and by using opioid drugs first, together with non-opioid and multimodal analgesia techniques. A simple and practical flowchart at the bedside is presented in Fig. 18.4.

Regarding sedation, a target RASS of 0/−1 is recommended for all ICU patients, with the use of deep sedation reserved only for patients with specific indications (e.g., early ARDS patients, requiring neuromuscular blocking or prone positioning). In particular, intensivists should consider the specific indication and individual goal of sedation and the pharmacokinetics/pharmacodynamics of each drug used. Non-benzodiazepine drugs, such as propofol or dexmedetomidine, have to be preferred. The need for sedation varies widely among different patients and with the illness course, and it has to be defined among "deep sedation", "cooperative/awake sedation," and "no sedation," always preferring superficial levels of sedation and promoting early mobilization. The use of containment measures in episodes of severe agitation has to be performed in this order: first verbal, then pharmacological, and finally physical, considering that neuroactive drugs should not be administered in excess as a form of "chemical immobilization." In the sedation flowchart (Fig. 18.5), it is clear that defining a target and evaluating the actual level of sedation or agitation with validated tools are absolute priorities. The choice of the specific sedative drug, albeit important, comes only after a clinical reasoning focused on managing the organic/metabolic causes and the problems that may be caused by adjustable invasive devices.

Recommendations about delirium are prescribed first to identify modifiable risk factors (Fig. 18.6) and to detect regularly the appearance of delirium by using the CAM-ICU. In case of delirium appearance, it is indicated to use a non-pharmacological protocol first, along with the suspension or decreasing of

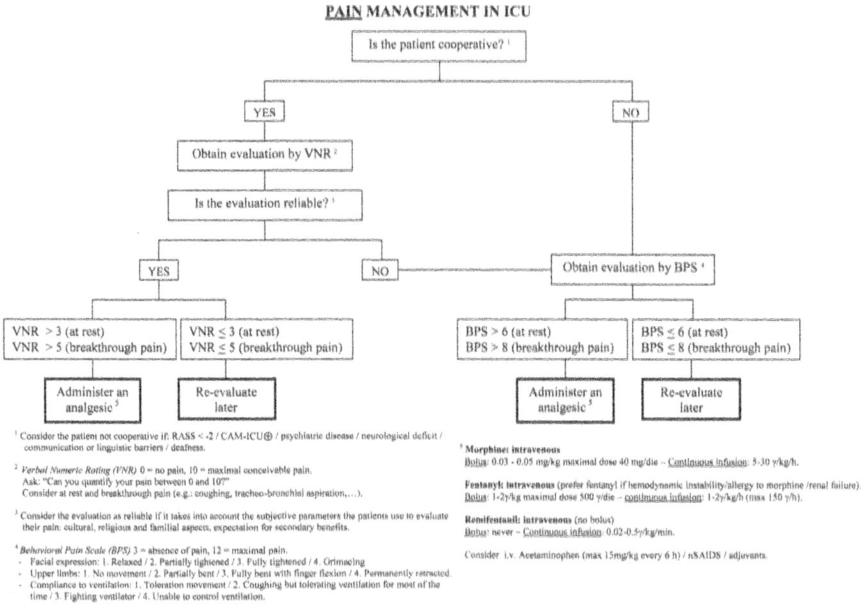

Fig. 18.4 This flowchart can be used at the bedside, to adequately manage pain in critically ill patients

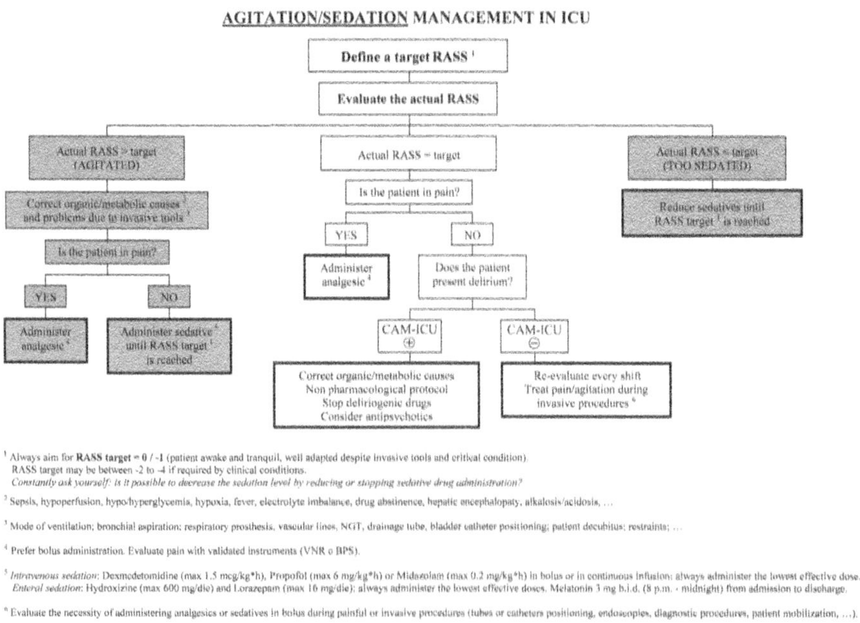

Fig. 18.5 This flowchart can be used at the bedside, to adequately manage agitation symptoms and to titrate sedative therapy for critically ill patients

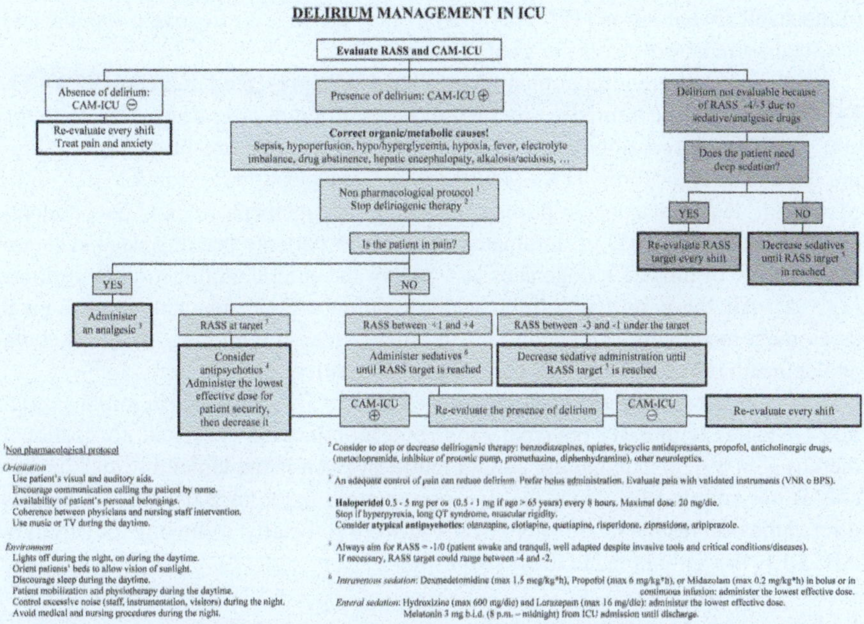

Fig. 18.6 This flowchart can be used at the bedside, to timely manage delirium in ICU

deliriogenic therapies, and then to select the most appropriate drug (haloperidol, atypical antipsychotics, or dexmedetomidine; avoid the use of benzodiazepines) and titer its dose to the lowest effective dose.

18.5 Sedation Protocols Presented in Literature

Beyond the choice of the specific drug [66–68], the most frequently used method for administering sedatives is the continuous intravenous route, because of its pharmacokinetic properties [63]. Intravenous infusions present predictable and easy to handle onset/offset properties, justifying the search for an early goal-directed sedation strategy [69]. Although these characteristics are necessary in short ICU stays, they may be useless, or even dangerous, for patients requiring more than 3 days of mechanical ventilation [27]. When using potent drugs, it is easy to incur in overadministration albeit goals are established and adequate [25]. Moreover, daily awakening trials produce far-from-physiological neurological fluctuations [70], and continuous deep sedation does not permit patients to recall factual memories, which has been proven effective in preventing PTSD [71].

If continuous intravenous infusion is used, the daily interruption of sedatives and analgesics is recommended in order to reduce the total administered dosage and to perform a spontaneous breathing trial, if allowed by the respiratory condition of the patient. The purpose is to reduce the development of complications and the duration of mechanical ventilation [17]. This strategy may prove less effective if specific and ICU team-shared protocols are used [72].

Many quite different sedation protocols have been presented in literature [10, 73, 74]. Some of them essentially rely on the use of different drug doses [75], with the aim to different sedation levels [56, 76]. Other protocols are based on nursing-implemented algorithms [13, 77–79] or on analgesia-first sedation [21, 80]. Moreover, tested ways to optimize sedation management in ICU are patient-controlled sedation [81] or automated sedation in patients needing deep sedation [82], the use of inhaled halogenates [83, 84], or the enteral administration of drugs [28, 85]. All these protocols rely on the continuous and adequate neurological assessment made with validated tools, in order to measure not only pain, agitation, and delirium but also level of consciousness and patient mobilization.

The most promising protocol, in terms of efficacy, recommends to join the sedation strategies with early physiotherapy [86], mobilization [87], and occupational therapy [88, 89], also engaging patient families. Even if implementing such protocols is not simple [90], from the first presentation made in 2010 [91, 92], it has offered the best results in terms of effectiveness [93]. Briefly, following the acronym ABCDEF, the authors made these suggestions:

- Assess, prevent, and manage pain.
- Both spontaneous awakening trial and spontaneous breathing trial.
- Choice of analgesia and sedation.
- Delirium: assess, prevent, and manage.
- Early mobility and exercise (goal-directed early mobilization).
- Family engagement and empowerment.

18.6 Special Circumstances

Regarding ARDS patients needing extracorporeal life support systems (ECLS), there is a gray area about sedation, where safety aspects and the ability to positively influence recovery must be balanced. Patients on ECLS have numerous risk factors to develop both delirium during the ICU stay and PTSD after discharge. Hyperactive delirium or agitation can be life-threatening for these patients, so that a consequent monitoring and a symptomatic therapy of stress, anxiety, delirium, pain, and insomnia is essential to safely achieve a target RASS of 0. The higher level of alertness allows the patient to actively partake in physical exercises [94] that is considered a feasible and safe goal [95, 96]. International guidelines recommend a strict definition of sedation targets for patients on ECLS, including frequent clinical monitoring and continuous adjustment of the level of sedation required [4].

Positioning therapy has been demonstrated effective in ameliorating prognosis of severe ARDS patients. It is used for prophylaxis and treatment of respiratory dysfunctions and requires an individual sedation target. Changes of the position frequently represent a challenge for the symptomatic treatment of anxiety, stress, and pain. Therefore, a symptom-orientated therapy should be adapted for changing demands during positioning therapy. Though a deep sedation may be indicated for patient repositioning [97], an excessive sedation should be avoided through the use of objective tools based on EEG analysis, as previously described.

The use of non-depolarizing neuromuscular blockers in patients with severe ARDS is suggested during the first 48 ICU hours. Despite this practice, it is suggested not to routinely increase the dose of sedatives, when accompanied by an infusion of opiates, even in patients subjected to permissive hypercapnia [98]. To control respiratory rate, fentanyl is recommended as the analgesic of choice in patients with hemodynamic instability, bronchial asthma, or COPD, with respect to the other opiates. Methadone via the enteral route could be used in patients receiving opiates for more than 5 days, but still needing mechanical ventilation. Once tracheostomy is performed, it is advisable to consider a decrease in sedative and analgesic regimens.

After the hyperacute phase of respiratory failure, a defined sedation and analgesia monitoring and dose adjustment protocol is recommended, to shorten the weaning process. This protocol should include daily evaluation of sedation, an awakening test and a spontaneous breathing test. It is advisable not to use benzodiazepines in the withdrawal of MV. Dexmedetomidine is recommended in case of weaning difficulties, in patients with withdrawal syndrome, or after failed attempts of weaning secondary to agitation and delirium [67]. Low-dose remifentanil in continuous infusion is another effective alternative during weaning process. Music therapy is a possible non-pharmacological adjuvant to sedation [99]. Melatonin supplementation could be useful to decrease the need for sedative drugs, then shortening the ventilation length [100], and to restore the sleep-wake rhythm.

References

1. Sessler CN, Varney K (2008) Patient-focused sedation and analgesia in the ICU. Chest 133(2):552–565. doi:10.1378/chest.07-2026
2. Pandharipande PP, Girard TD, Jackson JC, Morandi A, Thompson JL, Pun BT, Brummel NE, Hughes CG, Vasilevskis EE, Shintani AK, Moons KG, Geevarghese SK, Canonico A, Hopkins RO, Bernard GR, Dittus RS, Ely EW (2013) Long-term cognitive impairment after critical illness. N Engl J Med 369(14):1306–1316. doi:10.1056/NEJMoa1301372
3. Fraser GL, Riker RR (2007) Sedation and analgesia in the critically ill adult. Curr Opin Anaesthesiol 20(2):119–123. doi:10.1097/ACO.0b013e32808255b4
4. Baron R, Binder A, Biniek R, Braune S, Buerkle H, Dall P, Demirakca S, Eckardt R, Eggers V, Eichler I, Fietze I, Freys S, Frund A, Garten L, Gohrbandt B, Harth I, Hartl W, Heppner HJ, Horter J, Huth R, Janssens U, Jungk C, Kaeuper KM, Kessler P, Kleinschmidt S, Kochanek M, Kumpf M, Meiser A, Mueller A, Orth M, Putensen C, Roth B, Schaefer M, Schaefers R, Schellongowski P, Schindler M, Schmitt R, Scholz J, Schroeder S, Schwarzmann G, Spies C, Stingele R, Tonner P, Trieschmann U, Tryba M, Wappler F, Waydhas C, Weiss B, Weisshaar G (2015) Evidence and consensus based guideline for the management of delirium, analgesia, and sedation in intensive care medicine. Revision 2015 (DAS-Guideline 2015) - short version. Ger Med Sci GMS E-Journal 13:Doc19. doi:10.3205/000223
5. Barr J, Fraser GL, Puntillo K, Ely EW, Gelinas C, Dasta JF, Davidson JE, Devlin JW, Kress JP, Joffe AM, Coursin DB, Herr DL, Tung A, Robinson BR, Fontaine DK, Ramsay MA, Riker RR, Sessler CN, Pun B, Skrobik Y, Jaeschke R (2013) Clinical practice guidelines for

the management of pain, agitation, and delirium in adult patients in the intensive care unit. Crit Care Med 41(1):263–306. doi:10.1097/CCM.0b013e3182783b72
6. Celis-Rodriguez E, Birchenall C, de la Cal MA, Castorena Arellano G, Hernandez A, Ceraso D, Diaz Cortes JC, Duenas Castell C, Jimenez EJ, Meza JC, Munoz Martinez T, Sosa Garcia JO, Pacheco Tovar C, Palizas F, Pardo Oviedo JM, Pinilla DI, Raffan-Sanabria F, Raimondi N, Righy Shinotsuka C, Suarez M, Ugarte S, Rubiano S (2013) Clinical practice guidelines for evidence-based management of sedoanalgesia in critically ill adult patients. Med Intensiva/Sociedad Espanola de Medicina Intensiva y Unidades Coronarias 37(8):519–574. doi:10.1016/j.medin.2013.04.001
7. Ice CJ, Personett HA, Frazee EN, Dierkhising RA, Kashyap R, Oeckler RA (2016) Risk factors for dexmedetomidine-associated hemodynamic instability in noncardiac intensive care unit patients. Anesth Analg 122(2):462–469. doi:10.1213/ANE.0000000000001125
8. Nseir S, Makris D, Mathieu D, Durocher A, Marquette CH (2010) Intensive care unit-acquired infection as a side effect of sedation. Crit Care 14(2):R30
9. Pisani MA, Murphy TE, Araujo KL, Slattum P, Van Ness PH, Inouye SK (2009) Benzodiazepine and opioid use and the duration of intensive care unit delirium in an older population. Crit Care Med 37(1):177–183. doi:10.1097/CCM.0b013e318192fcf9
10. Jackson DL, Proudfoot CW, Cann KF, Walsh T (2010) A systematic review of the impact of sedation practice in the ICU on resource use, costs and patient safety. Crit Care 14(2):R59. doi:10.1186/cc8956
11. Riker RR, Fraser GL (2005) Adverse events associated with sedatives, analgesics, and other drugs that provide patient comfort in the intensive care unit. Pharmacotherapy 25(5 Pt 2):8S–18S
12. Cigada M, Corbella D, Mistraletti G, Forster CR, Tommasino C, Morabito A, Iapichino G (2008) Conscious sedation in the critically ill ventilated patient. J Crit Care 23(3):349–353. doi:10.1016/j.jcrc.2007.04.003
13. De Jonghe B, Bastuji-Garin S, Fangio P, Lacherade JC, Jabot J, Appere-De-Vecchi C, Rocha N, Outin H (2005) Sedation algorithm in critically ill patients without acute brain injury. Crit Care Med 33(1):120–127
14. Shehabi Y, Bellomo R, Reade MC, Bailey M, Bass F, Howe B, McArthur C, Seppelt IM, Webb S, Weisbrodt L (2012) Early intensive care sedation predicts long-term mortality in ventilated critically ill patients. Am J Respir Crit Care Med 186(8):724–731. doi:10.1164/rccm.201203-0522OC
15. Shehabi Y, Chan L, Kadiman S, Alias A, Ismail WN, Tan MA, Khoo TM, Ali SB, Saman MA, Shaltut A, Tan CC, Yong CY, Bailey M (2013) Sedation depth and long-term mortality in mechanically ventilated critically ill adults: a prospective longitudinal multicentre cohort study. Intensive Care Med 39(5):910–918. doi:10.1007/s00134-013-2830-2
16. Kress JP, Pohlman AS, O'Connor MF, Hall JB (2000) Daily interruption of sedative infusions in critically ill patients undergoing mechanical ventilation. N Engl J Med 342(20):1471–1477. doi:10.1056/NEJM200005183422002
17. Girard TD, Kress JP, Fuchs BD, Thomason JW, Schweickert WD, Pun BT, Taichman DB, Dunn JG, Pohlman AS, Kinniry PA, Jackson JC, Canonico AE, Light RW, Shintani AK, Thompson JL, Gordon SM, Hall JB, Dittus RS, Bernard GR, Ely EW (2008) Efficacy and safety of a paired sedation and ventilator weaning protocol for mechanically ventilated patients in intensive care (Awakening and Breathing Controlled trial): a randomised controlled trial. Lancet 371(9607):126–134. doi:10.1016/S0140-6736(08)60105-1
18. Breen D, Karabinis A, Malbrain M, Morais R, Albrecht S, Jarnvig IL, Parkinson P, Kirkham AJ (2005) Decreased duration of mechanical ventilation when comparing analgesia-based sedation using remifentanil with standard hypnotic-based sedation for up to 10 days in intensive care unit patients: a randomised trial [ISRCTN47583497]. Crit Care 9(3):R200–R210. doi:10.1186/cc3495
19. Spies C, Macguill M, Heymann A, Ganea C, Krahne D, Assman A, Kosiek HR, Scholtz K, Wernecke KD, Martin J (2011) A prospective, randomized, double-blind, multicenter study

comparing remifentanil with fentanyl in mechanically ventilated patients. Intensive Care Med 37(3):469–476. doi:10.1007/s00134-010-2100-5

20. Tan JA, Ho KM (2009) Use of remifentanil as a sedative agent in critically ill adult patients: a meta-analysis. Anaesthesia 64(12):1342–1352. doi:10.1111/j.1365-2044.2009.06129.x
21. Strom T, Martinussen T, Toft P (2010) A protocol of no sedation for critically ill patients receiving mechanical ventilation: a randomised trial. Lancet 375(9713):475–480. doi:10.1016/S0140-6736(09)62072-9
22. Chevron V, Menard JF, Richard JC, Girault C, Leroy J, Bonmarchand G (1998) Unplanned extubation: risk factors of development and predictive criteria for reintubation. Crit Care Med 26(6):1049–1053
23. Guttormson JL, Chlan L, Weinert C, Savik K (2010) Factors influencing nurse sedation practices with mechanically ventilated patients: a U.S. national survey. Intensive Crit Care Nurs Off J Br Assoc Crit Care Nurses 26(1):44–50. doi:10.1016/j.iccn.2009.10.004
24. Goodwin H, Lewin JJ, Mirski MA (2012) 'Cooperative sedation': optimizing comfort while maximizing systemic and neurological function. Crit Care 16(2):217. doi:10.1186/cc11231
25. Martin J, Franck M, Fischer M, Spies C (2006) Sedation and analgesia in German intensive care units: how is it done in reality? Results of a patient-based survey of analgesia and sedation. Intensive Care Med 32(8):1137–1142. doi:10.1007/s00134-006-0214-6
26. Payen JF, Chanques G, Mantz J, Hercule C, Auriant I, Leguillou JL, Binhas M, Genty C, Rolland C, Bosson JL (2007) Current practices in sedation and analgesia for mechanically ventilated critically ill patients: a prospective multicenter patient-based study. Anesthesiology 106 (4):687–695; quiz 891-682. doi:10.1097/01.anes.0000264747.09017.da
27. Devlin JW (2008) The pharmacology of oversedation in mechanically ventilated adults. Curr Opin Crit Care 14(4):403–407. doi:10.1097/MCC.0b013e32830280b3
28. Mistraletti G, Mantovani ES, Cadringher P, Cerri B, Corbella D, Umbrello M, Anania S, Andrighi E, Barello S, Di Carlo A, Martinetti F, Formenti P, Spanu P, Iapichino G (2013) Enteral vs. intravenous ICU sedation management: study protocol for a randomized controlled trial. Trials 14:92. doi:10.1186/1745-6215-14-92
29. Granja C, Gomes E, Amaro A, Ribeiro O, Jones C, Carneiro A, Costa-Pereira A (2008) Understanding posttraumatic stress disorder-related symptoms after critical care: the early illness amnesia hypothesis. Crit Care Med 36(10):2801–2809. doi:10.1097/CCM.0b013e318186a3e7
30. Robinson BR, Berube M, Barr J, Riker R, Gelinas C (2013) Psychometric analysis of subjective sedation scales in critically ill adults. Crit Care Med 41(9 Suppl 1):S16–S29. doi:10.1097/CCM.0b013e3182a16879
31. Payen JF, Bru O, Bosson JL, Lagrasta A, Novel E, Deschaux I, Lavagne P, Jacquot C (2001) Assessing pain in critically ill sedated patients by using a behavioral pain scale. Crit Care Med 29(12):2258–2263
32. Gelinas C, Fillion L, Puntillo KA, Viens C, Fortier M (2006) Validation of the critical-care pain observation tool in adult patients. Am J Crit Care Off Publ Am Assoc Crit-Care Nurses 15(4):420–427
33. Sessler CN, Gosnell MS, Grap MJ, Brophy GM, O'Neal PV, Keane KA, Tesoro EP, Elswick RK (2002) The Richmond Agitation-Sedation Scale: validity and reliability in adult intensive care unit patients. Am J Respir Crit Care Med 166(10):1338–1344. doi:10.1164/rccm.2107138
34. Riker RR, Picard JT, Fraser GL (1999) Prospective evaluation of the Sedation-Agitation Scale for adult critically ill patients. Crit Care Med 27(7):1325–1329
35. Ely EW, Margolin R, Francis J, May L, Truman B, Dittus R, Speroff T, Gautam S, Bernard GR, Inouye SK (2001) Evaluation of delirium in critically ill patients: validation of the Confusion Assessment Method for the Intensive Care Unit (CAM-ICU). Crit Care Med 29(7):1370–1379
36. Bergeron N, Dubois MJ, Dumont M, Dial S, Skrobik Y (2001) Intensive Care Delirium Screening Checklist: evaluation of a new screening tool. Intensive Care Med 27(5):859–864

37. Aissaoui Y, Zeggwagh AA, Zekraoui A, Abidi K, Abouqal R (2005) Validation of a behavioral pain scale in critically ill, sedated, and mechanically ventilated patients. Anesth Analg 101(5):1470–1476. doi:10.1213/01.ANE.0000182331.68722.FF
38. Ahlers SJ, van der Veen AM, van Dijk M, Tibboel D, Knibbe CA (2010) The use of the behavioral pain scale to assess pain in conscious sedated patients. Anesth Analg 110(1):127–133. doi:10.1213/ANE.0b013e3181c3119e
39. Pun BT, Gordon SM, Peterson JF, Shintani AK, Jackson JC, Foss J, Harding SD, Bernard GR, Dittus RS, Ely EW (2005) Large-scale implementation of sedation and delirium monitoring in the intensive care unit: a report from two medical centers. Crit Care Med 33(6):1199–1205
40. Morandi A, Pandharipande P, Trabucchi M, Rozzini R, Mistraletti G, Trompeo AC, Gregoretti C, Gattinoni L, Ranieri MV, Brochard L, Annane D, Putensen C, Guenther U, Fuentes P, Tobar E, Anzueto AR, Esteban A, Skrobik Y, Salluh JI, Soares M, Granja C, Stubhaug A, de Rooij SE, Ely EW (2008) Understanding international differences in terminology for delirium and other types of acute brain dysfunction in critically ill patients. Intensive Care Med 34(10):1907–1915. doi:10.1007/s00134-008-1177-6
41. Spronk PE, Riekerk B, Hofhuis J, Rommes JH (2009) Occurrence of delirium is severely underestimated in the ICU during daily care. Intensive Care Med 35(7):1276–1280. doi:10.1007/s00134-009-1466-8
42. Vasilevskis EE, Han JH, Hughes CG, Ely EW (2012) Epidemiology and risk factors for delirium across hospital settings. Best Pract Res Clin Anaesthesiol 26(3):277–287. doi:10.1016/j.bpa.2012.07.003
43. Pisani MA, Kong SY, Kasl SV, Murphy TE, Araujo KL, Van Ness PH (2009) Days of delirium are associated with 1-year mortality in an older intensive care unit population. Am J Respir Crit Care Med 180(11):1092–1097. doi:10.1164/rccm.200904-0537OC
44. Ely EW, Shintani A, Truman B, Speroff T, Gordon SM, Harrell FE Jr, Inouye SK, Bernard GR, Dittus RS (2004) Delirium as a predictor of mortality in mechanically ventilated patients in the intensive care unit. JAMA J Am Med Assoc 291(14):1753–1762. doi:10.1001/jama.291.14.1753
45. Mistraletti G, Pelosi P, Mantovani ES, Berardino M, Gregoretti C (2012) Delirium: clinical approach and prevention. Best Pract Res Clin Anaesthesiol 26(3):311–326. doi:10.1016/j.bpa.2012.07.001
46. Devlin JW, Fong JJ, Schumaker G, O'Connor H, Ruthazer R, Garpestad E (2007) Use of a validated delirium assessment tool improves the ability of physicians to identify delirium in medical intensive care unit patients. Crit Care Med 35 (12):2721–2724; quiz 2725
47. Strom T, Toft P (2011) Time to wake up the patients in the ICU: a crazy idea or common sense? Minerva Anestesiol 77(1):59–63
48. Sessler CN, Grap MJ, Ramsay MA (2008) Evaluating and monitoring analgesia and sedation in the intensive care unit. Crit Care 12(Suppl 3):S2. doi:10.1186/cc6148
49. Haenggi M, Ypparila-Wolters H, Buerki S, Schlauri R, Korhonen I, Takala J, Jakob SM (2009) Auditory event-related potentials, bispectral index, and entropy for the discrimination of different levels of sedation in intensive care unit patients. Anesth Analg 109(3):807–816. doi:10.1213/ane.0b013e3181acc85d
50. Walsh TS, Lapinlampi TP, Ramsay P, Sarkela MO, Uutela K, Viertio-Oja HE (2011) Responsiveness of the frontal EMG for monitoring the sedation state of critically ill patients. Br J Anaesth 107(5):710–718. doi:10.1093/bja/aer228
51. Mondello E, Siliotti R, Gravino E, Coluzzi F, David T, Sinardi AU (2005) Sedation monitoring in ICU. Minerva Anestesiol 71(9):487–496
52. LeBlanc JM, Dasta JF, Pruchnicki MC, Gerlach A, Cook C (2012) Bispectral index values, sedation-agitation scores, and plasma Lorazepam concentrations in critically ill surgical patients. Am J Crit Care Off Publ Am Assoc Crit Care Nurses 21(2):99–105. doi:10.4037/ajcc2012777
53. Masica AL, Girard TD, Wilkinson GR, Thomason JW, Truman Pun B, Nair UB, Light RW, Canonico AE, Dunn J, Pandharipande P, Shintani AK, Ely EW (2007) Clinical sedation

scores as indicators of sedative and analgesic drug exposure in intensive care unit patients. Am J Geriatr Pharmacother 5(3):218–231. doi:10.1016/j.amjopharm.2007.10.005
54. Mistraletti G, Taverna M, Sabbatini G, Carloni E, Bolgiaghi L, Pirrone M, Cigada M, Destrebecq AL, Carli F, Iapichino G (2009) Actigraphic monitoring in critically ill patients: preliminary results toward an "observation-guided sedation". J Crit Care 24(4):563–567. doi:10.1016/j.jcrc.2009.05.006
55. Grap MJ, Hamilton VA, McNallen A, Ketchum JM, Best AM, Arief NY, Wetzel PA (2011) Actigraphy: analyzing patient movement. Heart Lung J Crit Care 40(3):e52–e59. doi:10.1016/j.hrtlng.2009.12.013
56. Patel SB, Kress JP (2012) Sedation and analgesia in the mechanically ventilated patient. Am J Respir Crit Care Med 185(5):486–497. doi:10.1164/rccm.201102-0273CI
57. Ramsay MA, Savege TM, Simpson BR, Goodwin R (1974) Controlled sedation with alphaxalone-alphadolone. Br Med J 2(5920):656–659
58. Reschreiter H, Maiden M, Kapila A (2008) Sedation practice in the intensive care unit: a UK national survey. Crit Care 12(6):R152. doi:10.1186/cc7141
59. De Jonghe B, Cook D, Appere-De-Vecchi C, Guyatt G, Meade M, Outin H (2000) Using and understanding sedation scoring systems: a systematic review. Intensive Care Med 26(3):275–285
60. McGrane S, Pandharipande PP (2012) Sedation in the intensive care unit. Minerva Anestesiol 78(3):369–380
61. Mirski MA, LeDroux SN, Lewin JJ 3rd, Thompson CB, Mirski KT, Griswold M (2010) Validity and reliability of an intuitive conscious sedation scoring tool: the nursing instrument for the communication of sedation. Crit Care Med 38(8):1674–1684. doi:10.1097/CCM.0b013e3181e7c73e
62. De Jonghe B, Cook D, Griffith L, Appere-de-Vecchi C, Guyatt G, Theron V, Vagnerre A, Outin H (2003) Adaptation to the Intensive Care Environment (ATICE): development and validation of a new sedation assessment instrument. Crit Care Med 31(9):2344–2354. doi:10.1097/01.CCM.0000084850.16444.94
63. Brush DR, Kress JP (2009) Sedation and analgesia for the mechanically ventilated patient. Clin Chest Med 30 (1):131–141, ix. doi:10.1016/j.ccm.2008.09.001
64. Brown EN, Lydic R, Schiff ND (2010) General anesthesia, sleep, and coma. N Engl J Med 363(27):2638–2650. doi:10.1056/NEJMra0808281
65. Girardis M, Cantaroni C, Savoia G, Melotti R, Conti G (2016) A critical appraisal of the quality of analgosedation guidelines in critically ill patients. Minerva Anestesiol 82(2):230–235
66. Pandharipande PP, Pun BT, Herr DL, Maze M, Girard TD, Miller RR, Shintani AK, Thompson JL, Jackson JC, Deppen SA, Stiles RA, Dittus RS, Bernard GR, Ely EW (2007) Effect of sedation with dexmedetomidine vs lorazepam on acute brain dysfunction in mechanically ventilated patients: the MENDS randomized controlled trial. JAMA 298(22):2644–2653. doi:10.1001/jama.298.22.2644
67. Riker RR, Shehabi Y, Bokesch PM, Ceraso D, Wisemandle W, Koura F, Whitten P, Margolis BD, Byrne DW, Ely EW, Rocha MG (2009) Dexmedetomidine vs midazolam for sedation of critically ill patients: a randomized trial. JAMA 301(5):489–499. doi:10.1001/jama.2009.56
68. Jakob SM, Ruokonen E, Grounds RM, Sarapohja T, Garratt C, Pocock SJ, Bratty JR, Takala J (2012) Dexmedetomidine vs midazolam or propofol for sedation during prolonged mechanical ventilation: two randomized controlled trials. JAMA 307(11):1151–1160. doi:10.1001/jama.2012.304
69. Shehabi Y, Bellomo R, Reade MC, Bailey M, Bass F, Howe B, McArthur C, Murray L, Seppelt IM, Webb S, Weisbrodt L (2013) Early goal-directed sedation versus standard sedation in mechanically ventilated critically ill patients: a pilot study*. Crit Care Med 41(8):1983–1991. doi:10.1097/CCM.0b013e31828a437d
70. Svenningsen H, Egerod I, Videbech P, Christensen D, Frydenberg M, Tonnesen EK (2013) Fluctuations in sedation levels may contribute to delirium in ICU patients. Acta Anaesthesiol Scand 57(3):288–293. doi:10.1111/aas.12048

71. Jones C, Griffiths RD, Humphris G, Skirrow PM (2001) Memory, delusions, and the development of acute posttraumatic stress disorder-related symptoms after intensive care. Crit Care Med 29(3):573–580
72. Mehta S, Burry L, Cook D, Fergusson D, Steinberg M, Granton J, Herridge M, Ferguson N, Devlin J, Tanios M, Dodek P, Fowler R, Burns K, Jacka M, Olafson K, Skrobik Y, Hebert P, Sabri E, Meade M (2012) Daily sedation interruption in mechanically ventilated critically ill patients cared for with a sedation protocol: a randomized controlled trial. JAMA 308(19):1985–1992
73. Schweickert WD, Kress JP (2008) Strategies to optimize analgesia and sedation. Crit Care 12(Suppl 3):S6. doi:10.1186/cc6151
74. Sessler CN, Pedram S (2009) Protocolized and target-based sedation and analgesia in the ICU. Crit Care Clin 25 (3):489–513, viii. doi:10.1016/j.ccc.2009.03.001
75. Zhou Y, Jin X, Kang Y, Liang G, Liu T, Deng N (2014) Midazolam and propofol used alone or sequentially for long-term sedation in critically ill, mechanically ventilated patients: a prospective, randomized study. Crit Care 18(3):R122. doi:10.1186/cc13922
76. Samuelson KA, Lundberg D, Fridlund B (2008) Light vs. heavy sedation during mechanical ventilation after oesophagectomy–a pilot experimental study focusing on memory. Acta Anaesthesiol Scand 52(8):1116–1123. doi:10.1111/j.1399-6576.2008.01702.x
77. de Wit M, Gennings C, Jenvey WI, Epstein SK (2008) Randomized trial comparing daily interruption of sedation and nursing-implemented sedation algorithm in medical intensive care unit patients. Crit Care 12(3):R70. doi:10.1186/cc6908
78. Quenot JP, Ladoire S, Devoucoux F, Doise JM, Cailliod R, Cunin N, Aube H, Blettery B, Charles PE (2007) Effect of a nurse-implemented sedation protocol on the incidence of ventilator-associated pneumonia. Crit Care Med 35(9):2031–2036
79. Arias-Rivera S, Sanchez-Sanchez Mdel M, Santos-Diaz R, Gallardo-Murillo J, Sanchez-Izquierdo R, Frutos-Vivar F, Ferguson ND, Esteban A (2008) Effect of a nursing-implemented sedation protocol on weaning outcome. Crit Care Med 36(7):2054–2060. doi:10.1097/CCM.0b013e31817bfd60
80. Wilhelm W, Kreuer S (2008) The place for short-acting opioids: special emphasis on remifentanil. Crit Care 12(Suppl 3):S5. doi:10.1186/cc6152
81. Chlan LL, Weinert CR, Skaar DJ, Tracy MF (2010) Patient-controlled sedation: a novel approach to sedation management for mechanically ventilated patients. Chest 138(5):1045–1053. doi:10.1378/chest.09-2615
82. Le Guen M, Liu N, Bourgeois E, Chazot T, Sessler DI, Rouby JJ, Fischler M (2013) Automated sedation outperforms manual administration of propofol and remifentanil in critically ill patients with deep sedation: a randomized phase II trial. Intensive Care Med 39(3):454–462. doi:10.1007/s00134-012-2762-2
83. Mesnil M, Capdevila X, Bringuier S, Trine PO, Falquet Y, Charbit J, Roustan JP, Chanques G, Jaber S (2011) Long-term sedation in intensive care unit: a randomized comparison between inhaled sevoflurane and intravenous propofol or midazolam. Intensive Care Med 37(6):933–941. doi:10.1007/s00134-011-2187-3
84. Migliari M, Bellani G, Rona R, Isgro S, Vergnano B, Mauri T, Patroniti N, Pesenti A, Foti G (2009) Short-term evaluation of sedation with sevoflurane administered by the anesthetic conserving device in critically ill patients. Intensive Care Med 35(7):1240–1246. doi:10.1007/s00134-009-1414-7
85. Wanzuita R, Poli-de-Figueiredo LF, Pfuetzenreiter F, Cavalcanti AB, Westphal GA (2012) Replacement of fentanyl infusion by enteral methadone decreases the weaning time from mechanical ventilation: a randomized controlled trial. Crit Care 16(2):R49. doi:10.1186/cc11250
86. Balas MC, Burke WJ, Gannon D, Cohen MZ, Colburn L, Bevil C, Franz D, Olsen KM, Ely EW, Vasilevskis EE (2013) Implementing the awakening and breathing coordination, delirium monitoring/management, and early exercise/mobility bundle into everyday care: opportunities, challenges, and lessons learned for implementing the ICU Pain, Agitation, and Delirium Guidelines. Crit Care Med 41(9 Suppl 1):S116–S127. doi:10.1097/CCM.0b013e3182a17064

87. Morris PE, Goad A, Thompson C, Taylor K, Harry B, Passmore L, Ross A, Anderson L, Baker S, Sanchez M, Penley L, Howard A, Dixon L, Leach S, Small R, Hite RD, Haponik E (2008) Early intensive care unit mobility therapy in the treatment of acute respiratory failure. Crit Care Med 36(8):2238–2243. doi:10.1097/CCM.0b013e318180b90e
88. Llano-Diez M, Renaud G, Andersson M, Marrero HG, Cacciani N, Engquist H, Corpeno R, Artemenko K, Bergquist J, Larsson L (2012) Mechanisms underlying ICU muscle wasting and effects of passive mechanical loading. Crit Care 16(5):R209. doi:10.1186/cc11841
89. Schweickert WD, Pohlman MC, Pohlman AS, Nigos C, Pawlik AJ, Esbrook CL, Spears L, Miller M, Franczyk M, Deprizio D, Schmidt GA, Bowman A, Barr R, McCallister KE, Hall JB, Kress JP (2009) Early physical and occupational therapy in mechanically ventilated, critically ill patients: a randomised controlled trial. Lancet 373(9678):1874–1882. doi:10.1016/S0140-6736(09)60658-9
90. Hodgson C, Bellomo R, Berney S, Bailey M, Buhr H, Denehy L, Harrold M, Higgins A, Presneill J, Saxena M, Skinner E, Young P, Webb S (2015) Early mobilization and recovery in mechanically ventilated patients in the ICU: a bi-national, multi-centre, prospective cohort study. Crit Care 19:81. doi:10.1186/s13054-015-0765-4
91. Vasilevskis EE, Ely EW, Speroff T, Pun BT, Boehm L, Dittus RS (2010) Reducing iatrogenic risks: ICU-acquired delirium and weakness–crossing the quality chasm. Chest 138(5):1224–1233. doi:10.1378/chest.10-0466
92. Pandharipande P, Banerjee A, McGrane S, Ely EW (2010) Liberation and animation for ventilated ICU patients: the ABCDE bundle for the back-end of critical care. Crit Care 14(3):157. doi:10.1186/cc8999
93. Balas MC, Vasilevskis EE, Olsen KM, Schmid KK, Shostrom V, Cohen MZ, Peitz G, Gannon DE, Sisson J, Sullivan J, Stothert JC, Lazure J, Nuss SL, Jawa RS, Freihaut F, Ely EW, Burke WJ (2014) Effectiveness and safety of the awakening and breathing coordination, delirium monitoring/management, and early exercise/mobility bundle. Crit Care Med 42(5):1024–1036. doi:10.1097/CCM.0000000000000129
94. Rahimi RA, Skrzat J, Reddy DR, Zanni JM, Fan E, Stephens RS, Needham DM (2013) Physical rehabilitation of patients in the intensive care unit requiring extracorporeal membrane oxygenation: a small case series. Phys Ther 93(2):248–255. doi:10.2522/ptj.20120336
95. Del Sorbo L, Pisani L, Filippini C, Fanelli V, Fasano L, Terragni P, Dell'Amore A, Urbino R, Mascia L, Evangelista A, Antro C, D'Amato R, Sucre MJ, Simonetti U, Persico P, Nava S, Ranieri VM (2015) Extracorporeal Co2 removal in hypercapnic patients at risk of noninvasive ventilation failure: a matched cohort study with historical control. Crit Care Med 43(1):120–127. doi:10.1097/CCM.0000000000000607
96. Fuehner T, Kuehn C, Hadem J, Wiesner O, Gottlieb J, Tudorache I, Olsson KM, Greer M, Sommer W, Welte T, Haverich A, Hoeper MM, Warnecke G (2012) Extracorporeal membrane oxygenation in awake patients as bridge to lung transplantation. Am J Respir Crit Care Med 185(7):763–768. doi:10.1164/rccm.201109-1599OC
97. Kredel M, Bischof L, Wurmb TE, Roewer N, Muellenbach RM (2014) Combination of positioning therapy and venovenous extracorporeal membrane oxygenation in ARDS patients. Perfusion 29(2):171–177. doi:10.1177/0267659113502834
98. Cheng IW, Eisner MD, Thompson BT, Ware LB, Matthay MA (2005) Acute effects of tidal volume strategy on hemodynamics, fluid balance, and sedation in acute lung injury. Crit Care Med 33(1):63–70 discussion 239-240
99. Chlan LL, Weinert CR, Heiderscheit A, Tracy MF, Skaar DJ, Guttormson JL, Savik K (2013) Effects of patient-directed music intervention on anxiety and sedative exposure in critically ill patients receiving mechanical ventilatory support: a randomized clinical trial. JAMA 309(22):2335–2344. doi:10.1001/jama.2013.5670
100. Mistraletti G, Umbrello M, Sabbatini G, Miori S, Taverna M, Cerri B, Mantovani ES, Formenti P, Spanu P, D'Agostino A, Salini S, Morabito A, Fraschini F, Reiter RJ, Iapichino G (2015) Melatonin reduces the need for sedation in ICU patients: a randomized controlled trial. Minerva Anestesiol 81(12):1298–1310

Acute Respiratory Distress Syndrome in Children

19

Martin C.J. Kneyber

19.1 Introduction

A wide array of insults can lead to respiratory failure in children. Its most severe form – acute respiratory distress syndrome (ARDS) – was originally described by Ashbaugh in 1967 [9]. His description included criteria that remained the cornerstone for the diagnosis for decades, which included a PaO_2/FiO_2 ratio of less than 300 mmHg; diffuse, bilateral chest radiograph appearances; an identifiable insult within 7 days of the onset of ARDS; and well-preserved left ventricular function as demonstrated by a pulmonary capillary wedge pressure of less than 18 mmHg. This initial description included the word 'adult', although the disease appeared to be similar to a certain degree as to what was seen in paediatric critical care [70]. Similar to adults, paediatric ARDS (PARDS) occurs after pulmonary and extra-pulmonary insults. This chapter discusses the current understanding of PARDS and its similarities and differences with adults.

19.2 Epidemiology of Paediatric ARDS

For long, despite its inherent limitations, paediatric critical care practitioners have adopted the North American-European Consensus Conference (NAECC) definition of ARDS established in 1994 to describe and study the epidemiology of ARDS in children [15]. Using this adult-based definition, the incidence of ARDS in children

M.C.J. Kneyber, MD, PhD, FCCM
Department of Paediatrics, Division of Paediatric Critical Care Medicine,
Beatrix Children's Hospital, University Medical Center Groningen,
Internal postal code CA 80, 9700, RB, Groningen, The Netherlands

Critical Care, Anaesthesiology, Peri-operative & Emergency medicine (CAPE),
The University of Groningen, Groningen, The Netherlands
e-mail: m.c.j.kneyber@umcg.nl

D. Chiumello (ed.), *Acute Respiratory Distress Syndrome (ARDS)*,
DOI 10.1007/978-3-319-41852-0_19

varies between two and ten cases per 100,000 per year (Table 19.1) [17, 34, 46, 72, 80, 95, 156, 159]. In contrast, population-based studies in the USA, Europe, Australia and New Zealand using the NAECC definition indicate that the incidence of ARDS in the adult population ranges from 17.9 to 81.0 per 100,000 person-years [16, 92, 97, 123]. Thus, it appears that the susceptibility to ARDS may be age dependent. Importantly, it cannot be ruled out that the incidence may be underestimated as paediatric critical care physicians tend to describe the patient by diagnosis rather than ARDS [80]. Despite this, the prevalence of PARDS varies between 1.4 and 3.4 of all patients admitted to the paediatric intensive care unit (PICU) when estimated from the paediatric critical care perspective (Table 19.1). This number may increase up to approximately 7–10% of all children who are mechanically ventilated [80, 95]. Pulmonary ARDS in children is usually caused by a viral or bacterial pneumonia, whereas systemic infection or (major) trauma is a common cause of extra-pulmonary PARDS [29, 80].

PARDS is associated with significant but at the same time variable mortality rates. Numerous small and large observational and epidemiological studies of children with PARDS indicate mortality rates of 15–75% [126]. Mortality rates may be the lowest in children without comorbidities [95]. A recent systematic review of all published PARDS studies suggested that the mortality was higher in non-Western countries [126]. Remarkably, there appeared to be a decrease in mortality rates over time, especially when paediatric data reported before 1994 was taken into account (Fig. 19.1) [126]. The possible decrease in mortality may be explained by differences in patient population, changes in ventilatory management of children with PARDS over time or institutional variation in management of PARDS. For instance, some group of investigators reported relatively low mortality rates when lung-protective ventilation (LPV) strategies were applied [6, 116]. Furthermore, the use of high-frequency oscillatory ventilation (HFOV) is much more common in the paediatric population, potentially biasing the observations on mortality [7, 11, 95].

Various risk factors predicting mortality during the acute phase of PARDS have been identified, including the presence of immunodeficiency, non-pulmonary sepsis, older age, H1N1 influenza or multiple organ failure upon diagnosis of PARDS [50, 120]. The highest mortality rates (e.g. over 90%) have been reported in children with haematologic malignancies and disseminated intravascular coagulation or who have undergone bone marrow transplant [19, 42, 74]. Investigators have also observed that the degree of oxygenation impairment was associated with increased mortality in various patient cohorts [120]. Although predictive for patient outcome, commonly used metrics of oxygenation such as the PaO_2/FiO_2 ratio, oxygenation index, alveolar–arterial oxygen gradient, arterial–alveolar oxygen ratio and paediatric lung injury score necessitate arterial PaO_2. Alternatively, observational studies have shown that provided SpO_2 is less than 98%; the SpO_2/FiO_2 ratio, oxygen saturation index (OSI) and non-invasive paediatric lung injury score are validated non-invasive scores to estimate patient outcome [77, 79, 141]. Others have suggested that patient outcome may also be predicted by the end-tidal alveolar dead space fraction or the dead space to tidal volume ratio in PARDS [103] [58].

Table 19.1 Summary of studies reporting paediatric acute respiratory distress syndrome (PARDS) using the North American-European Consensus Conference (NAECC) definition

	Dahlem et al. [34]	Zimmerman et al. [159]	Bindl et al. [17]	Erickson et al. [46, 46]	Kneyber et al. [80]	Hu et al. [72]	Yu et al. [156]	Lopez-Fernandez et al. [95]
Study period	2 years (1998–1999)	1 year (1999–2000)	3 months (1997, 2001, 2004)	1 year (2004–2005)	2 years (2004–2006)	1 year (2005–2006)	1 year (2004–2005)	1 year (2010–2001)
Country	The Netherlands	The USA	Germany	Australia, New Zealand	The Netherlands	China	China	Spain
Design	Prospective	Prospective	Survey	Prospective	Retrospective	Prospective	Prospective	Prospective
Sites	Single centre	Multicentre	Multicentre	Multicentre	Single centre	Multicentre	Multicentre	Multicentre
Inclusion	NAECC + MV		NAECC + MV	NAECC + MV	NAECC + MV	NAECC	NAECC	NAECC + MV
PaO_2/FiO_2	≤ 200	≤ 200	≤ 200	≤ 200	≤ 200	Unknown	≤ 200	≤ 200
Age	0–18 years	½–15 years	1 month–18 years	< 16 years	< 18 years	1 month–15 years	1 month–15 years	1 month–15 years
Incidence (per 100,000 per year)	Not reported	9.5	3.2	2.6	2.2	Not reported	Not reported	3.9
Prevalence (percentage of PICU admissions	Not reported	Not reported	Not reported	1.9	3.4	2.6	1.4	1.4

NAECC North American-European Consensus Conference, *MV* mechanical ventilation

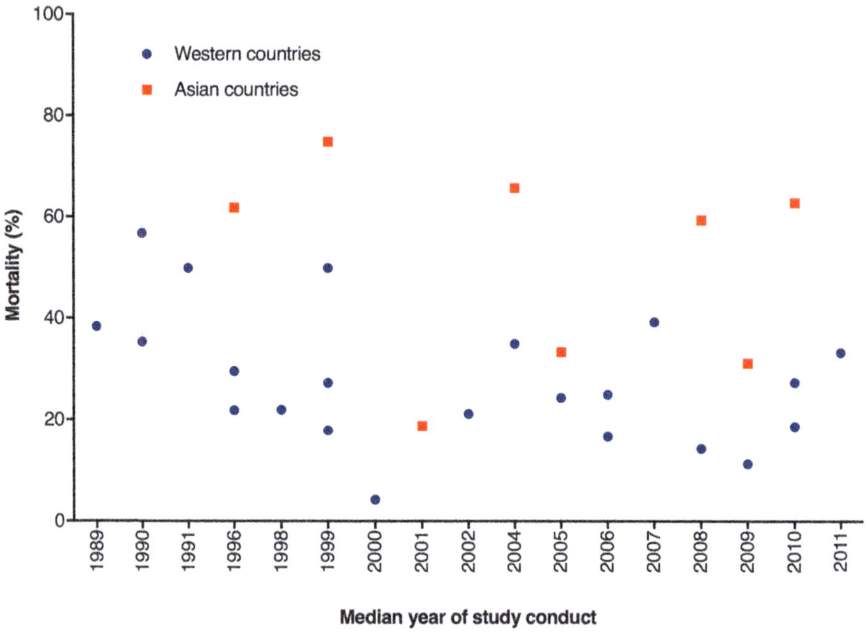

Fig. 19.1 Summary of mortality rates as function of time in children with acute respiratory distress syndrome (ARDS)

The role of biomarkers in predicting disease severity and outcome such as epithelial markers such as KL-6 and surfactant protein D, endothelial markers such as von Willebrand factor and Ang-2, coagulation and fibrinolysis markers and markers for inflammation is little studied and therefore remains inconclusive [104].

19.3 A New Definition for ARDS in Children

In 2015, the Pediatric Acute Lung Injury Consensus Conference (PALICC) developed a paediatric-specific definition for ARDS in children. This initiative was fuelled by the lack of a paediatric context in both the original NAECC definition of ARDS and its revised definition, the Berlin definition. By purely focusing on lung injury in adults, differences between children and adults related to risk factors, aetiologies and pathophysiology most likely have been overlooked.

The new definition of PARDS (Table 19.2) mirrors the Berlin definition in two ways, being timing of onset and exclusion of patients with cardiac failure or fluid overload that may explain the respiratory failure. Importantly, paediatric patients with causes of acute hypoxaemia that are unique to the perinatal period such as prematurity-related lung disease, perinatal lung injury (e.g. meconium aspiration syndrome, pneumonia and sepsis acquired during delivery) or other congenital abnormalities (e.g. congenital diaphragmatic hernia or alveolar capillary dysplasia)

Table 19.2 Definition of paediatric acute respiratory distress syndrome (PARDS) according to the Pediatric Acute Lung Injury Consensus Conference (PALICC)

Age	Exclude patients with perinatal-related lung disease			
Timing	Within 7 days of known clinical insult			
Origin of oedema	Respiratory failure not fully explained by cardiac failure or fluid overload			
Chest imaging	Chest imaging findings of new infiltrate(s) consistent with acute pulmonary parenchymal disease			
Oxygenation	**Invasive mechanical ventilation**			**Non-invasive mechanical ventilation**
	Mild	Moderate	Severe	PARDS (no severity stratification)
	$4 \leq OI < 8$ $5 \leq OSI < 7.5$[1]	$8 \leq OI < 16$ $7.5 \leq OSI < 12.3$[1]	$OI \geq 16$ $OSI \geq 12.3$[1]	Full face-mask bi-level ventilation or CPAP $\geq 5\ cmH_20$ PF ratio ≤ 300 SF ratio ≤ 264[1]
Special populations				
Cyanotic heart disease	Standard criteria above for age, timing and origin of oedema with chest imaging with an acute deterioration in oxygenation not explained by underlying cardiac disease[2]			
Chronic lung disease	Standard criteria above for age, timing and origin of oedema with chest imaging consistent with new infiltrate and acute deterioration in oxygenation from baseline which meet oxygenation criteria above[3]			
Left ventricular dysfunction	Standard criteria for age, timing and origin of oedema with chest imaging changes consistent with new infiltrate and acute deterioration in oxygenation which meet criteria above not explained by left ventricular dysfunction			

OI oxygenation index = (FiO_2* mean airway pressure)/PaO_2

OSI oxygen saturation index = (FiO_2* mean airway pressure)/SpO_2

[1]Use PaO_2-based metric when available. If PaO_2 is not available, the OSI or SF ratio may only be calculated when $SpO_2 \leq 97\%$

[2]ARDS severity groups stratified by OI or OSI is not applicable for children with chronic lung disease on chronic ventilation or for children with cyanotic congenital heart disease

[3]ARDS severity groups stratified by OI or OSI should not be applied to children with chronic lung disease who normally receive invasive mechanical ventilation or children with cyanotic congenital heart disease

were excluded from the definition. As in adults, in order to qualify for PARDS, the symptoms of hypoxaemia and radiographic changes have to occur within 7 days of a known clinical insult. Noticeably, children with left ventricular heart dysfunction or congenital heart disease that fulfil all other PARDS criteria have PARDS if the acute hypoxaemia and new chest imaging changes cannot be explained by acute left ventricular heart failure or fluid overload. This is a huge improvement of the new PARDS definition over other pre-existing definitions.

There are two major differences between the Berlin definition and the PARDS definition; these are related to chest radiograph appearances and the metrics for oxygenation. Unlike the Berlin definition, diagnosis of PARDS requires the need for at least one consolidation on chest radiograph rather than mandating the need for bilateral consolidations. The rationale for this is the low sensitivity of chest radiography to detect (subtle) changes in consolidation, atelectasis or oedema and the poor correlation between consolidations on chest CT scanning and chest radiography [20, 66, 93] [24, 27, 37, 55]. In addition, the presence of bilateral infiltrates provided minimal predictive value for outcome in acute respiratory failure in both children and adults [76, 97, 98].

Aside from this, paediatric critical care practitioners also critiqued both definitions for including the PaO_2/FiO_2 ratio; this metric of oxygenation does not take ventilator settings or mode of ventilation (e.g. HFOV) into account. In addition, there is an increased use of pulse oximetry in children as a substitute for children without an indwelling arterial line, thereby creating an additional problem to the criteria requiring arterial blood gas measurement. Hence, the OI is incorporated in the PARDS definition. Based on a derivation set of two data sets from the USA and Australia/New Zealand, the following cut-off points were derived: OI 4–8 (mild PARDS), 8–16 (moderate PARDS) and > 16 (severe PARDS) [78]. Data from six other centres was used as a validation set, showing increased mortality with increasing PARDS severity, thereby supporting the substitution of OI for PaO_2/FiO_2. For patients without indwelling arterial lines, the oxygen saturation index (OSI) is used as an alternative provided that the SpO_2 is 97% or less [78]. The OSI uses the SpO_2 rather than the PaO_2.

19.4 Pathobiology of Paediatric ARDS

ARDS can originate either from a direct pulmonary insult (i.e. pulmonary ARDS) such as a viral pneumonia or from extra-pulmonary insults such as sepsis (i.e. extra-pulmonary ARDS). The pathobiology of ARDS is a complex process, characterised by increased alveolo-capillary permeability, lung epithelial and endothelial injury and the accumulation of protein-rich oedema fluid during the acute phase of disease [146]. Surfactant homeostasis and haemostatic balance are altered. Much of the understanding of the pathobiology has come from clinical studies in adults or experimental models mimicking the adult clinical situation. Some of these underlying pathophysiological mechanisms are probably shared between children and adults, but it should also be appreciated that there are areas of significant difference including lung growth and development during (early) childhood, immune response and surfactant homeostasis. For instance, the lung parenchyma undergoes substantial structural remodelling and growth during childhood. In the neonatal period, the peripheral airspaces are subdivided by short and blunt tissue ridges into an increasing number of very shallow alveoli. It is by the age of 18 months that the lungs have developed into an adultlike structure [23]. After this period, the number of alveoli continues to grow through adolescence.

There are important differences in the immune response between infants and adults that are likely relevant [153]. In general, the immune system of a child < 1 year of age is relatively immature, including broad deficits in both innate and adaptive immunity [151]. Neonatal PMNs and monocytes function to a lesser degree compared with adults, with decreased chemotactic responses for as long as 1–2 years [54, 91, 100, 110]. Adaptive immunity is also different between young children and adults. At birth, the immune system has a strong T helper 2, anti-inflammatory predisposition with little ability of peripheral mononuclear cells to produce tumour necrosis factor alpha or other pro-inflammatory mediators compared with adults [13, 90]. In addition, at birth, T cells are biased towards regulatory T cells, thereby potentially suppressing the innate immune response [57, 157]. This anti-inflammatory predisposition may persist during early childhood [150]. Only a few studies have examined the role of immune responses in PARDS. Associations between elevated serum levels and interleukin (IL)-6 and PARDS and soluble intercellular adhesion molecule 1 with increased risk of death and/or prolonged duration of mechanical ventilation have been demonstrated in two small paediatric studies [44, 53]. Another small study showed an association of a genetic variant in the IL-1 receptor antagonist gene with ARDS in children with community-acquired pneumonia [114]. More recently, an association between markers of endothelial (angiopoetin 2) and pulmonary epithelial (soluble receptor for advanced glycation end products) injury and mortality in PARDS has been shown, especially in direct lung injury [152].

19.5 Mechanical Ventilation for Paediatric ARDS

Mechanical ventilation (MV) is clearly of benefit for children with ARDS although there are many questions that require study (Fig. 19.2) [81]. Both controlled and assisted modes of ventilation are used by paediatric critical care practitioners, irrespective of the size of the breath (pressure versus volume). However, superiority of one mode over the other has not been demonstrated [122]. This also applies to the

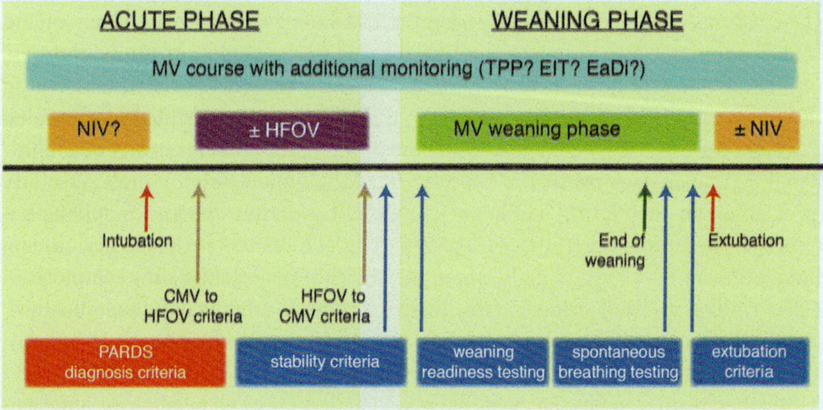

Fig. 19.2 Graphic summary of issues in the ventilatory management of paediatric acute respiratory distress syndrome (PARDS) (Reprinted with permission from Kneyber et al. [81])

use of ventilator modes that allow the patient to trigger the machine breath. Adult data has suggested that patient–ventilator asynchrony (i.e. no synchronisation between patient's demand and the delivered breaths) is associated with increased morbidity, but paediatric data is lacking [40]. Neurally adjusted ventilatory assist (NAVA) uses the electrical activity signal of the diaphragm to trigger inspiration. So far, paediatric experience with this alternative mode of triggering is limited. Piastra and colleagues showed that infants recovering from severe ARDS had a shorter duration of respiratory support when they were weaned with NAVA compared with pressure support ventilation [118].

MV may also exacerbate or even initiate lung injury and has therefore been identified as a predictor for poor outcome [131]. The development of this so-called ventilator-induced lung injury (VILI) has led to the concept of lung-protective ventilation (LPV). In brief, LPV encompasses the delivery of small tidal volume (Vt) to avoid end-inspiratory overdistension (i.e. volutrauma) and the application of a certain level of positive end-expiratory pressure (PEEP) to prevent repetitive opening and closure of alveoli (atelectrauma). The issue of LPV in PARDS is the subject of scientific debate. A large randomised controlled trial (RCT) in adult patients with ARDS according to the NAECC criteria showed improved patient outcome with 6 mL/kg ideal body weight (IBW) compared with 12 mL/kg/IBW [108]. However, other adult studies could not demonstrate a positive effect on mortality when 7 mL/kg IBW was compared with 10 mL/kg IBW [117]. Subsequent meta-analyses concluded that a Vt ≤ 10 mL/kg per predicted body weight was associated with higher survival [21, 22]. To date, a paediatric counterpart of the ARDS Network trial has not been performed. Remarkably however is the data coming from observational studies, showing an inverse or no relationship between Vt and mortality in children [46, 76](20) (Table 19.3). A systematic review of the available paediatric data could also not identify a specific threshold when Vt could be considered safe, irrespective of the presence of ARDS [39]. Experimental work has shown that very young animals were less susceptible to VILI compared with adult animals when subjected to injurious ventilation with supra-physiologic Vt (i.e. 30–40 mL/kg body weight) [84]. All of this challenges the role of volutrauma in PARDS. Various explanations may be proposed, including the incorrect measurement of Vt. The ventilator overestimates the Vt delivered to the patient in young children, signifying the need for correct measurement near the Y-piece of the patient circuit in children below 10–15 kg [25]. In addition, in adults, the Vt is calculated by predicted body weight for age, height and gender. In paediatric practice Vt is usually calculated by actual body weight. A paediatric counterpart of the ARDS Network trial is eagerly awaited, although such a trial seems very unlikely for various reasons including the need for a large sample size (i.e. > 500 patients) [82]. Interestingly, paediatric critical care practitioners may have already found the solution in targeting the optimal Vt in PARDS. Unlike in adult critical care, there is a large tendency to use pressure-controlled (PC) ventilation instead of volume-controlled (VC) ventilation. In contrast with the paediatric data showing an inverse relationship between tidal volume and mortality, these same studies did confirm an association between inspiratory pressures and mortality (Table 19.3). This is in line with the assumption that the patient with a more severe lung injury characterised by small residual inflatable lung volume

Table 19.3 Summary of studies reporting on ventilation practices and outcomes in paediatric acute respiratory distress syndrome (PARDS)

Reference	Study design	Age (years)	Type of lung disease	*N*	PaO_2/FiO_2 ratio	Overall mortality (%)	Median Vt (mL/kg)	Findings
Flori [52]	Prospective, multicentre	<18 years	ALI (67% ARDS)	320	161 ± 74[1]	22%	10	No association between Vt and mortality
Erickson [46]	Prospective, multicentre	<16 years	ALI	117	Not reported	35%	8.0	High Vt associated with lower mortality. Higher mortality with high inspiratory pressures
Albuali [6]	Retrospective, single centre Two periods	<17 years	ALI 79.2% ARDS)	164	153 ± 59.9 (P1), 139.2 ± 53.1 (P2)[1]	28%	10.2 ± 1.7 vs 8.1 ± 1.4[1]	High Vt associated with higher mortality after adjusting for disease severity, ventilator settings and use of HFOV.
Khemani [75]	Retrospective, single centre	<18 years	AHRF (48% ALI/ARDS)	389	138 (83–192)[1]	20%	7	High Vt associated with lower mortality. Higher mortality with high inspiratory pressures

(continued)

Table 19.3 (continued)

Reference	Study design	Age (years)	Type of lung disease	*N*	PaO_2/FiO_2 ratio	Overall mortality (%)	Median Vt (mL/kg)	Findings
Hu [72]	Retrospective, multicentre	<16 years	AHRF (11.2% ALI, 66.3% ARDS)	461	115 (76–168)[1]	41.6% (AHRF) 43.5% (ARDS)	8.8	No association between Vt and mortality at cut-off of 7 or 8 mL/kg
Zhu [158]	Prospective, multicentre	<18 years	AHRF (92.3% ALI, 78.6% ARDS	439	141 (106–192)	18.5% (AHRF), 32.2% (ARDS)	7.7	No association between Vt and mortality in children > 1 year, lower mortality with higher Vt in children < 1 year

[1] Mean ± standard deviation, [2]median (25–75 interquartile range). *ALI* acute lung injury; *AHRF* acute hypoxaemic respiratory failure, *y* year, *OR* odds ratio, *Vt* tidal volume

available for alveolar ventilation and therefore gas exchange (which is also known as the baby lung concept) should receive tidal volumes below physiologic values [56]. Patient subgroup analysis from the ARDS Network trial showed that only patients with poor respiratory system compliance at study entry had a benefit in terms of survival when randomised to the 6 mL/kg study arm [41]. This observation suggests strongly that physicians tend to use lower Vt resulting in higher inspiratory airway pressures in the sicker patients (i.e. patients with lower respiratory system compliance) at the onset of ARDS and mechanical ventilation. This latter observation is in alignment with the data from the other paediatric observational study showing that patients with higher initial lung injury scores were ventilated by smaller tidal volumes and showed worse outcome [76]. This goes along with the concept of keeping lung tissue strain (the ratio between inflated volume and functional residual capacity) low in order to protect the lung [94]. Reanalysis of adult data also showed the importance of limiting the driving pressure (i.e. the ratio of Vt of compliance at a zero-flow state) in ARDS [30]. However, given the absence of paediatric data, no recommendation can be made on the upper limit of the plateau pressure that is allowable. The same applies to the level of PEEP. Levels of PEEP should be set to prevent lung unit collapse at expiration and to avoid tidal recruitment at each breath cycle (collapse–opening–recollapse injury). Although adult data indicated that higher levels of PEEP may be associated with lower mortality, such issues remain to be resolved in paediatrics. Remarkably, paediatric physicians tend to tolerate a higher level of FiO_2 instead of turning up the PEEP because they worry about haemodynamic consequences.

From a theoretical perspective, high-frequency oscillatory ventilation (HFOV) is an ideal LPV mode [83]. With HFOV, a continuous distending pressure (CDP) is generated maintaining lung volume, with superimposed small oscillations in a frequency range of 5–15 Hz allowing for gas exchange. Paediatric critical care practitioners cherish HFOV despite the lack of scientific evidence. To date, there has been only one randomised controlled trial comparing high-frequency oscillatory ventilation to conventional mechanical ventilation in 70 children with diffuse alveolar disease and/or air leak syndrome [8]. This study showed that HFOV utilising an aggressive volume recruitment strategy resulted in a significant improvement in oxygenation and a decreased requirement for supplemental oxygen at 30 days. However, 30-day mortality was not changed in this particular trial. A meta-analysis of all six paediatric and adult clinical trials demonstrated improved mortality in patients randomised to HFOV [133]. However, two large randomised studies in adults with moderate-to-severe (early) ARDS troubled the discussion on HFOV in PARDS [49, 155]. Whereas in the OSCillation for ARDS (OSCAR) trial no difference in 30-day mortality was observed, and the OSCILLation for ARDS Treated Early (OSCILLATE) trial was prematurely stopped (after the 500 patient analyses) by the steering committee because of a significantly higher in-hospital (47% vs 35%) and 60-day mortality (47% vs 38%) in the HFOV group. In the absence of paediatric trials, a post hoc analysis of data of paediatric patients enrolled in a protocolised sedation trial showed similar mortality rates but prolonged duration of MV among patients managed with HFOV, calling for a paediatric RCT to examine the role of HFOV in PARDS [12].

Weaning from the ventilator should start as early as possible, although no paediatric data is available identifying a specific threshold when to start and how to do the weaning itself. Also, at present no paediatric criteria have been validated to discriminate extubation success and failure as well as commonly used adult parameters to monitor weaning including the rapid shallow breathing index (RSBI) [109]. The same applies to the application of spontaneous breathing trials (SBT) and extubation readiness test (ERT). It is unclear what the optimal SBT in PARDS is (i.e. using either continuous positive airway pressure (CPAP), a low level of pressure support ventilation or T-piece ventilation).

Non-invasive positive pressure ventilation (NPPV) is increasingly being used to treat respiratory failure from a variety of aetiologies in children, including paediatric ARDS [124]. Despite this growing, there is much uncertainty about the indications, strategies and effects on patient outcome for the use of NPPV, especially in paediatric ARDS [47, 128]. There are several paediatric prospective and retrospective cohort studies describing the use of NPPV for acute respiratory failure, but most include a heterogeneous population that includes mild-to-severe ARDS. Thus, it remains the subject of debate if NPPV actually prevents the need for endotracheal intubation. Observational studies indicated that the median intubation rate for children with severe PARDS is 57% [47]. In only one randomised controlled trial of 50 children with acute hypoxaemia respiratory failure, the intubation rate was significantly lower (28% vs 60%, $p = 0.045$) when NPPV was compared with standard care. However, this particular study included also patients with mild PARDS.

19.5.1 Extracorporeal Life Support

Extracorporeal life support (ECLS) is a modified form of cardiopulmonary bypass. During ECLS, blood is pumped through an extracorporeal circuit containing a membrane oxygenator in which O_2 is added and CO_2 removed from blood, which is then returned to the patient. An increasing number of paediatric patients with respiratory failure are managed with veno-venous or veno-arterial ECLS despite the absence of a great deal of data showing improved patient outcome [36]. No randomised trials have been performed in PARDS, making it difficult to determine the efficacy of ECLS. In one retrospective study, it was found that the use of ECLS was associated with a reduced mortality in paediatric acute respiratory failure [63]. Thus, ECLS should be considered in severe PARDS where the cause of the respiratory failure is believed to be reversible [36].

19.6 Pulmonary Specific Treatment of PARDS

The pathophysiologic and clinical features have triggered many investigators to study numerous pharmacological approaches to ARDS in critically ill adults [127]. Few of these approaches have been explored in critically ill children. As a consequence, much of the routine treatment for PARDS is based on data from adults or paediatric anecdotal experiences (Table 19.4). Despite this lack of scientific

Table 19.4 Summary of studies reporting on the use of pulmonary specific ancillary treatment in paediatric acute respiratory distress syndrome (PARDS)

Reference	Number of patients Disease	Intervention	Findings and conclusions
Exogenous surfactant			
Willson et al. [22]	$N = 42$ Acute hypoxaemic respiratory failure (OI >7)	Calf surfactant vs air placebo	Improved oxygenation, decreased ventilation time and shorter PICU stays
Willson et al. [24]	$N = 153$ Acute lung injury (OI > 7)	Calf surfactant vs air placebo	Improved oxygenation and decreased mortality. No difference in ventilator-free days (primary study outcome)
Willson et al. [25]	$N = 109$ Direct lung injury only	Pneumosurf vs air placebo	No effect on oxygenation or mortality
Thomas et al. [26]	$N = 165$ Acute hypoxaemic respiratory failure	Lucinactant (synthetic surfactant) vs air placebo	Improved oxygenation, but no effect on mortality, length of ventilation or length of stay
Nitric oxide			
Day et al. [33]	$N = 22$ Acute bilateral lung disease	10 ppm iNO vs control	Improved OI and PVRI, but not mortality
Dobyns et al. [34]	$N = 108$ AHRF	10 ppm iNO vs control	Improved OI and PVRI, but not mortality
Ibrahim et al. [35]	$N = 32$ ARDS	5 ppm iNO ± prone positioning vs control	Improved OI, but not mortality
Prone positioning			
Curley et al. [73]	$N = 102$ Acute lung injury (PaO_2/FiO_2 ratio ≤ 300 mmHg)	Prone positioning for 20 hours vs standard therapy	Improved oxygenation, no effect on ventilator-free days or mortality

evidence, many pulmonary-specific therapies including inhaled nitric oxide (iNO), surfactant or steroids are used in daily practice [124, 125].

19.6.1 Exogenous Surfactant

Animal studies, uncontrolled case reports and case series suggested a potential benefit to exogenous surfactant replacement therapy in PARDS [136]. However, clinical trials of exogenous surfactant outside of the neonatal population provided mixed results. Nonrandomised studies showed improved oxygenation but no effect on mortality in paediatric patients with moderate-to-severe ARDS according to the NAECC criteria. Calf lung surfactant (calfactant) was compared to placebo in a large, multicentre, randomised, placebo-controlled, masked trial in 153 children with acute lung injury [148]. Surfactant administration significantly improved oxygenation and reduced mortality (19% vs 36%) compared with placebo. However, this beneficial effect of surfactant disappeared after adjusting for immunocompromised state in multivariate analysis. The same group of investigators joined an international, multicentre, placebo-controlled trial comparing calfactant with placebo in both adult and paediatric patients with direct lung injury [149]. The trial utilised a novel form of surfactant, which was twice as concentrated as traditional calfactant. However, the trial was stopped prematurely due to futility. Recent attempts on identifying a possible role for exogenous surfactant through a multinational, prospective, blinded, randomised, controlled phase II trial of intratracheal instillation trial using a synthetic formulation of surfactant (lucinactant) among infants less than 2 years of age also showed no effect on patient outcome [140].

19.6.1.1 Nitric Oxide

The main effect of nitric oxide (NO) is smooth muscle relaxation by increasing intracellular cGMP. Vasodilation mainly occurs in areas that are adequately ventilated causing blood to shunt away from poorly ventilated areas [119]. Its use in ARDS may therefore be considered to reduce ventilation/perfusion mismatch by reducing dead space ventilation and, thereby, improving oxygenation. The clinical response to iNO has been reported in various (individual) case series, demonstrating a rapid improvement in oxygenation even with a concentration as low as 1 part per million (ppm) [1, 111, 129, 138]. Day and co-workers compared the effects of 10 ppm iNO in ten paediatric patients with acute bilateral lung disease requiring a positive end-expiratory pressure (PEEP) > 6 cmH_2O and a fraction of inspired oxygen (FiO_2) > 0.5 for > 12 h with 12 control patients [38]. Although there was an immediate, but unsustained improvement in pulmonary vascular resistance and systemic oxygenation defined by the OI, no beneficial effect on mortality was observed although this study was not designed to assess mortality. Dobyns et al. performed a prospective, multicentre, placebo-controlled RCT of 108 children > 1 month of age with severe acute hypoxaemic respiratory failure (i.e. OI > 15) randomised to iNO 10 ppm ($N = 53$ children) or control ($N = 55$) [43]. Patients with a congenital heart defect or after cardiac surgery were not included in this study, and nearly half of the patients suffered from underlying diseases (i.e. chronic lung disease or immunodeficiency). The positive effect of iNO on oxygenation was confirmed in just about half of the patients. Mortality was comparable between the two groups, although again this trial was also not designed to assess this. Subgroup analysis revealed a possible beneficial effect of iNO in immunocompromised patients and those with severe hypoxaemia (i.e. OI > 25), although the small sample size in these analyses precludes the robustness of these findings. Ibrahim et al. randomised 32 children aged 2 months–10 years with severe ARDS ($PaO_2/FiO_2 \leq 200$ mmHg, positive inspiratory pressure ≥ 30 cmH_2O and a $FiO_2 \geq 0.5$) to one of the three groups: (1) 24 h of iNO at 5 ppm in the prone position, (2) 24 h of iNO at 5 ppm in the supine position or (3) no iNO in the prone position [73]. In line with the two other studies, these investigators observed a significant improvement in oxygenation, but not in mortality. It may thus be concluded that although iNO improves oxygenation in PARDS, it does not positively affect patient outcomes. This conclusion is strengthened by the outcome of a Cochrane analysis of 604 children and adults with ARDS [3]. Oxygenation was improved, but there was no improvement in mortality, duration of mechanical ventilation, ventilator-free days or length of intensive care unit (ICU) or hospital stay in the iNO cohort [3]. Additionally, there appeared to be an increased occurrence of renal impairment in patients managed with iNO. Therefore, the use of iNO for PARDS should only be considered in patients with documented pulmonary hypertension or severe right ventricular dysfunction [99]. In patients with intractable hypoxaemia, iNO may be considered as rescue therapy from or as a bridge to extracorporeal life support (ECLS).

19.6.1.2 Corticosteroids

ARDS is characterised by an overwhelming inflammatory process [102]. Paediatric data on the effectiveness of steroids is limited to the case series, including the use of methylprednisolone (initial loading dose 5 mg/kg and subsequent maintenance therapy for 2 weeks of 2 mg/kg every 6 h) in a 12-month-old infant with late ARDS, and a case series of six children treated with high-dose steroids [60, 65, 68, 101]. To date, no RCTs have been performed investigating the efficacy of glucocorticoids in PARDS. The role of glucocorticoids as therapy for PARDS remains to be determined. Studies performed in adults with ARDS also fail to provide a clear answer. In fact, two systematic reviews of published adult data reported conflicting results [115, 137].

19.6.1.3 Other Pharmacological Therapies

Inhaled prostaglandin I_2, a natural pulmonary vasodilator, may be considered in a similar manner as iNO [35, 71, 113]. Dahlem observed a significant median improvement of 26% in the OI following nebulisation of 30 ng/kg/min epoprostenol, but the effect on patient outcome remains unknown [35]. To date, the effect of inhaled beta-adrenergic receptor agonists as the current adult evidence discourages the use of β2-agonist among ARDS patients, heliox, N-acetylcysteine or other drugs such as of ipratropium bromide, dornase alpha outside the cystic fibrosis population, plasminogen activators, fibrinolytics or other anticoagulants on patient outcome that remains to be established [2, 107, 130, 154].

19.6.2 Non-pharmacological Interventions

19.6.2.1 Prone Positioning

Preliminary data in children with acute lung injury subjected to prone positioning showed improved oxygenation without serious adverse events [136]. To date, only one RCT has been performed in children to investigate the efficacy of prone positioning on patient outcome [32]. In this particular study, $N = 102$ patients with acute lung injury were randomised to prone position for 20 h each day or supine. Despite the significant improvement in oxygenation, the study was stopped at the planned interim analysis on the basis of futility. Prone positioning did not exert a beneficial effect on ventilator-free days, all-cause mortality, time to recovery from lung injury, the number of organ-failure-free days, cognitive function or overall health. However, the drawback of this trial was that it was not limited to paediatric patients with severe PARDS. A meta-analysis of adult ARDS patients showed that the effect of prone positioning was the greatest in patients with severe disease, i.e. a $PaO_2/FiO_2 < 100$ mmHg [132]. This conclusion was supported by the adult PROSEVA trial, showing a significant improvement in mortality in patients with severe ARDS (i.e. $PaO_2/FiO_2 < 150$ mmHg [64].

19.6.2.2 Endotracheal Suctioning

Maintaining a patent airway is essential to the safe care of any mechanically ventilated patient, thereby making it one of the most performed interventions despite the lack of scientific evidence including in PARDS [28, 59, 106]. Also, the technique used to perform endotracheal suctioning also requires further study. So far, no RCT evaluating the effect of a closed versus open suctioning on patient outcome in PARDS is available. However, a drop in dynamic compliance and expired Vt indicative of a loss of lung volume may occur during open suctioning, thereby favouring closed suctioning systems [10, 105].

19.6.2.3 Chest Physiotherapy

The use of chest physiotherapy for airway clearance and sputum evacuation in mechanically ventilated children cannot be considered standard of care [86]. The efficacy of chest physiotherapy for PARDS also has not been tested in a single RCT to date.

19.6.3 Non-pulmonary Specific Treatment

19.6.3.1 Sedation

Use of sedatives in children supported on mechanical ventilation is highly common despite lacking sound scientific evidence for this practice [142]. So far, there is no data specifically focusing on PARDS patients. Two recent trials did not confirm a beneficial effect of either protocolised sedation or a daily interruption of sedation on patient outcome [33, 144]. Both trials however did also include patients other than those with PARDS.

19.6.3.2 Neuromuscular Blockade

High-quality evidence to guide the use of neuromuscular blockade (NMB) in children with PARDS supported by mechanical ventilation is lacking. Papazian and colleagues showed improved 90-day survival and increased time off the ventilator without increased muscular weakness associated with early use of NMB in N = 340 adults with severe ARDS ($PaO_2/FiO_2 < 150$) in a multicentre double-blind randomised controlled trial [112]. It is unclear if such beneficial effects of NMB can also be seen in PARDS.

19.6.3.3 Fluid Management

Increased extravascular lung water has been associated with poor outcomes in adults with ARDS [31]. Furthermore, the NHLBI Fluid and Catheter Treatment Trial (FACTT) demonstrated decreased duration of mechanical ventilation, ICU length of stay and improved oxygenation with a conservative fluid strategy (i.e. CVP < 4 mmHg or pulmonary artery occlusion pressure < 8 mmHg) compared to a liberal fluid strategy (i.e. CVP 10–14 mmHg or PAOP 14–18 mmHg) in adults with acute lung injury in whom underlying shock had been reversed [139]. Such trials are lacking in PARDS. Observational prospective and retrospectively collected data have suggested though that increasing fluid balance in children with acute lung injury is associated with worse outcomes, including worsening of oxygenation, prolonged duration of mechanical ventilation and increased mortality, persisting after adjusting for severity of illness [51, 121, 143]. One study of 27 children with PARDS reported significantly lower extravascular lung water at baseline in survivors as compared to non-survivors [96]. This extravascular lung water was correlated with fluid overload, suggesting the need for restrictive fluid management.

As it cannot be ruled out that fluid balance is a proxy for greater severity of illness, the optimal fluid management in PARDS needs to be established. As such, there is no paediatric data related to the best choice of fluid for PARDS or the timing of using continuous renal replacement therapy (CRRT) to reduce fluid overload in PARDS. Greater fluid overload at the initiation of CRRT, after adjusting for illness severity, has been associated with increased mortality in critically ill children [61, 134]. Disappointingly, there is limited data reporting on the best method to determine adequate intravascular status in patients with PARDS in order to prevent fluid overload [89].

19.6.3.4 Transfusion

Red blood cell (RBC) transfusions are very common in critically ill children, despite the fact that a large randomised study confirmed an equivalent effect of a restrictive transfusion strategy (i.e. only transfusing when the haemoglobin is ≤ 7.0 g/dL) compared to a liberal transfusion strategy in haemodynamically stable patients [87]. This observation also held true for patients with respiratory failure, including PARDS. However, there have been no RCTs evaluating RBC transfusion thresholds specifically focusing on PARDS.

19.7 Monitoring of PARDS

It is obvious that patients with PARDS need the minimal monitoring routinely used in children admitted to the paediatric intensive care unit (PICU), including continuous monitoring of cardiac and respiratory rates, pulse oximetry and blood pressure [45]. Ventilatory monitoring should at least include respiratory system mechanics such as exhaled Vt and inspiratory pressures delivered to the patient. However, the peak inspiratory pressure is largely influenced by the resistance of endotracheal tube and airways and is therefore a poor surrogate for pressures applied to the alveoli in the context of using a ventilatory mode that does not incorporate a zero-flow state. Adult data has shown that there is a poor correlation between the plateau pressure and the transpulmonary pressure (Ptp). Ptp (i.e. the difference between the alveolar and the pleural pressure) reflects lung strain, but this requires the use of an oesophageal catheter [4]. So far, no paediatric data has shown improved outcome when oesophageal manometry is routinely applied in ventilated PARDS patients. In contrast, oesophageal manometry-guided PEEP setting resulted in improved oxygenation and respiratory compliance over the first 72 hours in adult ARDS patients compared with PEEP setting according to the ARDSnet PEEP/FiO_2 protocol [135].

Ventilators should also display flow-time, pressure-time and volume-time curves as they provide simple and useful information [45]. The expiratory phase examination allows for the detection of dynamic hyperinflation (inspiration occurring while expiration flow is not null) and expiratory flow limitation, a condition that may occur especially during ventilation with high respiratory rate for compensation of low tidal volumes and relatively long inspiratory time. Also, high expiratory flow during early expiration is a sign of poor compliance, with a fast time constant. Asymmetry between inspiratory and expiratory volume may suggests air leak from the respiratory system. Noisy expiratory and inspiratory flow may suggest the presence of tracheal secretions [88]. Finally, patient ventilator asynchrony may be identified by observing ventilator waveforms, although this is not the most superior method of detecting PVA [18, 26]. The location of measurement of flow and tidal volume is important. Vt measured at the proximal airway with a pneumotachograph was found to be different from those measured at the ventilator, especially in infants and small children [5, 25, 69].

Quasi-static pressure–volume (PV) loop is the reference method to evaluate the compliance of the respiratory system; monitoring this loop has been proposed as tool to identify the lower inflection point (LIP) of the PV loop and to set the level of PEEP. However, the technique is complex and the patient needs to be deeply sedated or paralyzed, the interpretation of the loop is difficult and there are no clinical benefits of this monitoring reported in adult ARDS. Also, data in PARDS is lacking. Alternatively, the dynamic pressure-volume loop may be used for patient monitoring, but these loops are very much influenced by the resistance of the respiratory system including endotracheal tube [67]. Dynamic pressure-volume loops should therefore be interpreted with caution. Furthermore, evaluating the dynamic compliance (i.e. the ratio of exhaled tidal volume divided by the driving pressure) mandates a zero-flow state, the absence of patient effort, precise measurement of the Vt and no or minimal leakage around the ETT. The suitability of other various parameters for PARDS has not been evaluated, including the 'stress index' (i.e. the shape of the airway pressure curve during inspiration), measuring of intrinsic PEEP (PEEPi) when expiratory flow is limited, oesophageal manometry to calculate transpulmonary pressure at the end of in- and expiration or calculate work of breathing, measuring respiratory drive by P0.1 and the electrical activity of the diaphragm (EADi) [62]. Although continuous monitoring of end-tidal CO_2 is recommended to assess the accuracy of ventilation support, it is unclear if incorporating volumetric capnography improves PARDS outcome. Furthermore, end-tidal CO_2 cannot be used as a reliable surrogate for arterial or capillary CO_2 until a correction method is validated [75]. Peripheral venous blood gas also does not accurately predict arterial gas.

Chest radiography is initially important to establish the diagnosis of PARDS; however, the optimal frequency of radiograph control in children with PARDS is not established. Chest CT scan may be necessary in PARDS to help with the aetiological diagnosis or to diagnose certain complications but not as routine monitoring tool. Lung ultrasonography is a simple, radiation-free, easily accessible and validated method to evaluate pleural effusion in adults and children [145]. It is increasingly used in adults with ARDS to detect lung complications and to evaluate lung recruitment [93, 145]. Data in children with PARDS are not available.

19.8 Outcome of Paediatric ARDS

Despite increasing indications that there are significant long-term consequences in adult survivors of ARDS, the long-term consequences of PARDS in children remain largely unknown. Multiple studies of adult survivors of ARDS reported adverse long-term effects, including decreased lung function, reduced quality of life and diminished neurocognitive functioning that impacts daily living [120]. The few paediatric studies examining pulmonary function in PARDS survivors are small series with pulmonary function test (PFT) assessments performed at highly variable times after hospital discharge [14, 48, 147]. However, despite the inherent limitations, these uncontrolled studies have indicated abnormalities in PFT persisting for up to 12 years after hospital discharge in a heterogeneous group of PARDS survivors [120]. Importantly, parents also reported more lung problems in a group of 1–6 year olds 3–6 months after discharge from the PICU [85]. These studies underscore that pulmonary function impairments representing both obstructive and restrictive disease do occur in PARDS survivors, necessitating the need for structural follow-up. Recent studies have also begun to focus on the acquisition of new physical deficits and effects on quality of life, mental health and family functioning although these studies are not limited to PARDS patients only [120]. Thus, long-term neuropsychological and cognitive outcomes in children who survive PARDS have not yet been adequately examined.

Conclusions

It may thus be concluded that although PARDS may be relatively uncommon in children admitted to the PICU, its development has important implications for patient outcome including high mortality among specific subgroups. Based upon the available literature and the PALICC recommendations, Table 19.5 summarises current directions for the management of children with PARDS. It is important to recognise that the paucity of data in PARDS lends itself to many avenues of study generating novel and much needed, vital data. Only with a concerted effort, and worldwide collaboration, it will be possible to improve the care of children with PARDS.

Table 19.5 Recommendations on the clinical approach to paediatric acute respiratory distress syndrome (PARDS)

Approach	Recommendation
Mechanical ventilation	
Mode of ventilation	No recommendation can be made
Tidal volume	Target tidal volume in physiologic range Keep tidal volume < 10 mL/kg No recommendation on optimal Vt
Inspiratory pressures	Keep inspiratory pressure ≤ 32 cmH_2O in the absence of transpulmonary pressure measurements
Positive end-expiratory pressure	Set end-expiratory pressure taking oxygen delivery, respiratory system compliance and haemodynamics in account No recommendation on optimal PEEP
Lung recruitment	No recommendation on if and how lung recruitment should be done
High-frequency oscillatory ventilation	May be considered in case of refractory hypoxaemia
Non-invasive ventilation	Non-invasive bi-level ventilation may be considered as first-line mode of support in patients with mild-to-moderate lung injury
Oxygenation	No recommendation on optimal target of oxygenation; SpO_2 88–92% should be considered when severe disease
Ventilation	No recommendation on optimal target of ventilation; permissive hypercapnia should be considered when severe disease
Extracorporeal life support	Consider for patients with severe ARDS where the cause of the respiratory failure is reversible or as bridge to lung transplantation
Weaning	As soon as possible No recommendation on optimal weaning approach
Extubation readiness testing	No recommendation on optimal extubation readiness testing
Pulmonary specific ancillary treatment	
Inhaled nitric oxide	Not for routine use, only as bridge to extracorporeal life support or in patients with documented pulmonary hypertension or severe right ventricular dysfunction
Exogenous surfactant	Not recommended
Prone positioning	Not recommended, may be considered in patients with severe disease
Non-pulmonary specific ancillary treatment	
Sedation and analgesia	Minimal, yet effective, targeted sedation is recommended, titrated using validated sedation scores
Neuromuscular blockade	May be considered in patients with severe disease
Fluid management	Goal-directed fluid management is recommended, aimed at preventing a positive fluid balance
Transfusion	Only transfuse if the haemoglobin is < 7.0 g/dL, unless haemodynamically unstable (then transfuse if < 10 g/dL)

References

1. Abman SH, Griebel JL, Parker DK, Schmidt JM, Swanton D, Kinsella JP (1994) Acute effects of inhaled nitric oxide in children with severe hypoxemic respiratory failure. J Pediatr 124(6):881–888
2. Adhikari N, Burns KE, Meade MO (2004) Pharmacologic therapies for adults with acute lung injury and acute respiratory distress syndrome. Cochrane Database Syst Rev 4:CD004477. doi:10.1002/14651858.CD004477.pub2
3. Afshari A, Brok J, Moller AM, Wetterslev J (2010) Inhaled nitric oxide for acute respiratory distress syndrome (ARDS) and acute lung injury in children and adults. Cochrane Database Syst Rev 7:CD002787. doi:10.1002/14651858.CD002787.pub2
4. Akoumianaki E, Maggiore SM, Valenza F, Bellani G, Jubran A, Loring SH, Pelosi P, Talmor D, Grasso S, Chiumello D, Guerin C, Patroniti N, Ranieri VM, Gattinoni L, Nava S, Terragni PP, Pesenti A, Tobin M, Mancebo J, Brochard L (2014) The application of esophageal pressure measurement in patients with respiratory failure. Am J Respir Crit Care Med 189(5):520–531. doi:10.1164/rccm.201312-2193CI
5. Al-Majed SI, Thompson JE, Watson KF, Randolph AG (2004) Effect of lung compliance and endotracheal tube leakage on measurement of tidal volume. Crit Care 8 (6):R398–R402. doi:cc2954 [pii] 6 1186/cc2954 [doi]
6. Albuali WH, Singh RN, Fraser DD, Seabrook JA, Kavanagh BP, Parshuram CS, Komecki A (2007) Have changes in ventilation practice improved outcome in children with acute lung injury? Pediatr Crit Care Med 8(4):324–330
7. Anton N, Joffe KM, Joffe AR (2003) Inability to predict outcome of acute respiratory distress syndrome in children when using high frequency oscillation. Intensive Care Med 29(10):1763–1769. doi:10.1007/s00134-003-1928-3
8. Arnold JH, Hanson JH, Toro-Figuero LO, Gutierrez J, Berens RJ, Anglin DL (1994) Prospective, randomized comparison of high-frequency oscillatory ventilation and conventional mechanical ventilation in pediatric respiratory failure. Crit Care Med 22(10):1530–1539
9. Ashbaugh DG, Bigelow DB, Petty TL, Levine BE (1967) Acute respiratory distress in adults. Lancet 2(7511):319–323
10. Avena MJ, de Carvalho WB, Beppu OS (2003) Evaluation of oxygenation, ventilation and respiratory mechanics before and after endotracheal suction in mechanically ventilated children. Rev Assoc Med Bras 49(2):156–161
11. Babbitt CJ, Cooper MC, Nussbaum E, Liao E, Levine GK, Randhawa IS (2012) High-frequency oscillatory ventilation in pediatric acute hypoxemic respiratory failure: disease-specific morbidity survival analysis. Lung 190(6):685–690. doi:10.1007/s00408-012-9417-5
12. Bateman ST, Borasino S, Asaro LA, Cheifetz IM, Diane S, Wypij D, Curley MA, Investigators RS (2016) Early High-Frequency Oscillatory Ventilation in Pediatric Acute Respiratory Failure. A Propensity Score Analysis. Am J Respir Crit Care Med 193(5):495–503. doi:10.1164/rccm.201507-1381OC
13. Belderbos ME, van Bleek GM, Levy O, Blanken MO, Houben ML, Schuijff L, Kimpen JL, Bont L (2009) Skewed pattern of Toll-like receptor 4-mediated cytokine production in human neonatal blood: low LPS-induced IL-12p70 and high IL-10 persist throughout the first month of life. Clin Immunol 133 (2):228–237. doi:S1521-6616(09)00729-3 [pii] 15 1016/j.clim.2009.07.003
14. Ben-Abraham R, Weinbroum AA, Roizin H, Efrati O, Augarten A, Harel R, Moreh O, Barzilay Z, Paret G (2002) Long-term assessment of pulmonary function tests in pediatric survivors of acute respiratory distress syndrome. Med Sci Monit 8(3):CR153–CR157
15. Bernard GR, Artigas A, Brigham KL, Carlet J, Falke K, Hudson L, Lamy M, LeGall JR, Morris A, Spragg R (1994) The American-European Consensus Conference on ARDS. Definitions, mechanisms, relevant outcomes, and clinical trial coordination. AmJRespirCrit Care Med 149(3 Pt 1):818–824

16. Bersten AD, Edibam C, Hunt T, Moran J, Australian, New Zealand Intensive Care Society Clinical Trials G (2002) Incidence and mortality of acute lung injury and the acute respiratory distress syndrome in three Australian States. Am J Respir Crit Care Med 165(4):443–448. doi:10.1164/ajrccm.165.4.2101124
17. Bindl L, Dresbach K, Lentze MJ (2005) Incidence of acute respiratory distress syndrome in German children and adolescents: a population-based study. Crit Care Med 33(1):209–312
18. Blokpoel RG, Burgerhof JG, Markhorst DG, Kneyber MC (2016) Patient-Ventilator asynchrony during assisted ventilation in children. Pediatr Crit Care Med 17(5):e204–e211. doi:10.1097/PCC.0000000000000669
19. Bojko T, Notterman DA, Greenwald BM, De Bruin WJ, Magid MS, Godwin T (1995) Acute hypoxemic respiratory failure in children following bone marrow transplantation: an outcome and pathologic study. Crit Care Med 23(4):755–759
20. Bombino M, Gattinoni L, Pesenti A, Pistolesi M, Miniati M (1991) The value of portable chest roentgenography in adult respiratory distress syndrome. Comparison with computed tomography. Chest 100(3):762–769
21. Brower RG, Rubenfeld GD (2003) Lung-protective ventilation strategies in acute lung injury. Crit Care Med 31(4 Suppl):S312–S316. doi:10.1097/01.CCM.0000057909.18362.F6
22. Burns KE, Adhikari NK, Slutsky AS, Guyatt GH, Villar J, Zhang H, Zhou Q, Cook DJ, Stewart TE, Meade MO (2011) Pressure and volume limited ventilation for the ventilatory management of patients with acute lung injury: a systematic review and meta-analysis. PLoS One 6(1):e14623. doi:10.1371/journal.pone.0014623
23. Burri PH (2006) Structural aspects of postnatal lung development - alveolar formation and growth. Biol Neonate 89(4):313–322. doi:10.1159/000092868
24. Caironi P, Langer T, Gattinoni L, Caironi P, Langer T, Gattinoni L (2008) Acute lung injury/acute respiratory distress syndrome pathophysiology: what we have learned from computed tomography scanning. Curr Opin Crit Care 14 (1):64–69. doi: http://dx.doi.org/10.1097/MCC.0b013e3282f42d8c
25. Cannon ML, Cornell J, Tripp-Hamel DS, Gentile MA, Hubble CL, Meliones JN, Cheifetz IM (2000) Tidal volumes for ventilated infants should be determined with a pneumotachometer placed at the endotracheal tube. Am J Respir Crit Care Med 162(6):2109–2112
26. Colombo D, Cammarota G, Alemani M, Carenzo L, Barra FL, Vaschetto R, Slutsky AS, Della Corte F, Navalesi P (2011) Efficacy of ventilator waveforms observation in detecting patient-ventilator asynchrony. Crit Care Med 39 (11):2452–2457. doi:10.1097/CCM.0b013e318225753c
27. Constantin JM, Grasso S, Chanques G, Aufort S, Futier E, Sebbane M, Jung B, Gallix B, Bazin JE, Rouby JJ, Jaber S, Constantin J-M, Grasso S, Chanques G, Aufort S, Futier E, Sebbane M, Jung B, Gallix B, Bazin JE, Rouby J-J, Jaber S (2010) Lung morphology predicts response to recruitment maneuver in patients with acute respiratory distress syndrome. Crit Care Med 38 (4):1108–1117. doi: http://dx.doi.org/10.1097/CCM.0b013e3181d451ec
28. Copnell B, Fergusson D (1995) Endotracheal suctioning: time-worn ritual or timely intervention? American journal of critical care : an official publication. Am Assoc Crit Care Nurses 4(2):100–105
29. Cornfield DN (2013) Acute respiratory distress syndrome in children: physiology and management. Curr Opin Pediatr 25(3):338–343. doi:10.1097/MOP.0b013e328360bbe7
30. Costa EL, Slutsky AS, Amato MB (2015) Driving pressure as a key ventilation variable. N Engl J Med 372(21):2072. doi:10.1056/NEJMc1503487
31. Craig TR, Duffy MJ, Shyamsundar M, McDowell C, McLaughlin B, Elborn JS, McAuley DF (2010) Extravascular lung water indexed to predicted body weight is a novel predictor of intensive care unit mortality in patients with acute lung injury. Crit Care Med 38(1):114–120. doi:10.1097/CCM.0b013e3181b43050
32. Curley MA, Hibberd PL, Fineman LD, Wypij D, Shih MC, Thompson JE, Grant MJ, Barr FE, Cvijanovich NZ, Sorce L, Luckett PM, Matthay MA, Arnold JH (2005) Effect of prone positioning on clinical outcomes in children with acute lung injury: a randomized controlled trial. JAMA 294(2):229–237

33. Curley MA, Wypij D, Matthay MA, Investigators RS (2015) Sedation protocol for critically ill pediatric patients--reply. JAMA 313(17):1754–1755. doi:10.1001/jama.2015.3462
34. Dahlem P, van Aalderen WM, Hamaker ME, Dijkgraaf MG, Bos AP (2003) Incidence and short-term outcome of acute lung injury in mechanically ventilated children. Eur Respir J 22(6):980–985
35. Dahlem P, Van Aalderen WMC, De Neef M, Dijkgraaf MGW, Bos AP (2004) Randomized controlled trial of aerosolized prostacyclin therapy in children with acute lung injury. Crit Care Med 32:1055–1060
36. Dalton HJ, Macrae DJ, Pediatric Acute Lung Injury Consensus Conference G (2015) Extracorporeal support in children with pediatric acute respiratory distress syndrome: proceedings from the Pediatric Acute Lung Injury Consensus Conference. Pediatr Crit Care Med 16(5 Suppl 1):S111–S117. doi:10.1097/PCC.0000000000000439
37. David M, Karmrodt J, Bletz C, David S, Herweling A, Kauczor HU, Markstaller K, David M, Karmrodt J, Bletz C, David S, Herweling A, Kauczor H-U, Markstaller K (2005) Analysis of atelectasis, ventilated, and hyperinflated lung during mechanical ventilation by dynamic CT. Chest 128(5):3757–3770
38. Day RW, Allen EM, Witte MK (1997) A randomized, controlled study of the 1-h and 24-h effects of inhaled nitric oxide therapy in children with acute hypoxemic respiratory failure. Chest 112:1324–1331
39. de Jager P, Burgerhof JG, van Heerde M, Albers MJ, Markhorst DG, Kneyber MC (2014) Tidal volume and mortality in mechanically ventilated children: a systematic review and meta-analysis of observational studies*. Crit Care Med 42(12):2461–2472. doi:10.1097/CCM.0000000000000546
40. de Wit M, Miller KB, Green DA, Ostman HE, Gennings C, Epstein SK (2009) Ineffective triggering predicts increased duration of mechanical ventilation. Crit Care Med 37(10):2740–2745
41. Deans KJ, Minneci PC, Suffredini AF, Danner RL, Hoffman WD, Ciu X, Klein HG, Schechter AN, Banks SM, Eichacker PQ, Natanson C (2007) Randomization in clinical trials of titrated therapies: unintended consequences of using fixed treatment protocols. Crit Care Med 35(6):1509–1516. doi:10.1097/01.CCM.0000266584.40715.A6
42. DeBruin W, Notterman DA, Magid M, Godwin T, Johnston S (1992) Acute hypoxemic respiratory failure in infants and children: clinical and pathologic characteristics. Crit Care Med 20(9):1223–1234
43. Dobyns EL, Cornfield DN, Anas NG, Fortenberry JD, Tasker RC, Lynch A, Liu P, Eells PL, Griebel J, Baier M, Kinsella JP, Abman SH (1999a) Multicenter randomized controlled trial of the effects of inhaled nitric oxide therapy on gas exchange in children with acute hypoxemic respiratory failure. J Pediatr 134:406–412
44. Dobyns EL, Eells PL, Griebel JL, Abman SH (1999b) Elevated plasma endothelin-1 and cytokine levels in children with severe acute respiratory distress syndrome. J Pediatr 135(2 Pt 1):246–249
45. Emeriaud G, Newth CJ, Pediatric Acute Lung Injury Consensus Conference G (2015) Monitoring of children with pediatric acute respiratory distress syndrome: proceedings from the Pediatric Acute Lung Injury Consensus Conference. Pediatr Crit Care Med 16(5 Suppl 1):S86–101. doi:10.1097/PCC.0000000000000436
46. Erickson S, Schibler A, Numa A, Nuthall G, Yung M, Pascoe E, Wilkins B (2007a) Acute lung injury in pediatric intensive care in Australia and New Zealand: a prospective, multicenter, observational study. PediatrCrit Care Med 8(4):317–323
47. Essouri S, Carroll C, Pediatric Acute Lung Injury Consensus Conference G (2015) Noninvasive support and ventilation for pediatric acute respiratory distress syndrome: proceedings from the Pediatric Acute Lung Injury Consensus Conference. Pediatr Crit Care Med 16(5 Suppl 1):S102–S110. doi:10.1097/PCC.0000000000000437
48. Fanconi S, Kraemer R, Weber J, Tschaeppeler H, Pfenninger J (1985) Long-term sequelae in children surviving adult respiratory distress syndrome. J Pediatr 106(2):218–222
49. Ferguson ND, Cook DJ, Guyatt GH, Mehta S, Hand L, Austin P, Zhou Q, Matte A, Walter SD, Lamontagne F, Granton JT, Arabi YM, Arroliga AC, Stewart TE, Slutsky AS, Meade MO,

Investigators OT, Canadian Critical Care Trials G (2013) High-frequency oscillation in early acute respiratory distress syndrome. N Engl J Med 368(9):795–805. doi:10.1056/NEJMoa1215554

50. Flori H, Dahmer MK, Sapru A, Quasney MW, Pediatric Acute Lung Injury Consensus Conference G (2015) Comorbidities and assessment of severity of pediatric acute respiratory distress syndrome: proceedings from the Pediatric Acute Lung Injury Consensus Conference. Pediatr Crit Care Med 16(5 Suppl 1):S41–S50. doi:10.1097/PCC.0000000000000430
51. Flori HR, Church G, Liu KD, Gildengorin G, Matthay MA (2011) Positive fluid balance is associated with higher mortality and prolonged mechanical ventilation in pediatric patients with acute lung injury. Crit Care Res Pract 2011:854142. doi:10.1155/2011/854142
52. Flori HR, Glidden DV, Rutherford GW, Matthay M (2005) Pediatric acute lung injury: prospective evaluation of risk factors associated with mortality. Am J Respir Crit Care Med 171:995–1001
53. Flori HR, Ware LB, Glidden D, Matthay MA (2003) Early elevation of plasma soluble intercellular adhesion molecule-1 in pediatric acute lung injury identifies patients at increased risk of death and prolonged mechanical ventilation. Pediatr Crit Care Med 4(3):315–321. doi:10.1097/01.PCC.0000074583.27727.8E
54. Fox SE, Lu W, Maheshwari A, Christensen RD, Calhoun DA (2005) The effects and comparative differences of neutrophil specific chemokines on neutrophil chemotaxis of the neonate. Cytokine 29(3):135–140. doi:10.1016/j.cyto.2004.10.007
55. Gattinoni L, Caironi P, Pelosi P, Goodman LR (2001) What has computed tomography taught us about the acute respiratory distress syndrome? Am J Respir Crit Care Med 164(9):1701–1711
56. Gattinoni L, Pesenti A (2005) The concept of "baby lung". Intensive Care Med 31(6):776–784. doi:10.1007/s00134-005-2627-z
57. Ghazal P, Dickinson P, Smith CL (2013) Early life response to infection. Curr Opin Infect Dis 26(3):213–218. doi:10.1097/QCO.0b013e32835fb8bf
58. Ghuman AK, Newth CJ, Khemani RG (2012) The association between the end tidal alveolar dead space fraction and mortality in pediatric acute hypoxemic respiratory failure. Pediatr Crit Care Med 13(1):11–15. doi:10.1097/PCC.0b013e3182192c42
59. Gilbert M (1999) Assessing the need for endotracheal suction. Paediatr Nurs 11(1):14–17
60. Goh AY, Sekaran D, Roziah M (1999) Corticosteroid rescue in late paediatric acute respiratory distress syndrome. Respirology 4:295–297
61. Goldstein SL, Somers MJ, Baum MA, Symons JM, Brophy PD, Blowey D, Bunchman TE, Baker C, Mottes T, McAfee N, Barnett J, Morrison G, Rogers K, Fortenberry JD (2005) Pediatric patients with multi-organ dysfunction syndrome receiving continuous renal replacement therapy. Kidney Int 67(2):653–658. doi:10.1111/j.1523-1755.2005.67121.x
62. Grasso S, Stripoli T, De Michele M, Bruno F, Moschetta M, Angelelli G, Munno I, Ruggiero V, Anaclerio R, Cafarelli A, Driessen B, Fiore T (2007) ARDSnet ventilatory protocol and alveolar hyperinflation: role of positive end-expiratory pressure. Am J Respir Crit Care Med 176 (8):761–767. doi:200702-193OC [pii] 65 1164/rccm.200702-193OC
63. Green TP, Timmons OD, Fackler JC, Moler FW, Thompson AE, Sweeney MF (1996) The impact of extracorporeal membrane oxygenation on survival in pediatric patients with acute respiratory failure. Pediatric Critical Care Study Group. Crit Care Med 24(2):323–329
64. Guerin C, Reignier J, Richard JC, Beuret P, Gacouin A, Boulain T, Mercier E, Badet M, Mercat A, Baudin O, Clavel M, Chatellier D, Jaber S, Rosselli S, Mancebo J, Sirodot M, Hilbert G, Bengler C, Richecoeur J, Gainnier M, Bayle F, Bourdin G, Leray V, Girard R, Baboi L, Ayzac L, Group PS (2013) Prone positioning in severe acute respiratory distress syndrome. N Engl J Med 368(23):2159–2168. doi:10.1056/NEJMoa1214103
65. Guglani L, Jain S, Lodha R (2006) Methylprednisolone therapy in a child with unresolving ARDS. Indian Pediatr 43(7):639–642
66. Halperin BD, Feeley TW, Mihm FG, Chiles C, Guthaner DF, Blank NE (1985) Evaluation of the portable chest roentgenogram for quantitating extravascular lung water in critically ill adults. Chest 88(5):649–652

67. Harris RS (2005) Pressure-volume curves of the respiratory system. Respir Care 50(1):78–98 discussion 98-79
68. Haselton DJ, Klekamp JG, Christman BW, Barr FE (2000) Use of high-dose corticosteroids and high-frequency oscillatory ventilation for treatment of a child with diffuse alveolar hemorrhage after bone marrow transplantation: case report and review of the literature. Crit Care Med 28:245–248
69. Heulitt MJ, Thurman TL, Holt SJ, Jo CH, Simpson P (2009) Reliability of displayed tidal volume in infants and children during dual-controlled ventilation. Pediatr Crit Care Med 10(6):661–667. doi:10.1097/PCC.0b013e3181bb2b2b
70. Holbrook PR, Taylor G, Pollack MM, Fields AI (1980) Adult respiratory distress syndrome in children. Pediatr Clin N Am 27(3):677–685
71. Howard LS, Morrell NW (2005) New therapeutic agents for pulmonary vascular disease. Paediatr Respir Rev 6(4):285–291. doi:10.1016/j.prrv.2005.09.006
72. Hu X, Qian S, Xu F, Huang B, Zhou D, Wang Y, Li C, Fan X, Lu Z, Sun B, Chinese Collaborative Study Group for Pediatric Respiratory F (2010) Incidence, management and mortality of acute hypoxemic respiratory failure and acute respiratory distress syndrome from a prospective study of Chinese paediatric intensive care network. Acta Paediatr 99(5):715–721. doi:10.1111/j.1651-2227.2010.01685.x
73. Ibrahim TS, El-Mohamady H (2007) Inhaled nitric oxide and prone position: How far they can improve oxygenation in pediatric patients with acute respiratory distress syndrome? J Med Sci 7:390–395
74. Keenan HT, Bratton SL, Martin LD, Crawford SW, Weiss NS (2000) Outcome of children who require mechanical ventilatory support after bone marrow transplantation. Crit Care Med 28(3):830–835
75. Khemani RG, Celikkaya EB, Shelton CR, Kale D, Ross PA, Wetzel RC, Newth CJ (2013) Algorithms to estimate PaCO2 and pH using non invasive parameters for children with Hypoxemic Respiratory Failure. Respir Care. 59(8):1248–1257. doi:respcare.02806 [pii] 79 4187/respcare.02806
76. Khemani RG, Conti D, Alonzo TA, Bart RD 3rd, Newth CJ (2009a) Effect of tidal volume in children with acute hypoxemic respiratory failure. Intensive Care Med 35(8):1428–1437. doi:10.1007/s00134-009-1527-z
77. Khemani RG, Patel NR, Bart RD 3rd, Newth CJ (2009c) Comparison of the pulse oximetric saturation/fraction of inspired oxygen ratio and the PaO2/fraction of inspired oxygen ratio in children. Chest 135(3):662–668. doi:10.1378/chest.08-2239
78. Khemani RG, Rubin S, Belani S, Leung D, Erickson S, Smith LS, Zimmerman JJ, Newth CJ (2015) Pulse oximetry vs. PaO2 metrics in mechanically ventilated children: Berlin definition of ARDS and mortality risk. Intensive Care Med 41(1):94–102. doi:10.1007/s00134-014-3486-2
79. Khemani RG, Thomas NJ, Venkatachalam V, Scimeme JP, Berutti T, Schneider JB, Ross PA, Willson DF, Hall MW, Newth CJ (2012) Comparison of SpO2 to PaO_2 based markers of lung disease severity for children with acute lung injury. Crit Care Med 40(4):1309–1316. doi:10.1097/CCM.0b013e31823bc61b
80. Kneyber MC, Brouwers AG, Caris JA, Chedamni S, Plotz FB (2008) Acute respiratory distress syndrome: is it underrecognized in the pediatric intensive care unit? Intensive Care Med 34(4):751–754. doi:10.1007/s00134-008-1029-4
81. Kneyber MC, Jouvet PA, Rimensberger PC (2014a) How to manage ventilation in pediatric acute respiratory distress syndrome? Intensive Care Med 40(12):1924–1926. doi:10.1007/s00134-014-3498-y
82. Kneyber MC, Rimensberger PC (2012) The need for and feasibility of a pediatric ventilation trial: reflections on a survey among pediatric intensivists. Pediatr Crit Care Med. doi:10.1097/PCC.0b013e31824fbc37
83. Kneyber MC, van Heerde M, Markhorst DG (2012) Reflections on pediatric high-frequency oscillatory ventilation from a physiologic perspective. Respir Care 57 (9):1496–1504. doi:rc01571r1kneyber [pii] 89 4187/respcare.01571

84. Kneyber MC, Zhang H, Slutsky AS (2014b) Ventilator-induced lung injury. Similarity and differences between children and adults. Am J Respir Crit Care Med 190(3):258–265. doi:10.1164/rccm.201401-0168CP
85. Knoester H, Bronner MB, Bos AP, Grootenhuis MA (2008) Quality of life in children three and nine months after discharge from a paediatric intensive care unit: a prospective cohort study. Health Qual Life Outcomes 6:21. doi:10.1186/1477-7525-6-21
86. Krause MF, Hoehn T (2000) Chest physiotherapy in mechanically ventilated children: a review. Crit Care Med 28(5):1648–1651
87. Lacroix J, Hebert PC, Hutchison JS, Hume HA, Tucci M, Ducruet T, Gauvin F, Collet JP, Toledano BJ, Robillard P, Joffe A, Biarent D, Meert K, Peters MJ (2007) Transfusion strategies for patients in pediatric intensive care units. N Engl J Med 356(16):1609–1619
88. Leclerc F, Riou Y, Martinot A, Deschildre A, Neve V, Hue V, Fourier C (1996) Use of the flow-volume loop to detect secretions in ventilated children. Intensive Care Med 22(1):88
89. Lemson J, Nusmeier A, van der Hoeven JG (2011) Advanced hemodynamic monitoring in critically ill children. Pediatrics 128(3):560–571. doi:10.1542/peds.2010-2920
90. Levy O, Zarember KA, Roy RM, Cywes C, Godowski PJ, Wessels MR (2004) Selective impairment of TLR-mediated innate immunity in human newborns: neonatal blood plasma reduces monocyte TNF-alpha induction by bacterial lipopeptides, lipopolysaccharide, and imiquimod, but preserves the response to R-848. J Immunol 173 (7):4627–4634. doi:173/7/4627 [pii]
91. Lewis DB, Wilson CB (2006) Developmental immunology and role of host defenses in fetal and neonatal susceptibility to infection. In: Remington JS, Klein JO, Wilson CB (eds) Infectious diseases of the fetus and newborn infant. Elsevier Saunders, Philadelphia, pp 87–210
92. Li G, Malinchoc M, Cartin-Ceba R, Venkata CV, Kor DJ, Peters SG, Hubmayr RD, Gajic O (2011) Eight-year trend of acute respiratory distress syndrome: a population-based study in Olmsted County, Minnesota. Am J Respir Crit Care Med 183(1):59–66. doi:10.1164/rccm.201003-0436OC
93. Lichtenstein D, Goldstein I, Mourgeon E, Cluzel P, Grenier P, Rouby JJ (2004a) Comparative diagnostic performances of auscultation, chest radiography, and lung ultrasonography in acute respiratory distress syndrome. Anesthesiology 100(1):9–15
94. Liu Q, Li W, Zeng QS, Zhong NS, Chen RC (2013) Lung stress and strain during mechanical ventilation in animals with and without pulmonary acute respiratory distress syndrome. J Surg Res 181 (2):300–307. doi: 102.1016/j.jss.2012.07.010. S0022-4804(12)00643-9 [pii]
95. Lopez-Fernandez Y, Azagra AM, de la Oliva P, Modesto V, Sanchez JI, Parrilla J, Arroyo MJ, Reyes SB, Pons-Odena M, Lopez-Herce J, Fernandez RL, Kacmarek RM, Villar J, Pediatric Acute Lung Injury E, Natural History N (2012) Pediatric Acute Lung Injury Epidemiology and Natural History study: Incidence and outcome of the acute respiratory distress syndrome in children. Crit Care Med 40(12):3238–3245. doi:10.1097/CCM.0b013e318260caa3
96. Lubrano R, Cecchetti C, Elli M, Tomasello C, Guido G, Di Nardo M, Masciangelo R, Pasotti E, Barbieri MA, Bellelli E, Pirozzi N (2011) Prognostic value of extravascular lung water index in critically ill children with acute respiratory failure. Intensive Care Med 37(1):124–131. doi:10.1007/s00134-010-2047-6
97. Luhr OR, Antonsen K, Karlsson M, Aardal S, Thorsteinsson A, Frostell CG, Bonde J (1999a) Incidence and mortality after acute respiratory failure and acute respiratory distress syndrome in Sweden, Denmark, and Iceland. The ARF Study Group. Am J Respir Crit Care Med 159(6):1849–1861. doi:10.1164/ajrccm.159.6.9808136
98. Luhr OR, Karlsson M, Thorsteinsson A, Rylander C, Frostell CG (2000) The impact of respiratory variables on mortality in non-ARDS and ARDS patients requiring mechanical ventilation. Intensive Care Med 26(5):508–517
99. Macrae DJ, Field D, Mercier JC, Moller J, Stiris T, Biban P, Cornick P, Goldman A, Gothberg S, Gustafsson LE, Hammer J, Lonnqvist PA, Sanchez-Luna M, Sedin G, Subhedar N (2004) Inhaled nitric oxide therapy in neonates and children: reaching a European consensus. Intensive Care Med 30:372–380. doi:10.1007/s00134-003-2122-3

100. Marodi L, Csorba S, Nagy B (1980) Chemotactic and random movement of human newborn monocytes. Eur J Pediatr 135(1):73–75
101. Martinot A, Fourier C, Cremer R, Hue V, Deschildre A, Leclerc F (1997) Short-course, high-dose corticosteroid treatment in six children with late ARDS. Pediatr Pulmonol 23: 314–316
102. Matthay MA, Ware LB, Zimmerman GA (2012) The acute respiratory distress syndrome. J Clin Invest 122(8):2731–2740. doi:10.1172/JCI60331
103. McSwain SD, Hamel DS, Smith PB, Gentile MA, Srinivasan S, Meliones JN, Cheifetz IM (2010) End-tidal and arterial carbon dioxide measurements correlate across all levels of physiologic dead space. Respir Care 55(3):288–293
104. Moreira A, Sapru A, Rimensberger PC (2016) What's new about circulating biomarkers in pediatric acute lung disease. Intensive Care Med 42(5):803–805. doi:10.1007/s00134-016-4304-9
105. Morrow B, Futter M, Argent A (2006) Effect of endotracheal suction on lung dynamics in mechanically-ventilated paediatric patients. Aust J Physiot 52(2):121–126
106. Morrow BM, Argent AC (2008) A comprehensive review of pediatric endotracheal suctioning: effects, indications, and clinical practice. Pediatr Crit Care Med 9(5):465–477. doi:10.1097/PCC.0b013e31818499cc
107. Nawab US, Touch SM, Irwin-Sherman T, Blackson TJ, Greenspan JS, Zhu G, Shaffer TH, Wolfson MR (2005) Heliox attenuates lung inflammation and structural alterations in acute lung injury. Pediatr Pulmonol 40(6):524–532. doi:10.1002/ppul.20304
108. Network A (2000) Ventilation with lower tidal volumes as compared with traditional tidal volumes for acute lung injury and the acute respiratory distress syndrome. The Acute Respiratory Distress Syndrome Network. N Engl J Med 342(18):1301–1308
109. Newth CJ, Venkataraman S, Willson DF, Meert KL, Harrison R, Dean JM, Pollack M, Zimmerman J, Anand KJ, Carcillo JA, Nicholson CE, Eunice Shriver Kennedy National Institute of Child H, Human Development Collaborative Pediatric Critical Care Research N (2009) Weaning and extubation readiness in pediatric patients. Pediatr Crit Care Med 10(1):1–11. doi:10.1097/PCC.0b013e318193724d
110. Nussbaum C, Sperandio M (2011) Innate immune cell recruitment in the fetus and neonate. J Reprod Immunol 90(1):74–81. doi:10.1016/j.jri.2011.01.022
111. Okamoto K, Hamaguchi M, Kukita I, Kikuta K, Sato T (1998) Efficacy of inhaled nitric oxide in children with ARDS. Chest 114(3):827–833
112. Papazian L, Forel JM, Gacouin A, Penot-Ragon C, Perrin G, Loundou A, Jaber S, Arnal JM, Perez D, Seghboyan JM, Constantin JM, Courant P, Lefrant JY, Guerin C, Prat G, Morange S, Roch A, Investigators AS (2010) Neuromuscular blockers in early acute respiratory distress syndrome. N Engl J Med 363(12):1107–1116. doi:10.1056/NEJMoa1005372
113. Pappert D, Busch T, Gerlach H, Lewandowski K, Radermacher P, Rossaint R (1995) Aerosolized prostacyclin versus inhaled nitric oxide in children with severe acute respiratory distress syndrome. Anesthesiology 82:1507–1511
114. Patwari PP, O'Cain P, Goodman DM, Smith M, Krushkal J, Liu C, Somes G, Quasney MW, Dahmer MK (2008) Interleukin-1 receptor antagonist intron 2 variable number of tandem repeats polymorphism and respiratory failure in children with community-acquired pneumonia. Pediatr Crit Care Med 9(6):553–559. doi:10.1097/PCC.0b013e31818d32f1
115. Peter JV, John P, Graham PL, Moran JL, George IA, Bersten A (2008) Corticosteroids in the prevention and treatment of acute respiratory distress syndrome (ARDS) in adults: meta-analysis. BMJ 336(7651):1006–1009. doi:10.1136/bmj.39537.939039.BE
116. Peters MJ, Tasker RC, Kiff KM, Yates R, Hatch DJ (1998) Acute hypoxemic respiratory failure in children: case mix and the utility of respiratory severity indices. Intensive Care Med 24(7):699–705
117. Petrucci N, De Feo C (2013) Lung protective ventilation strategy for the acute respiratory distress syndrome. Cochrane Database Syst Rev 2:CD003844. doi:10.1002/14651858.CD003844.pub4
118. Piastra M, De Luca D, Costa R, Pizza A, De Sanctis R, Marzano L, Biasucci D, Visconti F, Conti G (2014) Neurally adjusted ventilatory assist vs pressure support ventilation in infants

recovering from severe acute respiratory distress syndrome: nested study. J Crit Care 29(2):312 e311–312 e315. doi:10.1016/j.jcrc.2013.08.006
119. Puri N, Dellinger RP (2011) Inhaled nitric oxide and inhaled prostacyclin in acute respiratory distress syndrome: what is the evidence? Crit Care Clin 27(3):561–587. doi:10.1016/j.ccc.2011.05.001
120. Quasney MW, Lopez-Fernandez YM, Santschi M, Watson RS, Pediatric Acute Lung Injury Consensus Conference G (2015) The outcomes of children with pediatric acute respiratory distress syndrome: proceedings from the Pediatric Acute Lung Injury Consensus Conference. Pediatr Crit Care Med 16(5 Suppl 1):S118–S131. doi:10.1097/PCC.0000000000000438
121. Randolph AG, Forbes PW, Gedeit RG, Arnold JH, Wetzel RC, Luckett PM, O'Neil ME, Venkataraman ST, Meert KL, Cheifetz IM, Cox PN, Hanson JH (2005) Cumulative fluid intake minus output is not associated with ventilator weaning duration or extubation outcomes in children. PediatrCrit Care Med 6(6):642–647
122. Rimensberger PC, Cheifetz IM, Pediatric Acute Lung Injury Consensus Conference G (2015) Ventilatory support in children with pediatric acute respiratory distress syndrome: proceedings from the pediatric Acute Lung Injury Consensus Conference. Pediatr Crit Care Med 16(5_suppl Suppl 1):S51–S60. doi:10.1097/PCC.0000000000000433
123. Rubenfeld GD, Caldwell E, Peabody E, Weaver J, Martin DP, Neff M, Stern EJ, Hudson LD (2005) Incidence and outcomes of acute lung injury. N Engl J Med 353(16):1685–1693. doi:10.1056/NEJMoa050333
124. Santschi M, Jouvet P, Leclerc F, Gauvin F, Newth CJ, Carroll CL, Flori H, Tasker RC, Rimensberger PC, Randolph AG (2010) Acute lung injury in children: therapeutic practice and feasibility of international clinical trials. Pediatr Crit Care Med 11:681–689
125. Santschi M, Randolph AG, Rimensberger PC, Jouvet P, Pediatric Acute Lung Injury Mechanical Ventilation Investigators tPALI, Sepsis Investigators N, the European Society of P, Neonatal Intensive C (2013) Mechanical ventilation strategies in children with acute lung injury: a survey on stated practice pattern*. Pediatr Crit Care Med 14(7):e332–e337. doi:10.1097/PCC.0b013e31828a89a2
126. Schouten LR, Veltkamp F, Bos AP, van Woensel JB, Serpa Neto A, Schultz MJ, Wosten-van Asperen RM (2016) Incidence and mortality of acute respiratory distress syndrome in children: a systematic review and meta-analysis. Crit Care Med 44(4):819–829. doi:10.1097/CCM.0000000000001388
127. Shafeeq H, Lat I (2012) Pharmacotherapy for acute respiratory distress syndrome. Pharmacotherapy 32(10):943–957. doi:10.1002/j.1875-9114.2012.01115
128. Shah PS, Ohlsson A, Shah JP (2013) Continuous negative extrathoracic pressure or continuous positive airway pressure compared to conventional ventilation for acute hypoxaemic respiratory failure in children. Cochrane Database Syst Rev 11:CD003699. doi:10.1002/14651858.CD003699.pub4
129. Sheridan RL, Zapol WM, Ritz RH, Tompkins RG (1999) Low-dose inhaled nitric oxide in acutely burned children with profound respiratory failure. Surgery 126(5):856–862
130. Singh B, Tiwari AK, Singh K, Mommer SK, Ahmed A, Erwin PJ, Franco PM (2013) Beta-2-Agonist for the treatment of acute lung injury: a systematic review and meta-analysis. Respir Care. doi:10.4187/respcare.02571
131. Slutsky AS, Ranieri VM (2013) Ventilator-induced lung injury. N Engl J Med 369:2126–2136
132. Sud S, Friedrich JO, Taccone P, Polli F, Adhikari NK, Latini R, Pesenti A, Guerin C, Mancebo J, Curley MA, Fernandez R, Chan MC, Beuret P, Voggenreiter G, Sud M, Tognoni G, Gattinoni L (2010a) Prone ventilation reduces mortality in patients with acute respiratory failure and severe hypoxemia: systematic review and meta-analysis. Intensive Care Med 36(4):585–599. doi:10.1007/s00134-009-1748-1
133. Sud S, Sud M, Friedrich JO, Meade MO, Ferguson ND, Wunsch H, Adhikari NK (2010b) High frequency oscillation in patients with acute lung injury and acute respiratory distress syndrome (ARDS): systematic review and meta-analysis. BMJ 340:c2327
134. Sutherland SM, Zappitelli M, Alexander SR, Chua AN, Brophy PD, Bunchman TE, Hackbarth R, Somers MJ, Baum M, Symons JM, Flores FX, Benfield M, Askenazi D, Chand

D, Fortenberry JD, Mahan JD, McBryde K, Blowey D, Goldstein SL (2010) Fluid overload and mortality in children receiving continuous renal replacement therapy: the prospective pediatric continuous renal replacement therapy registry. Am J Kidney Dis: Off J National Kidney Foundation 55(2):316–325. doi:10.1053/j.ajkd.2009.10.048

135. Talmor D, Sarge T, Malhotra A, O'Donnell CR, Ritz R, Lisbon A, Novack V, Loring SH (2008) Mechanical ventilation guided by esophageal pressure in acute lung injury. N Engl J Med 359 (20):2095–2104.doi:NEJMoa0708638 [pii] 145 1056/NEJMoa0708638
136. Tamburro RF, Kneyber MC, Pediatric Acute Lung Injury Consensus Conference G (2015) Pulmonary specific ancillary treatment for pediatric acute respiratory distress syndrome: proceedings from the Pediatric Acute Lung Injury Consensus Conference. Pediatr Crit Care Med 16(5 Suppl 1):S61–S72. doi:10.1097/PCC.0000000000000434
137. Tang BM, Craig JC, Eslick GD, Seppelt I, McLean AS (2009) Use of corticosteroids in acute lung injury and acute respiratory distress syndrome: a systematic review and meta-analysis. Crit Care Med 37(5):1594–1603. doi:10.1097/CCM.0b013e31819fb507
138. Tang SF, Sherwood MC, Miller OI (1998) Randomised trial of three doses of inhaled nitric oxide in acute respiratory distress syndrome. Arch Dis Child 79(5):415–418
139. The National Heart L, Network BIARDSCT (2006) Comparison of two fluid-management strategies in acute lung injury. N Engl J Med 354(24):2564–2575. doi:10.1056/NEJMoa062200
140. Thomas NJ, Guardia CG, Moya FR, Cheifetz IM, Markovitz B, Cruces P, Barton P, Segal R, Simmons P, Randolph AG, Network P (2012) A pilot, randomized, controlled clinical trial of lucinactant, a peptide-containing synthetic surfactant, in infants with acute hypoxemic respiratory failure. Pediatr Crit Care Med 13(6):646–653. doi:10.1097/PCC.0b013e3182517bec
141. Thomas NJ, Shaffer ML, Willson DF, Shih MC, Curley MA (2010) Defining acute lung disease in children with the oxygenation saturation index. Pediatr Crit Care Med 11(1):12–17. doi:10.1097/PCC.0b013e3181b0653d
142. Valentine SL, Nadkarni VM, Curley MA, Pediatric Acute Lung Injury Consensus Conference G (2015) Nonpulmonary treatments for pediatric acute respiratory distress syndrome: proceedings from the Pediatric Acute Lung Injury Consensus Conference. Pediatr Crit Care Med 16(5 Suppl 1):S73–S85. doi:10.1097/PCC.0000000000000435
143. Valentine SL, Sapru A, Higgerson RA, Spinella PC, Flori HR, Graham DA, Brett M, Convery M, Christie LM, Karamessinis L, Randolph AG, Pediatric Acute Lung I Sepsis Investigator's N, Acute Respiratory Distress Syndrome Clinical Research N (2012) Fluid balance in critically ill children with acute lung injury. Crit Care Med 40(10):2883–2889. doi:10.1097/CCM.0b013e31825bc54d
144. Vet NJ, de Wildt SN, Verlaat CW, Knibbe CA, Mooij MG, van Woensel JB, van Rosmalen J, Tibboel D, de Hoog M (2016) A randomized controlled trial of daily sedation interruption in critically ill children. Intensive Care Med 42(2):233–244. doi:10.1007/s00134-015-4136-z
145. Volpicelli G, Elbarbary M, Blaivas M, Lichtenstein DA, Mathis G, Kirkpatrick AW, Melniker L, Gargani L, Noble VE, Via G, Dean A, Tsung JW, Soldati G, Copetti R, Bouhemad B, Reissig A, Agricola E, Rouby JJ, Arbelot C, Liteplo A, Sargsyan A, Silva F, Hoppmann R, Breitkreutz R, Seibel A, Neri L, Storti E, Petrovic T (2012) International evidence-based recommendations for point-of-care lung ultrasound. Intensive Care Med 38(4):577–591. doi:10.1007/s00134-012-2513-4
146. Ware LB, Matthay MA (2000) The acute respiratory distress syndrome. N Engl J Med 342(18):1334–1349. doi:10.1056/NEJM200005043421806
147. Weiss I, Ushay HM, DeBruin W, O'Loughlin J, Rosner I, Notterman D (1996) Respiratory and cardiac function in children after acute hypoxemic respiratory failure. Crit Care Med 24(1):148–154
148. Willson DF, Thomas NJ, Markovitz BP, Bauman LA, DiCarlo JV, Pon S, Jacobs BR, Jefferson LS, Conaway MR, Egan EA, Pediatric Acute Lung I, Sepsis I (2005) Effect of exogenous surfactant (calfactant) in pediatric acute lung injury: a randomized controlled trial. JAMA 293(4):470–476. doi:10.1001/jama.293.4.470

149. Willson DF, Thomas NJ, Tamburro R, Truemper E, Truwit J, Conaway M, Traul C, Egan EE, Pediatric Acute L, Sepsis Investigators N (2013) Pediatric calfactant in acute respiratory distress syndrome trial. Pediatr Crit Care Med 14(7):657–665. doi:10.1097/PCC.0b013e3182917b68
150. Wood JH, Partrick DA, Johnston RB Jr (2010) The inflammatory response to injury in children. Curr Opin Pediatr 22(3):315–320. doi:10.1097/MOP.0b013e328338da48
151. Wynn J, Cornell TT, Wong HR, Shanley TP, Wheeler DS (2010) The host response to sepsis and developmental impact. Pediatrics 125 (5):1031–1041. doi:peds.2009-3301 [pii] 162 1542/peds.2009-3301
152. Yehya N, Thomas NJ, Meyer NJ, Christie JD, Berg RA, Margulies SS (2016) Circulating markers of endothelial and alveolar epithelial dysfunction are associated with mortality in pediatric acute respiratory distress syndrome. Intensive Care Med 42(7):1137–1145. doi:10.1007/s00134-016-4352-1
153. Ygberg S, Nilsson A (2012) The developing immune system - from foetus to toddler. Acta Paediatr 101(2):120–127. doi:10.1111/j.1651-2227.2011.02494.x
154. Yilmaz S, Daglioglu K, Yildizdas D, Bayram I, Gumurdulu D, Polat S (2013) The effectiveness of heliox in acute respiratory distress syndrome. Annals Thoracic Med 8(1):46–52. doi:10.4103/1817-1737.105719
155. Young D, Lamb SE, Shah S, Mac Kenzie I, Tunnicliffe W, Lall R, Rowan K, Cuthbertson BH, Group OS (2013) High-frequency oscillation for acute respiratory distress syndrome. N Engl J Med 368(9):806–813. doi:10.1056/NEJMoa1215716
156. Yu WL, Lu ZJ, Wang Y, Shi LP, Kuang FW, Qian SY, Zeng QY, Xie MH, Zhang GY, Zhuang DY, Fan XM, Sun B, Collaborative Study Group of Pediatric Respiratory F (2009) The epidemiology of acute respiratory distress syndrome in pediatric intensive care units in China. Intensive Care Med 35(1):136–143. doi:10.1007/s00134-008-1254-x
157. Zhao J, Yang X, Auh SL, Kim KD, Tang H, Fu YX (2009) Do adaptive immune cells suppress or activate innate immunity? Trends Immunol 30(1):8–12. doi:10.1016/j.it.2008.10.003
158. Zhu Yan-feng, Xu Feng, Lu Xiu-lan, Wang Ying, Chen Jian-li, Chao Jian-xin, Zhou Xiao-wen, Zhang Jian-hui, Huang Yan-zhi, Yu Wen-liang, Xie Min-hui, Yan Chao-ying, Lu Zhu-jin, Sun Bo (2012) Chinese Collaborative Study Group for Pediatric Hypoxemic Respiratory Failure. Chinese Medical Journal 125(13):2265-2271.
159. Zimmerman JJ, Akhtar SR, Caldwell E, Rubenfeld GD (2009) Incidence and outcomes of pediatric acute lung injury. Pediatrics 124(1):87–95. doi:10.1542/peds.2007-2462

Pulmonary Infections in Acute Respiratory Distress Syndrome

20

Gianluigi Li Bassi, Tarek Sanussi, Paolo Pelosi, and Otavio Tavares Ranzani

20.1 Introduction

Hospital-acquired pulmonary infections, i.e., ventilator-associated tracheobronchitis (VAT) and ventilator-associated pneumonia (VAP), often complicate the course of acute respiratory distress syndrome (ARDS). The most common risk factors for VAP are greatly accentuated in ARDS, due to overwhelming injury of the lungs, impaired host defenses, and invasive interventions, necessary to stabilize and treat these patients. The risk factors for developing VAP during ARDS have been extensively investigated throughout the years. In particular, it has long been known that

G.L. Bassi, MD, PhD (✉)
Department of Pulmonary and Critical Care Medicine, Thorax Institute, Hospital Clínic, Calle Villarroel 170, Esc 6/8 Planta 2, 08036 Barcelona, Spain

Institut d'Investigacions Biomèdiques August Pi i Sunyer (IDIBAPS), Barcelona, Spain

Centro de Investigación Biomedica En Red- Enfermedades Respiratorias (CIBERES), Barcelona, Spain
e-mail: glibassi@clinic.cat

T. Sanussi, MD
Department of Pulmonary and Critical Care Medicine, Thorax Institute, Hospital Clínic, Calle Villarroel 170, Esc 6/8 Planta 2, 08036 Barcelona, Spain

Department of Surgical Sciences and Integrated Diagnostics; IRCCS AOU San Martino- IST, University of Genoa, Genoa, Italy

P. Pelosi, MD
Department of Surgical Sciences and Integrated Diagnostics; IRCCS AOU San Martino- IST, University of Genoa, Genoa, Italy

O.T. Ranzani, MD, MSc
Department of Pulmonary and Critical Care Medicine, Thorax Institute, Hospital Clínic, Calle Villarroel 170, Esc 6/8 Planta 2, 08036 Barcelona, Spain

Centro de Investigación Biomedica En Red- Enfermedades Respiratorias (CIBERES), Barcelona, Spain

D. Chiumello (ed.), *Acute Respiratory Distress Syndrome (ARDS)*,
DOI 10.1007/978-3-319-41852-0_20

the widespread injury of the lungs exponentially increases risks of iatrogenic pulmonary infections. In the early 1980s, Johanson WG first corroborated risk of VAP in a model of ARDS in baboons on invasive mechanical ventilation (MV) for several days [1, 2]. Briefly, sequential boluses of oleic acid were administered into the right atrium of the animals, until severe respiratory failure ensued. Colonization of the oropharynx by pathogenic enteric bacteria rapidly developed, within 24–48 h of MV, followed by pulmonary aspiration. Eventually, oropharyngeal pathogens overcame host's respiratory defenses and led to severe pneumonia, namely, ventilator-associated pneumonia.

In this chapter, we will provide a comprehensive appraisal on the epidemiology, pathophysiology, diagnosis, and prognosis of VAP in ARDS patients. In particular, we will address potential diagnostic challenges, preventive strategies, and treatments, and we will look at potential areas of investigation that should be further explored in future studies.

20.2 Incidence

Currently, incidence of VAP has decreased to approximately 10–15% or to an incidence density of 5–10 cases per 1000 ventilator days. Notably, in the last decade, the hospital data from the National Healthcare Safety Network have reported a steady decline in VAP [3, 4], likely due to better implementation of preventive bundles. Yet, these encouraging numbers should be interpreted with caution. Indeed, the true incidence of VAP is difficult to ascertain, particularly due to the well-known diagnostic challenges. Thus, as described in the next paragraphs, VAP incidence may be either overestimated when only diagnostic clinical signs are used, or underestimated when invasive diagnostic methods are used to sample distal pulmonary regions. Also, it is worthy to mention that epidemiology data from other reliable sources in the United States, i.e., the Medicare Patient Safety Monitoring System – which attains medical records from a random sample of hospitalized patients – have reported a steady incidence of VAP of approximately 10%, without any decrease throughout the years [5].

As for the incidence of VAP in patients with ARDS, several studies have consistently reported higher rates, ranging from 15 to 60% (Table 20.1). In particular, Chastre and collaborators [6] used cultures of bronchoalveolar lavage (BAL) fluids to diagnose VAP and found an incidence of 28% in patients without ARDS. Conversely, in patients with ARDS, VAP incidence increased up to 55%. Other investigators reported much lower VAP rates, sustaining disagreement in this field. Indeed, in a study by Sutherland et al., VAP incidence rate was 15%, likely, due to the use of broad-spectrum antibiotics, prior to BAL sampling. In conclusion, as reported in Table 20.1, it seems that ARDS patients, in comparison with other critically ill mechanically ventilated patients, are at higher risk for developing VAP.

Table 20.1 Epidemiology of ventilator-associated pneumonia in patients with acute respiratory distress syndrome

First author	Year	Incidence of VAP in ARDS patients	Incidence of VAP in no ARDS patients	Diagnostic methods	Journal
Markowicz	2000	49 out of 134 (36%)	173 out of 744 (23%)	PSB, BAL, or mini-BAL	*Am J Respir Crit Care Med Vol 161. pp. 1942–1948, 2000*
Meduri	1998	40 out of 94 (43%)	NA	Bilateral BAL	*Am J Respir Crit Care Med Vol 158. pp. 870–875, 1998*
Chastre	1998	31 out of 56 (55%)	53 out of 187 (28%)	PSB and BAL (before any change in antibiotic treatment)	*Am J Respir Crit Care Med Vol 157. pp. 1165–1172, 1998*
Delclaux	1997	24 out of 30 (60%)	NA	Mini-BAL	*Am J Respir Crit Care Med Vol. 156. pp. 1092–1098, 1997*
Sutherland	1995	16 out of 105 (15%)	NA	PSB, BAL	*Am J Respir Crit Care Med. 1995 Aug;152* [2]*:550–6.*

ARDS acute respiratory distress syndrome, *NA* not available, *VAP* ventilator-associated pneumonia

20.3 Morbidity and Mortality

ARDS is one of the most severe pulmonary diseases, leading to significant patient morbidity and healthcare burden [7]. Thus, it is expected that any iatrogenic complication that ensues during the course of ARDS may delay weaning from the MV, prolong the intensive care unit (ICU) stay, require additional treatments, and exponentially increase costs. In a recent international, multicenter, prospective cohort study of 2377 patients with ARDS, the median length of MV was 8 days (interquartile range (IQR), 4–16). Early studies have consistently reported a significant increase in duration of MV, when VAP occurred in ARDS patients. Chastre et al. found that in ARDS patients who developed VAP, the length of MV increased from 17 ± 19 to 34 ± 32 days, whereas Markowicz et al. found that in ARDS patients, the first episode of VAP did not occur until a mean length of MV of 11.7 ± 11.9 days. Interestingly, the mean duration of MV, for ARDS patients who did not develop VAP, was highly similar: 11.3 ± 9.1 days. Conversely, when they did develop VAP, the length of stay increased up to 33 ± 21 days.

It is fascinating that in early studies [6, 8], investigators failed to demonstrate any impact of VAP on mortality. Considering the clinical severity of ARDS, it is somewhat difficult to justify the lack of effect on mortality, when VAP complicates the course of the disease. Yet, several factors may explain these counterintuitive findings. First, in ARDS patients, the occurrence of VAP can be biased by the presence of competing events, specifically death or ICU discharge, which preclude VAP occurrence or dramatically changing its risk [9]. For instance, a highly severe ARDS patient, at high risk of VAP, could decease during the time on MV, but before the onset of VAP. Unfortunately, traditional methods of time-to-event analysis considered patients who died while on MV as non-informative censoring, resulting in biased estimates. Yet, in more recent analyses [10–12], patients have been considered under risk either up to the occurrence of VAP or until one of the other competing events occurred or until follow-up was completed. Thus, latest studies [10], in patients without ARDS, reported an attributable mortality of 10%. Also, it seems that surgical patients and with midrange severity of illness present the highest associated risk of mortality. To the best of our knowledge, no studies have been specifically assessed the attributable mortality of VAP in ARDS patients. Nevertheless, considering the severity of this condition, it is rationale to assume that VAP might unhinge the delicate clinical balance of these patients, and lead to worse outcome.

20.4 Pathogenesis

ARDS patients on MV often become colonized by exogenous pathogens acquired from healthcare personnel or, more commonly, by endogenous pathogens that colonize the gastrointestinal tract, oropharynx, tracheal tube, and proximal trachea. Several defense mechanisms prevent overwhelming colonization, i.e., cough, mucus clearance, and cellular and humoral immune responses. Yet, in ARDS patients, these defenses are impaired, because of the severe lung injury, comorbidities, and tracheal intubation. In the next paragraphs, several risk factors for the development of VAP will be described, with a specific focus on the specific risks and conditions that may occur in ARDS patients.

20.4.1 The Endotracheal Tube and Pulmonary Aspiration

The primary mechanism in the pathogenesis of VAP is through pulmonary aspiration of colonized oropharyngeal secretions across the high-volume low-pressure (HVLP) endotracheal tube (ETT) cuff. The HVLP cuff was designed in the late 1970s to closely monitor the pressure exerted against the trachea [13]. Yet, when HVLP cuffs are inflated within the trachea, folds are formed, because the cuff outer diameter is larger than the tracheal internal diameter [14]. In vitro studies have demonstrated that cuff outer diameter, length, and positive end-expiratory pressure (PEEP) are the main determinants of cuff sealing efficacy. Indeed, the larger the cuff the more folds form on its surface, promoting leakage across the folds (Fig. 20.1).

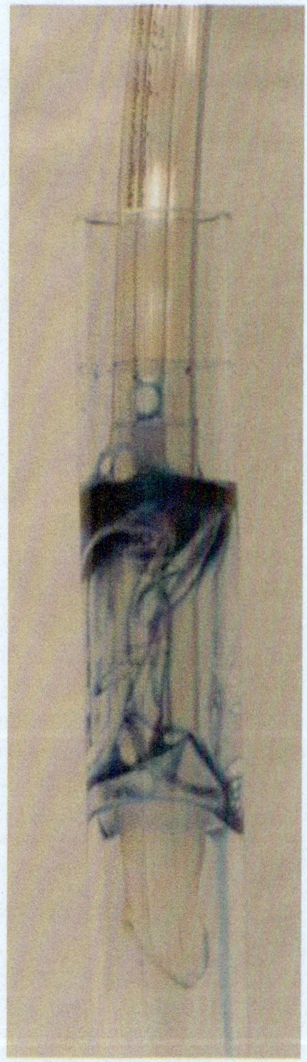

Fig. 20.1 High-volume low-pressure cuff inflated within an artificial translucent tracheal model. The tracheal model internal diameter is 20 mm, whereas the cuff outer diameter is 28 mm. Upon inflation, folds are formed on the cuff surface. Methylene blue is poured above the cuff to highlight leakage of fluid across the channels formed by the folds

Pathogens may also grow on the internal surface of the ETT, forming a complex structure called *biofilm* [15]. ETT biofilm is composed by sessile bacteria within a self-produced exopolysaccharide matrix and respiratory secretions [16–18]. It is still not fully elucidated the role of ETT biofilm in the pathogenesis of VAP. Shah and collaborators [19] demonstrated a close association between intraluminal narrowing of the ETT by biofilm/secretions and length of stay on MV. Given that ARDS patients present longer periods of MV, it is reasonable to assume that a large amount of biofilm builds up and constitutes a persistent source of infection for recurrent episodes of VAP.

20.4.2 Oropharyngeal Colonization

Overall, in critically ill patients on MV, the oral flora shifts early to a predominance of aerobic Gram-negative pathogens [20], *Pseudomonas aeruginosa*, and methicillin-resistant *Staphylococcus aureus* (MRSA). Comorbidities and inherent patient's characteristics such as alcohol abuse [21–23], diabetes [24, 25], and chronic obstructive pulmonary disease [26] increase risks of colonization by Gram-negative pathogens. ARDS patients present additional risk factors, because they require prolonged periods of MV and large amounts of antibiotics. The ETT is a foreign body, and after several days within the mouth, the salivary flow [27] and oral pH progressively decrease. This leads to an abnormal adherence of pathogens to the buccal epithelial cells [28]. These risks are amplified in patients with poor oral health upon intubation [29–31]. As mentioned above, oropharyngeal pathogens are ultimately aspirated into the airways and may ultimately cause VAP [32].

20.4.2.1 Gastrointestinal Tract

In the 1990s, several pivotal studies demonstrated that the stomach of ICU patients is colonized by pathogens, due to alkalinization of gastric contents by enteral nutrition and drugs for stress ulcer prophylaxis [33]. Commonly, ARDS patients are on enteral feeding and receive these prophylactic drugs that alter the gastric pH. Gastric pathogens may translocate into the oropharynx, due to the gastroesophageal reflux. In particular, prone position could increase risks for oropharyngeal colonization by gastric pathogens. To date, no studies have assessed gastroesophageal reflux in the prone position, but considering that in previous studies [34, 35], vomiting was a frequent complication, gastroesophageal reflux may be common in such position, particularly during enteral feeding.

20.4.3 Other Risk Factors

In ARDS patients, several other risk factors may play a role in the pathogenesis of VAP. ARDS patients require a high level of care throughout the day; as a result, the risks for cross transmission of pathogens from other patients are exponentially increased. This may be relevant in ICUs where patient-to-nurse ratios are higher than 1, where healthcare personnel are not adequately trained on infection control and preventive strategies, and where strict sterilization protocols and handwashing with alcohol-based solutions are not efficiently implemented.

Mucociliary clearance is one of the most important innate airway defense mechanisms to clear pathogens. In young, healthy nonsmokers, the mucociliary velocity ranges between 10 and 15 mm/min. Studies on intubated critically ill patients have confirmed a tenfold decrease in mucociliary clearance rate [36] and higher risks of VAP in patients with the slowest rates. In ARDS patients, several factors may affect mucus clearance rate. First, endotracheal intubation and the inflation of the cuff have shown a drastic decrease in mucus clearance rate within hours [37]. Second,

ARDS patients often require high concentration of oxygen, which is known to reduce mucus clearance rate in a dose-dependent fashion [38]. Finally, these patients often present markedly increased respiratory drive that impairs efficiency of commonly used humidifiers. Of note, even brief period of suboptimal humidification may depress cilia function [39].

Finally, investigators have found a temporary immunoparalysis early in the course of the critical illness and admission to the ICU [40], which is the results of various and heterogeneous inciting events like ARDS [41], severe trauma [42], and sepsis [43]. The immunoparalysis is aimed at counterbalancing the exaggerated inflammatory response with an anti-inflammatory milieu. Yet, during this period of immunodepression, the organism is unable to adequately respond to a second hit, increasing potential risks of acquiring iatrogenic infections, such as VAP.

20.4.4 Etiologic Agents

ARDS patients are at higher risk for developing VAP caused by *S. aureus*; non-glucose-fermenting Gram-negative bacilli, i.e., *P. aeruginosa*, *Acinetobacter baumannii*, and *Enterobacteriaceae*. Of note, in ARDS patients, antibiotics are profusely administered very early. As a result, antimicrobial causes a selective pressure over more susceptible bacteria, allowing potentially resistant bacteria to survive. In particular, Chastre et al. [6] compared VAP in patients with and without ARDS and found that methicillin-resistant *S. aureus* was isolated in 44% and 17% of the patients with or without ARDS, whereas Markowicz et al. [8] found that non-fermenting Gram-negative bacilli were more frequent in ARDS patients (47% vs. 33% in non-ARDS patients). Also, methicillin-susceptible *S. aureus* was less common in ARDS patients (3% vs. 15% in non-ARDS patients). In ARDS patients, VAP is often caused by multiple pathogens [44, 45]. Combes and colleagues [46] studied 124 ICU patients, of whom 65 (52%) had monomicrobial VAP and 59 (48%) had polymicrobial VAP. In most patients (34%), two different bacteria were isolated; however, up to four different bacteria coexisted in seven patients (6%). Interestingly, no differences were detected in mortality rates at 30 days between patients with polymicrobial or monomicrobial infection. Also, multiple episodes of VAP may occur in approximately 50% of the patients, which may be related to the prolonged stay in the ICU or substantial presence of ETT biofilm.

20.5 Prevention

VAP is an iatrogenic infection that, in ARDS patients, impairs morbidity and constitutes an important burden for the healthcare system. Therefore, preventive strategies should be applied to avoid the disease. To date, several preventive measures are available for all mechanically ventilated patients and are often grouped as a bundle

Table 20.2 Preventive bundle

Implementation of educational programs for caregivers and frequent performance feedbacks and compliance assessment Strict alcohol-based hand hygiene
Daily sedation vacation and implementation of weaning protocols
No ventilatory circuit tube changes unless the circuit is soiled or damaged
Use of tracheal tube with cuff made of novel materials
Use of silver-coated tracheal tube
Application of low-level PEEP during tracheal intubation
Aspiration of subglottic secretions
Internal cuff pressure maintained within the recommended range and carefully controlled during transport of patients outside ICU
Oral care with chlorhexidine
Avoid stress ulcer prophylaxis in very low-risk patients for gastrointestinal bleed, and consider the use of sucralfate when indicated
Semirecumbent patient positioning
SDD for patients requiring >48 h of mechanical ventilation

ICU intensive care unit, *PEEP* positive end-expiratory pressure, *SDD* selective digestive decontamination

(Table 20.2). Nevertheless, in the next paragraphs, the most important strategies aimed at preventing VAP in ARDS patients will be highlighted.

20.5.1 Patient Transport and Sedation

ARDS patients often require intrahospital transport out of the ICU for surgical procedures, imaging, and invasive interventions. However, transport out of the ICU has been associated with potential complications, primarily VAP [47]. Kollef et al. [48] studied 273 patients, who required at least one transport outside the ICU vs. 248 who did not. Of note, 66 (24.2%) of the transported patients developed VAP, compared with 11 (4.4%) of the patients who were not trasported outside (relative risk = 5.5; 95% confidence interval [CI] = 2.9–10.1; $p < 0.001$). Importantly, prior to the transport, clinicians and nursing staff should carefully check the internal pressure of the ETT cuff, particularly when the patient is expected to be maintained supine during diagnostic or therapeutic procedures; ventilator circuits should be carefully manipulated in order to prevent aspiration of colonized fluids from within the circuit. Also, sedation should be increased only if necessary to improve patient safety or for a specific test that requires immobility. Yet, sedation should be rapidly interrupted or lightened as soon as possible. Along the same line, even in patients with ARDS, daily interruption or lightening of sedation [49–51] and early mobilization [52] should be attempted to avoid severe impairment of respiratory defenses and prolonged intubation.

20.5.2 Extracorporeal Membrane Oxygenation and Tracheal Extubation

Tracheal intubation is the main risk factor for VAP and therefore should be avoided whenever possible or used for the shortest time possible. Very recently, extracorporeal membrane oxygenation (ECMO) has been used in awake ARDS patients who were extubated and allowed to breathe spontaneously [53]. In an interesting preliminary study, Hoeper MM et al. [54] studied six ARDS immunocompromised patients with only lung failure, who underwent an "awake ECMO" strategy, through extubation shortly after initiation of ECMO. Overall, 66% of the patients survived. Only one patient developed VAP, but after being re-intubated for complications. These fascinating results call for future larger studies to avoid tracheal intubation, which is the main culprit of the disease.

Novel Endotracheal Tubes In the latest years, several improvements in the design of ETT have been achieved, specifically to address HVLP cuff limitations. We recently demonstrated [14] that the main determinants in the design of ETT cuff for sealing effectiveness are the cuff material, outer diameter, length, and the internal cuff pressure. In particular, narrower cuffs form less folds, upon inflation within the trachea. Cuffs made of new materials such as polyurethane [55] have been developed and tested in laboratory and clinical trials. A few studies in medical ICU patients [56, 57] or cardiac surgical patients [58, 59] have shown that polyurethane cuffs reduce risks of developing VAP. Yet, in a recent multicenter study [60], cuffs composed of cylindrical polyvinyl chloride, cylindrical polyurethane, conical polyvinyl chloride, or conical polyurethane were compared for the prevention of tracheal colonization, and no differences were found. Importantly, the majority of aforementioned studies used novel ETTs in all patients, irrespective of their inherent risks of developing VAP. Conversely, we think that their use should only be limited to the patients at very high risk. In particular, to date, no studies have tested novel ETTs in ARDS patients, who present the highest risk factors for VAP.

In ARDS patients who are often ventilated with high level of positive end-expiratory pressure (PEEP), it could be assumed that aspiration of oropharyngeal secretions across the cuff is largely counterbalanced by PEEP. Lucangelo et al. [61] investigated the effects of 5–8 cmH_2O of PEEP in normoxemic ventilated patients. They showed a significant reduction in the rate of VAP (PEEP group 9.4%, control patients 25.4%, relative risk, 0.37; 95% CI = 0.15–0.84; $p = 0.017$). Thus, in the absence of major contraindication, a low level of PEEP should always be maintained in ARDS patients, even during the weaning period to avoid pulmonary aspiration. It is also very important to maintain the internal ETT cuff pressure between 25 and 30 cmH_2O to prevent aspiration of contaminated secretions into the lower airways or tracheal injury. Ideally, in ARDS patients at high risk of VAP, it would be advisable to use continuous control of internal cuff pressure, as demonstrated in previous studies [62–64], to reduce risks of unforeseen cuff deflation and pulmonary aspiration.

Some ETTs allow aspiration of colonized subglottic secretions above the cuff and potentially prevent macro-leakage into the trachea. A recent meta-analysis [65], pooling data from 17 randomized clinical trials of a total of 3369 patients, has shown that subglottic secretion drainage reduced the overall risk ratio (RR) for VAP by half (risk ratio, 0.58; 95% CI, 0.51–0.67; I2 = 0%). Most of the studies were conducted in post-cardiac surgery patients; thus, although this strategy seems highly effective, further evidence on ARDS patients is needed before wider use.

Finally, the use of ETT coated with antimicrobial agents such as silver [66] could be another promising strategy to prevent biofilm formation and repetitive episodes of VAP. Unfortunately, to date, only one large randomized clinical trial, the North American Silver-Coated Endotracheal Tube (NASCENT) randomized trial [67], evaluated benefits of a silver-coated vs. a conventional tube. They included patients with lower degrees of severity, and they found a lower incidence of microbiologically confirmed VAP (37/766 (4.8%) vs. 56/743 (7.5%); $p = 0.03$), for a relative risk reduction of 35.9%. Thus, the benefits of coated ETTs in ARDS patients at high risk of VAP should also be investigated in future studies.

Body Position Nowadays, most of the ICU patients are kept in the semirecumbent position, because intubated patients are at higher risk for gastropulmonary aspiration when placed in the supine position (0 degree), as compared with a semirecumbent position (45 degrees) [33, 68, 69]. One randomized trial [70] demonstrated a reduction in the incidence of VAP in patients positioned in the semirecumbent position, compared with patients completely supine. Interestingly, as clearly demonstrated by Guerin et al. [71] prone position is highly beneficial in ARDS patients. Theoretically, the prone position could also have VAP preventive effects, because patients, as soon as they are placed to the prone position, clear from the ETT and the mouth all secretions that are retained. A study by Ayzac [72] and collaborators retrospectively evaluated patients included in their early prone-supine study the impact on VAP. Unfortunately, they found that the cumulative probability of VAP was higher in the prone than in the supine position group (46.5% at 90 days in the prone position group and 33.5% in the supine position group ($p = 0.11$)).

20.6 Diagnosis

In mechanically ventilated patients, VAP is suspected when a new radiographic infiltrate develops with several unspecific clinical signs [73, 74] of pulmonary infection, such as fever or hypothermia, purulent secretions, and leukocytosis or leukopenia. Unfortunately, in ARDS patients, chest radiographs are difficult to interpret (Fig. 20.2), because bilateral infiltrates are already present, prior to the development of VAP. Also, it is difficult to differentiate among cardiogenic and non-cardiogenic pulmonary edema, pulmonary contusion, atelectasis, and pneumonia. A few studies appraised VAP diagnostic accuracy of portable chest radiographs in the ICU [75–79]. Wunderink et al. [78] demonstrated that in deceased patients with autopsy-proven VAP, no single radiographic sign had a diagnostic accuracy greater than 68%. In ARDS patients, not even the presence of air bronchograms or alveolar opacities improved VAP diagnostic accuracy.

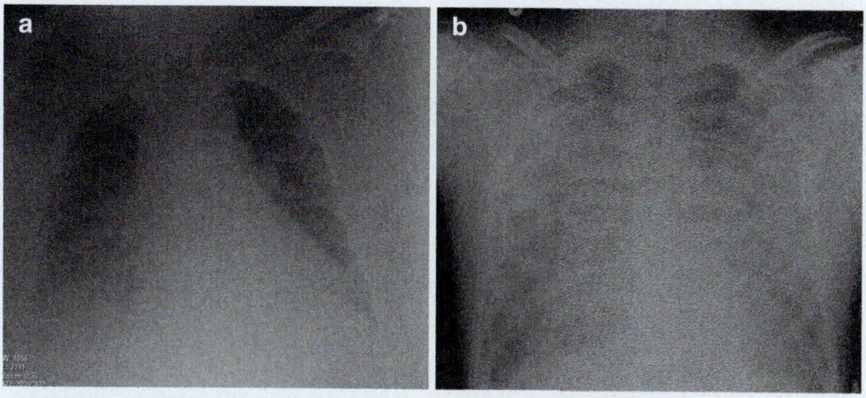

Correlation of radiologic signs with autopsy-proven pneumonia

Radiologic Sign	Sensitivity, %	Specificity, %	Positive, %	Negative
Air bronchogram	83.3	57.8	51.3	86
- Single	16.6	95.5	66.7	68
- Multiple	66.7	62.2	69.5	77
Silhouette	79.2	33.3	38.8	75
Alveolar infiltrate	87.5	25.6	39.6	78
- Unilateral	20.5	79.0	35.7	64
- Bilateral	66.7	46.5	41.0	86
Fissure Abutment	8.3	95.6	50.0	66
Atelectasis*	29.2	62.8	30.4	61

Fig. 20.2 The challenges in the diagnosis of ventilator-associated pneumonia through analyses of portable chest radiographs. A: patient who developed clinical signs of ventilator-associated pneumonia after 3 days of mechanical ventilation, and, at the chest radiograph, a new progressive pulmonary infiltrate was evident at the lower right lobe. B: patient with acute respiratory distress syndrome, who developed clinical signs of ventilator-associated pneumonia after 7 days of mechanical ventilation. Of note, due to the bilateral infiltrates, it is challenging to identify any new pulmonary infiltrate. At the bottom of the figure is reported specificity and sensitivity of radiologic signs corroborated by gross findings upon autopsy (From Wunderink et al. [78])

The Clinical Pulmonary Infection Score (CPIS) was developed to improve diagnostic accuracy [80]. CPIS comprises clinical variables, such as temperature, blood leukocyte count, volume and purulence of tracheal secretions, oxygenation, pulmonary radiographic findings, and semiquantitative culture of tracheal aspirate. In pivotal studies [80, 81], a CPIS value ≥ 6 was an accurate threshold to identify patients with VAP. Yet, in ARDS patients, the clinical value of CPIS remains to be validated.

In the latest guidelines for the management of patients with VAP [82], it is strongly recommended to obtain cultures of respiratory secretions from all patients with clinical suspicion of VAP. Nevertheless, considering that available evidence

[83–87] demonstrated that invasive quantitative sampling did not impact any clinical outcome, including mean duration of MV, ICU length of stay, or mortality [88], the specimens can be obtained non-invasively, and cultures can be performed semi-quantitatively. Many sampling procedures of respiratory secretions, such as endotracheal aspirates, BAL, and protected specimen brush (PSB), are available. Previous studies in patients with ARDS have used BAL, mini-BAL, and PSB to diagnose VAP. In addition, there are several microbiological techniques including Gram staining and intracellular organism count from specimens obtained via BAL. Each diagnostic technique has advantages, as well as limitations and provides different diagnostic specificity/sensitivity. Overall, qualitative cultures of endotracheal aspirates have, potentially, a high percentage of false-positive results, due to frequent bacterial colonization of the proximal airways. Conversely, quantitative cultures of distal samples have, theoretically, an improved specificity but worse sensitivity.

In an important study by Meduri and collaborators [89], the diagnostic accuracy of bilateral BAL sampling was assessed in ARDS patients with clinical suspicion of VAP. Among 55 bronchoscopies that yielded positive culture results, 33 (60%) had significant growth in only one lung. Bilateral growth in BAL samples was more likely to be polymicrobial, and with a bacterial growth $>10^5$ cfu/ml. The authors also corroborated changes in BAL accuracy, when antibiotics were administered before BAL sampling.

In conclusion, in ARDS patients with clinical suspicion of VAP, sampling of the lower respiratory tract is advisable to accurately diagnose VAP and appropriately use the most effective antibiotics, after microbiology results become available. Microbiological diagnosis of VAP is pivotal not only for determining whether a patient has VAP, but also for narrowing or discontinuing antimicrobial therapy as soon as possible. Considering that VAP in ARDS patients is multifocal, predominantly in lower lobes [90] and it is bilateral in 40% of the cases, non-bronchoscopic techniques are sufficiently reliable to obtain respiratory secretions. This also in light of the potential complications that may occur in ARDS patients during bronchoscopy.

20.7 Treatment

A major problem in the management of patients with suspicion of VAP is when to initiate antibiotics and the prospective susceptibility of the causative pathogens. The indiscriminate and empiric administration of antibiotics, following clinical suspicion, contributes to the emergence of multidrug-resistant (MDR) pathogens and exposes the patient to antibiotic-related adverse effects and higher costs [91]. On the other hand, it is mandatory to initiate prompt treatment of VAP to improve survival [92–95]. However, the choice of the initial antibiotic treatment is challenging, particularly in ARDS patients undergoing long-term antibiotic treatment before VAP

Table 20.3

Risk factors for ventilator-associated pneumonia caused by multi-drug resistant pathogens
Prior intravenous antibiotic use within 90 days
Septic shock upon diagnosis of VAP
ARDS preceding VAP
Five or more days of hospitalization prior to the occurrence of VAP
Acute renal replacement therapy prior to VAP onset
Risk factors for methicillin-resistant Staphylococcus aureus
Prior intravenous antibiotic use within 90 days
Risk factors for multi-drug resistant Pseudomonas aeruginosa
Prior intravenous antibiotic use within 90 days

ARDS acute respiratory distress syndrome, *VAP* ventilator-associated pneumonia

development [96]. Also, it is important to consider patient's inherent risk factors for MDR pathogens (Table 20.3) [82]. Finally, physicians should consider resistance patterns, which vary extremely among countries, regions, hospitals, and ICUs. Rello et al. [97] analyzed variations in VAP etiology among three Spanish ICUs and compared them with data collected in Paris. The authors concluded that VAP pathogens largely changed among the four clinical centers, with marked differences among the microorganisms isolated from the Spanish and French centers. Therefore, clinicians must be aware of the most common microorganisms in their own unit and antimicrobial susceptibility to avoid the administration of inadequate empiric antimicrobial therapy.

The latest guidelines emphasized the risks associated with ARDS for developing late-onset VAP, caused by MRSA and non-glucose-fermenting Gram-negative bacilli [6, 8]. Theoretically, ARDS patients are at very low risk of developing VAP caused by multi-susceptible pathogens, because they require antibiotic therapy for many days before the suspicion of VAP.

Thus, in summary, in ARDS patients, *P. aeruginosa* should always be covered, preferably with two antibiotics of different classes, particularly in units where >10% of Gram-negative isolates are resistant to an agent being considered for monotherapy, and in ICUs where local antimicrobial susceptibility rates are not available [98]. Likewise, ARDS patients are at high risk of developing MRSA VAP; thus, this pathogen should also be covered either with vancomycin or linezolid. A detailed description of antibiotic recommendations is reported in Table 20.4. Of note, after the results of antimicrobial susceptibility test become available, the therapy should always be readjusted, narrowed, or fully changed/withdrawn. Also, for highly resistant *Acinetobacter* spp. and carbapenem-resistant pathogens, intravenous polymyxins (colistin or polymyxin B) and inhaled colistin are highly recommended.

Table 20.4 Suggested empiric treatment options for clinically suspected ventilator-associated pneumonia in ARDS patients

Antibiotics for Gram-negative bacteria with anti-pseudomonal activity: β-lactam-based agents	Antibiotics for Gramnegative bacteria with anti-pseudomonal activity: non-β-lactam-based agents	Antibiotics for Gram-positive bacteria with MRSA activity
Anti-pseudomonal penicillins[1]	*Fluoroquinolones*	*Glycopeptides*[4]
Anti-pseudomonal penicillins[1] Piperacillin-tazobactam 4.5 g IV q6h[1]	Ciprofloxacin 400 mg IV q8h Levofloxacin 750 mg IV q24h	Vancomycin 15 mg/kg IV q8–12 h (consider a loading dose of 25–30 mg/kg × 1 for severe illness)
Or	*Or*	*Or*
Cephalosporins[1]	*Aminoglycosides*[4, 5]	*Oxazolidinones*
Cefepime 2 g IV q8h Ceftazidime 2 g IV q8h	Amikacin 15–20 mg/kg IV q24h Gentamicin 5–7 mg/kg IV q24h Tobramycin 5–7 mg/kg IV q24h	Linezolid 600 mg IV q12h
Or	*Or*	
Carbapenems[1]	*Polymyxind*[4, 6]	
Imipenem 500 mg IV q6h[2] Meropenem 1 g IV q8h	Colistin 5 mg/kg IV × 1 (loading dose) followed by 2.5 mg × (1.5 × CrCl + 30) IV q12h (maintenance dose) Polymyxin B 2.5–3.0 mg/kg/d divided into two daily IV doses	
Or		
Monobactams[3]		
Aztreonam 2 g IV q8h		

In patients with ARDS, based on the latest guidelines [82], double therapy against *P. aeruginosa* and coverage against MRSA are recommended. The initial doses may need further adjustment for patients with hepatic or renal dysfunction

CrCl creatinine clearance, *IV* intravenous, *MRSA* methicillin-resistant *Staphylococcus aureus*

[1]Extended infusions may be appropriate

[2]The dose may need to be lowered in patients weighing <70 kg to prevent seizures

[3]In the absence of other options, it is acceptable to use aztreonam as an adjunctive agent with another β-lactam-based agent because it has different targets within the bacterial cell wall

[4]Drug levels and adjustment of doses and/or intervals required

[5]On meta-analysis, aminoglycoside regimens were associated with lower clinical response rates with no differences in mortality

[6]Polymyxins should be reserved for settings where there is a high prevalence of multidrug resistance and local expertise in using this medication. Dosing is based on colistin base activity (CBA); for example, one million IU of colistin is equivalent to about 30 mg of CBA, which corresponds to about 80 mg of the prodrug colistimethate. Polymyxin B (1 mg = 10,000 units)

Adapted from [82]

Conclusions

In conclusion, VAP is a common complication in ARDS patients. In these patients, VAP developed later, and it is commonly caused by multidrug-resistant pathogens. Although VAP may not increase mortality in these patients, it prolongs the length of stay in the ICU, and constitutes an important burden for the healthcare systems. Significant efforts should be undertaken to avoid such iatrogenic complications, and future research should corroborate, specifically in ARDS patients, preventive and therapeutic benefits of novel devices and/or strategies.

References

1. Johanson WG, Holcomb JR, Coalson JJ (1982) Experimental diffuse alveolar damage in baboons. Am Rev Respir Dis 126:142–151
2. Campbell GD, Coalson JJ, Johanson WG (1984) The effect of bacterial superinfection on lung function after diffuse alveolar damage. Am Rev Respir Dis 129:974–978
3. Dudeck MA, Edwards JR, Allen-Bridson K, Gross C, Malpiedi PJ, Peterson KD, Pollock DA, Weiner LM, Sievert DM (2015) National Healthcare Safety Network report, data summary for 2013, Device-associated Module. Am J Infect Control 43:206–221
4. Dudeck MA, Weiner LM, Allen-Bridson K, Malpiedi PJ, Peterson KD, Pollock DA, Sievert DM, Edwards JR (2013) National Healthcare Safety Network (NHSN) report, data summary for 2012, Device-associated module. Am J Infect Control 41:1148–1166
5. Wang Y, Eldridge N, Metersky ML, Verzier NR, Meehan TP, Pandolfi MM, Foody JM, Ho SY, Galusha D, Kliman RE, Sonnenfeld N, Krumholz HM, Battles J (2014) National trends in patient safety for four common conditions, 2005-2011. N Engl J Med 370:341–351
6. Chastre J, Trouillet JL, Vuagnat A, Joly-Guillou ML, Clavier H, Dombret MC, Gibert C (1998) Nosocomial pneumonia in patients with acute respiratory distress syndrome. Am J Respir Crit Care Med 157:1165–1172
7. Bellani G, Laffey JG, Pham T, Fan E, Brochard L, Esteban A, Gattinoni L, Haren FV, Larsson A, McAuley DF, Ranieri M, Rubenfeld G, Thompson BT, Wrigge H, Slutsky AS, Pesenti A (2016) Epidemiology, Patterns of Care, and Mortality for Patients With Acute Respiratory Distress Syndrome in Intensive Care Units in 50 Countries. JAMA 315:788–800
8. Markowicz P, Wolff M, Djedaïni K, Cohen Y, Chastre J, Delclaux C, Merrer J, Herman B, Veber B, Fontaine A, Dreyfuss D (2000) Multicenter prospective study of ventilator-associated pneumonia during acute respiratory distress syndrome. Incidence, prognosis, and risk factors. ARDS Study Group. Am J Respir Crit Care Med 161:1942–1948
9. Wolkewitz M, Cooper BS, Bonten MJ, Barnett AG, Schumacher M (2014) Interpreting and comparing risks in the presence of competing events. BMJ 349:g5060
10. Melsen WG, Rovers MM, Groenwold RH, Bergmans DC, Camus C, Bauer TT, Hanisch EW, Klarin B, Koeman M, Krueger WA, Lacherade JC, Lorente L, Memish ZA, Morrow LE, Nardi G, van Nieuwenhoven CA, O'Keefe GE, Nakos G, Scannapieco FA, Seguin P, Staudinger T, Topeli A, Ferrer M, Bonten MJ (2013) Attributable mortality of ventilator-associated pneumonia: a meta-analysis of individual patient data from randomised prevention studies. Lancet Infect Dis 13:665–671
11. Bekaert M, Timsit JF, Vansteelandt S, Depuydt P, Vésin A, Garrouste-Orgeas M, Decruyenaere J, Clec'h C, Azoulay E, Benoit D (2011) Outcomerea Study Group: Attributable mortality of ventilator-associated pneumonia: a reappraisal using causal analysis. Am J Respir Crit Care Med 184:1133–1139
12. Timsit JF, Zahar JR, Chevret S (2011) Attributable mortality of ventilator-associated pneumonia. Curr Opin Crit Care 17:464–471
13. Nordin U (1977) The trachea and cuff-induced tracheal injury An experimental study on causative factors and prevention. Acta Otolaryngol Suppl 345:1–71
14. Li Bassi G, Ranzani OT, Marti JD, Giunta V, Luque N, Isetta V, Ferrer M, Farre R, Pimentel GL, Torres A (2013) An in vitro study to assess determinant features associated with fluid sealing in the design of endotracheal tube cuffs and exerted tracheal pressures. Crit Care Med 41:518–526

15. Inglis TJ, Millar MR, Jones JG, Robinson DA (1989) Tracheal tube biofilm as a source of bacterial colonization of the lung. J Clin Microbiol 27:2014–2018
16. De Souza PR, De Andrade D, Cabral DB, Watanabe E (2014) Endotracheal tube biofilm and ventilator-associated pneumonia with mechanical ventilation. Microsc Res Tech 77:305–312
17. Gil-Perotin S, Ramirez P, Marti V, Sahuquillo JM, Gonzalez E, Calleja I, Menendez R, Bonastre J (2012) Implications of endotracheal tube biofilm in ventilator-associated pneumonia response: a state of concept. Crit Care 16:R93
18. Wilson A, Gray D, Karakiozis J, Thomas J (2012) Advanced endotracheal tube biofilm stage, not duration of intubation, is related to pneumonia. J Trauma Acute Care Surg 72:916–923
19. Shah C, Kollef MH (2004) Endotracheal tube intraluminal volume loss among mechanically ventilated patients. Crit Care Med 32:120–125
20. Johanson WG, Pierce AK, Sanford JP, Thomas GD (1972) Nosocomial respiratory infections with gram-negative bacilli. The significance of colonization of the respiratory tract. Ann Intern Med 77:701–706
21. Golin V, Mimica IM, Mimica LM (1998) Oropharynx microbiota among alcoholics and non-alcoholics. Sao Paulo Med J 116:1727–1733
22. Fuxench-López Z, Ramírez-Ronda CH (1978) Pharyngeal flora in ambulatory alcoholic patients: prevalence of gram-negative bacilli. Arch Intern Med 138:1815–1816
23. Mackowiak PA, Martin RM, Jones SR, Smith JW (1978) Pharyngeal colonization by gram-negative bacilli in aspiration-prone persons. Arch Intern Med 138:1224–1227
24. Frandah W, Colmer-Hamood J, Mojazi Amiri H, Raj R, Nugent K (2013) Oropharyngeal flora in patients admitted to the medical intensive care unit: clinical factors and acid suppressive therapy. J Med Microbiol 62:778–784
25. Mackowiak PA, Martin RM, Smith JW (1979) The role of bacterial interference in the increased prevalence of oropharyngeal gram-negative bacilli among alcoholics and diabetics. Am Rev Respir Dis 120:589–593
26. Scannapieco FA, Bush RB, Paju S (2003) Associations between periodontal disease and risk for nosocomial bacterial pneumonia and chronic obstructive pulmonary disease. A systematic review. Ann Periodontol 8:54–69
27. Dennesen P, van der Ven A, Vlasveld M, Lokker L, Ramsay G, Kessels A, van den Keijbus P, van Nieuw AA, Veerman E (2003) Inadequate salivary flow and poor oral mucosal status in intubated intensive care unit patients. Crit Care Med 31:781–786
28. Ayars GH, Altman LC, Fretwell MD (1982) Effect of decreased salivation and pH on the adherence of Klebsiella species to human buccal epithelial cells. Infect Immun 38:179–182
29. Gibbons RJ, Etherden I (1986) Fibronectin-degrading enzymes in saliva and their relation to oral cleanliness. J Periodontal Res 21:386–395
30. Nakamura M, Slots J (1983) Salivary enzymes. Origin and relationship to periodontal disease. J Periodontal Res 18:559–569
31. Scannapieco FA (1999) Role of oral bacteria in respiratory infection. J Periodontol 70:793–802
32. Fourrier F, Duvivier B, Boutigny H, Roussel-Delvallez M, Chopin C (1998) Colonization of dental plaque: a source of nosocomial infections in intensive care unit patients. Crit Care Med 26:301–308
33. Torres A, El-Ebiary M, Soler N, Montón C, Fàbregas N, Hernández C (1996) Stomach as a source of colonization of the respiratory tract during mechanical ventilation: association with ventilator-associated pneumonia. Eur Respir J 9:1729–1735
34. Taccone P, Pesenti A, Latini R, Polli F, Vagginelli F, Mietto C, Caspani L, Raimondi F, Bordone G, Iapichino G, Mancebo J, Guérin C, Ayzac L, Blanch L, Fumagalli R, Tognoni G, Gattinoni L, Prone-Supine II (2009) Study Group: Prone positioning in patients with moderate and severe acute respiratory distress syndrome: a randomized controlled trial. JAMA 302:1977–1984
35. Gattinoni L, Tognoni G, Pesenti A, Taccone P, Mascheroni D, Labarta V, Malacrida R, Di Giulio P, Fumagalli R, Pelosi P, Brazzi L, Latini R (2001) Prone-Supine Study Group: Effect of prone positioning on the survival of patients with acute respiratory failure. N Engl J Med 345:568–573

36. Benjamin R, Chapman G, Kim C, Sackner M (1989) Removal of bronchial secretions by two-phase gas-liquid transport. *Chest* 95:658–663
37. Sackner MA, Hirsch J, Epstein S (1975) Effect of cuffed endotracheal tubes on tracheal mucous velocity. Chest 68:774–777
38. Sackner MA, Hirsch JA, Epstein S, Rywlin AM (1976) Effect of oxygen in graded concentrations upon tracheal mucous velocity. A study in anesthetized dogs. Chest 69:164–167
39. Hirsch JA, Tokayer JL, Robinson MJ, Sackner MA (1975) Effects of dry air and subsequent humidification on tracheal mucous velocity in dogs. J Appl Physiol 39:242–246
40. Leentjens J, Kox M, van der Hoeven JG, Netea MG, Pickkers P (2013) Immunotherapy for the adjunctive treatment of sepsis: from immunosuppression to immunostimulation. Time for a paradigm change? Am J Respir Crit Care Med 187:1287–1293
41. Headley AS, Tolley E, Meduri GU (1997) Infections and the inflammatory response in acute respiratory distress syndrome. Chest 111:1306–1321
42. Nakos G, Malamou-Mitsi VD, Lachana A, Karassavoglou A, Kitsiouli E, Agnandi N, Lekka ME (2002) Immunoparalysis in patients with severe trauma and the effect of inhaled interferon-gamma. Crit Care Med 30:1488–1494
43. Leentjens J, Kox M, van der Hoeven JG, Netea MG, Pickkers P. (2013) Immunotherapy for the adjunctive treatment of sepsis: from immunosuppression to immunostimulation. Time for a paradigm change? Am J Respir Crit Care Med 187:1287–93
44. Delclaux C, Roupie E, Blot F, Brochard L, Lemaire F, Brun-Buisson C (1997) Lower respiratory tract colonization and infection during severe acute respiratory distress syndrome: incidence and diagnosis. Am J Respir Crit Care Med 156:1092–1098
45. Fagon JY, Chastre J (2003) Diagnosis and treatment of nosocomial pneumonia in ALI/ARDS patients. Eur Respir J Suppl 42:77s–83s
46. Combes A, Figliolini C, Trouillet JL, Kassis N, Wolff M, Gibert C, Chastre J (2002) Incidence and outcome of polymicrobial ventilator-associated pneumonia. Chest 121:1618–1623
47. Schwebel C, Clec'h C, Magne S, Minet C, Garrouste-Orgeas M, Bonadona A, Dumenil AS, Jamali S, Kallel H, Goldgran-Toledano D, Marcotte G, Azoulay E, Darmon M, Ruckly S, Souweine B, Timsit JF (2013) OUTCOMEREA Study Group: Safety of intrahospital transport in ventilated critically ill patients: a multicenter cohort study*. Crit Care Med 41:1919–1928
48. Kollef MH, Von Harz B, Prentice D, Shapiro SD, Silver P, St John R, Trovillion E (1997) Patient transport from intensive care increases the risk of developing ventilator-associated pneumonia. Chest 112:765–773
49. Kress JP, Pohlman AS, O'Connor MF, Hall JB (2000) Daily interruption of sedative infusions in critically ill patients undergoing mechanical ventilation. N Engl J Med 342:1471–1477
50. Schweickert WD, Gehlbach BK, Pohlman AS, Hall JB, Kress JP (2004) Daily interruption of sedative infusions and complications of critical illness in mechanically ventilated patients. Crit Care Med 32:1272–1276
51. Strøm T, Martinussen T, Toft P (2010) A protocol of no sedation for critically ill patients receiving mechanical ventilation: a randomised trial. Lancet 375:475–480
52. Schweickert WD, Pohlman MC, Pohlman AS, Nigos C, Pawlik AJ, Esbrook CL, Spears L, Miller M, Franczyk M, Deprizio D, Schmidt GA, Bowman A, Barr R, McCallister KE, Hall JB, Kress JP (2009) Early physical and occupational therapy in mechanically ventilated, critically ill patients: a randomised controlled trial. Lancet 373:1874–1882
53. Langer T, Santini A, Bottino N, Crotti S, Batchinsky AI, Pesenti A, Gattinoni L (2016) "Awake" extracorporeal membrane oxygenation (ECMO): pathophysiology, technical considerations, and clinical pioneering. Crit Care 20:150
54. Hoeper MM, Wiesner O, Hadem J, Wahl O, Suhling H, Duesberg C, Sommer W, Warnecke G, Greer M, Boenisch O, Busch M, Kielstein JT, Schneider A, Haverich A, Welte T, Kühn C (2013) Extracorporeal membrane oxygenation instead of invasive mechanical ventilation in patients with acute respiratory distress syndrome. Intensive Care Med 39:2056–7.
55. Dullenkopf A, Gerber A, Weiss M (2003) Fluid leakage past tracheal tube cuffs: evaluation of the new Microcuff endotracheal tube. Intensive Care Med 29:1849–1853

56. Lorente L, Lecuona M, Jiménez A, Mora ML, Sierra A (2007) Influence of an endotracheal tube with polyurethane cuff and subglottic secretion drainage on pneumonia. Am J Respir Crit Care Med 176:1079–1083
57. Miller MA, Arndt JL, Konkle MA, Chenoweth CE, Iwashyna TJ, Flaherty KR, Hyzy RC (2011) A polyurethane cuffed endotracheal tube is associated with decreased rates of ventilator-associated pneumonia. J Crit Care 26:280–286
58. Poelaert J, Haentjens P, Blot S (2014) Association among duration of mechanical ventilation, cuff material of endotracheal tube, and postoperative nosocomial pneumonia in cardiac surgical patients: A prospective study. J Thorac Cardiovasc Surg 148:1622–1627
59. Poelaert J, Depuydt P, De Wolf A, Van de Velde S, Herck I, Blot S (2008) Polyurethane cuffed endotracheal tubes to prevent early postoperative pneumonia after cardiac surgery: a pilot study. J Thorac Cardiovasc Surg 135:771–776
60. Philippart F, Gaudry S, Quinquis L, Lau N, Ouanes I, Touati S, Nguyen JC, Branger C, Faibis F, Mastouri M, Forceville X, Abroug F, Ricard JD, Grabar S, Misset B (2015) TOP-Cuff Study Group: Randomized intubation with polyurethane or conical cuffs to prevent pneumonia in ventilated patients. Am J Respir Crit Care Med 191:637–645
61. Lucangelo U, Zin WA, Antonaglia V, Petrucci L, Viviani M, Buscema G, Borelli M, Berlot G (2008) Effect of positive expiratory pressure and type of tracheal cuff on the incidence of aspiration in mechanically ventilated patients in an intensive care unit. Crit Care Med 36:409–413
62. Nseir S, Zerimech F, Fournier C, Lubret R, Ramon P, Durocher A, Balduyck M (2011) Continuous control of tracheal cuff pressure and microaspiration of gastric contents in critically ill patients. Am J Respir Crit Care Med 184:1041–1047
63. Rouzé A, Nseir S (2013) Continuous control of tracheal cuff pressure for the prevention of ventilator-associated pneumonia in critically ill patients: where is the evidence? Curr Opin Crit Care 19:440–447
64. Valencia M, Ferrer M, Farre R, Navajas D, Badia JR, Nicolas JM, Torres A (2007) Automatic control of tracheal tube cuff pressure in ventilated patients in semirecumbent position: a randomized trial. Crit Care Med 35:1543–1549
65. Muscedere J, Rewa O, McKechnie K, Jiang X, Laporta D, Heyland DK (2011) Subglottic secretion drainage for the prevention of ventilator-associated pneumonia: a systematic review and meta-analysis. Crit Care Med 39:1985–1991
66. Høiby N, Bjarnsholt T, Moser C, Bassi GL, Coenye T, Donelli G, Hall-Stoodley L, Holá V, Imbert C, Kirketerp-Møller K, Lebeaux D, Oliver A, Ullmann AJ, Williams C (2014) ESCMID Study Group for Biofilms (ESGB) and Consulting External Expert Werner Zimmerli: ESCMID guideline for Markowicz 2015; i37–i40
67. Kollef MH, Afessa B, Anzueto A, Veremakis C, Kerr KM, Margolis BD, Craven DE, Roberts PR, Arroliga AC, Hubmayr RD, Restrepo MI, Auger WR, Schinner R (2008) NASCENT Investigation Group: Silver-coated endotracheal tubes and incidence of ventilator-associated pneumonia: the NASCENT randomized trial. JAMA 300:805–813
68. Torres A, Serra-Batlles J, Ros E, Piera C (1992) Puig de la Bellacasa J, Cobos A, Lomeña F, Rodríguez-Roisin R: Pulmonary aspiration of gastric contents in patients receiving mechanical ventilation: the effect of body position. Ann Intern Med 116:540–543
69. Orozco-Levi M, Torres A, Ferrer M (1995) Piera C, el-Ebiary M, de la Bellacasa JP, Rodriguez-Roisin R: Semirecumbent position protects from pulmonary aspiration but not completely from gastroesophageal reflux in mechanically ventilated patients. Am J Respir Crit Care Med 152:1387–1390
70. Drakulovic MB, Torres A, Bauer TT, Nicolas JM, Nogué S, Ferrer M (1999) Supine body position as a risk factor for nosocomial pneumonia in mechanically ventilated patients: a randomised trial. Lancet 354:1851–1858
71. Guérin C, Reignier J, Richard JC, Beuret P, Gacouin A, Boulain T, Mercier E, Badet M, Mercat A, Baudin O, Clavel M, Chatellier D, Jaber S, Rosselli S, Mancebo J, Sirodot M, Hilbert G, Bengler C, Richecoeur J, Gainnier M, Bayle F, Bourdin G, Leray V, Girard R, Baboi L, Ayzac L (2013) PROSEVA Study Group: Prone positioning in severe acute respiratory distress syndrome. N Engl J Med 368:2159–2168

72. Ayzac L, Girard R, Baboi L, Beuret P, Rabilloud M, Richard JC, Guérin C (2015) Ventilator-associated pneumonia in ARDS patients: the impact of prone positioning. A secondary analysis of the PROSEVA trial. Intensive Care Med 42:871–878
73. Tejerina E, Esteban A, Fernández-Segoviano P, Frutos-Vivar F, Aramburu J, Ballesteros D, Rodríguez-Barbero JM (2010) Accuracy of clinical definitions of ventilator-associated pneumonia: comparison with autopsy findings. J Crit Care 25:62–68
74. Fàbregas N, Ewig S, Torres A, El-Ebiary M, Ramirez J, de La Bellacasa JP, Bauer T, Cabello H (1999) Clinical diagnosis of ventilator associated pneumonia revisited: comparative validation using immediate post-mortem lung biopsies. Thorax 54:867–873
75. Andrews CP, Coalson JJ, Smith JD, Johanson WG (1981) Diagnosis of nosocomial bacterial pneumonia in acute, diffuse lung injury. Chest 80:254–258
76. Lefcoe MS, Fox GA, Leasa DJ, Sparrow RK, McCormack DG (1994) Accuracy of portable chest radiography in the critical care setting. Diagnosis of pneumonia based on quantitative cultures obtained from protected brush catheter. Chest 105:885–887
77. Wunderink RG (2000) Radiologic diagnosis of ventilator-associated pneumonia. Chest 117:188S–190S
78. Wunderink RG, Woldenberg LS, Zeiss J, Day CM, Ciemins J, Lacher DA (1992) The radiologic diagnosis of autopsy-proven ventilator-associated pneumonia. Chest 101:458–463
79. Meduri GU, Mauldin GL, Wunderink RG, Leeper KV, Jones CB, Tolley E, Mayhall G (1994) Causes of fever and pulmonary densities in patients with clinical manifestations of ventilator-associated pneumonia. Chest 106:221–235
80. Pugin J, Auckenthaler R, Mili N, Janssens JP, Lew PD, Suter PM (1991) Diagnosis of ventilator-associated pneumonia by bacteriologic analysis of bronchoscopic and nonbronchoscopic "blind" bronchoalveolar lavage fluid. Am Rev Respir Dis 143:1121–1129
81. Singh N, Rogers P, Atwood CW, Wagener MM, Yu VL (2000) Short-course empiric antibiotic therapy for patients with pulmonary infiltrates in the intensive care unit. A proposed solution for indiscriminate antibiotic prescription. Am J Respir Crit Care Med 162:505–511
82. Kalil AC, Metersky ML, Klompas M, Muscedere J, Sweeney DA, Palmer LB, Napolitano LM, O'Grady NP, Bartlett JG, Carratalà J, El Solh AA, Ewig S, Fey PD, File TM, Restrepo MI, Roberts JA, Waterer GW, Cruse P, Knight SL, Brozek JL (2016) Management of Adults With Hospital-acquired and Ventilator-associated Pneumonia: 2016 Clinical Practice Guidelines by the Infectious Diseases Society of America and the American Thoracic Society. Clin Infect Dis 63:575–582
83. Canadian Critical Care Trials Group (2006) A randomized trial of diagnostic techniques for ventilator-associated pneumonia. N Engl J Med 355:2619–2630
84. Sanchez-Nieto JM, Torres A, Garcia-Cordoba F, El-Ebiary M, Carrillo A, Ruiz J, Nuñez ML, Niederman M (1998) Impact of invasive and noninvasive quantitative culture sampling on outcome of ventilator-associated pneumonia: a pilot study. Am J Respir Crit Care Med 157:371–376
85. Solé Violán J, Fernández JA, Benítez AB, Cardeñosa Cendrero JA (2000) Rodríguez de Castro F: Impact of quantitative invasive diagnostic techniques in the management and outcome of mechanically ventilated patients with suspected pneumonia. Crit Care Med 28:2737–2741
86. Ruiz M, Torres A, Ewig S, Marcos MA, Alcón A, Lledó R, Asenjo MA, Maldonaldo A (2000) Noninvasive versus invasive microbial investigation in ventilator-associated pneumonia: evaluation of outcome. Am J Respir Crit Care Med 162:119–125
87. Fagon JY, Chastre J, Wolff M, Gervais C, Parer-Aubas S, Stéphan F, Similowski T, Mercat A, Diehl JL, Sollet JP, Tenaillon A (2000) Invasive and noninvasive strategies for management of suspected ventilator-associated pneumonia. A randomized trial. Ann Intern Med 132:621–630
88. Berton DC, Kalil AC, Teixeira PJ (2014) Quantitative versus qualitative cultures of respiratory secretions for clinical outcomes in patients with ventilator-associated pneumonia. Cochrane Database Syst Rev 10:CD006482
89. Meduri GU, Reddy RC, Stanley T, El-Zeky F (1998) Pneumonia in acute respiratory distress syndrome. A prospective evaluation of bilateral bronchoscopic sampling. Am J Respir Crit Care Med 158:870–875

90. Rouby JJ, Martin De Lassale E, Poete P, Nicolas MH, Bodin L, Jarlier V, Le Charpentier Y, Grosset J, Viars P (1992) Nosocomial bronchopneumonia in the critically ill. Histologic and bacteriologic aspects. Am Rev Respir Dis 146:1059–1066
91. Nair GB, Niederman MS (2015) Ventilator-associated pneumonia: present understanding and ongoing debates. Intensive Care Med 41:34–48
92. Kollef MH, Ward S, Sherman G, Prentice D, Schaiff R, Huey W, Fraser VJ (2000) Inadequate treatment of nosocomial infections is associated with certain empiric antibiotic choices. Crit Care Med 28:3456–3464
93. Iregui M, Ward S, Sherman G, Fraser VJ, Kollef MH (2002) Clinical importance of delays in the initiation of appropriate antibiotic treatment for ventilator-associated pneumonia. Chest 122:262–268
94. Luna CM, Aruj P, Niederman MS, Garzón J, Violi D, Prignoni A, Ríos F, Baquero S, Gando S (2006) Grupo Argentino de Estudio de la Neumonía Asociada al Respirador group: Appropriateness and delay to initiate therapy in ventilator-associated pneumonia. Eur Respir J 27:158–164
95. Kuti EL, Patel AA, Coleman CI (2008) Impact of inappropriate antibiotic therapy on mortality in patients with ventilator-associated pneumonia and blood stream infection: a meta-analysis. J Crit Care 23:91–100
96. Hanberger H, Garcia-Rodriguez JA, Gobernado M, Goossens H, Nilsson LE, Struelens MJ (1999) Antibiotic susceptibility among aerobic gram-negative bacilli in intensive care units in 5 European countries. French and Portuguese ICU Study Groups. JAMA 281:67–71
97. Rello J, Sa-Borges M, Correa H, Leal SR, Baraibar J (1999) Variations in etiology of ventilator-associated pneumonia across four treatment sites: implications for antimicrobial prescribing practices. Am J Respir Crit Care Med 160:608–613
98. Martin-Loeches I, Deja M, Koulenti D, Dimopoulos G, Marsh B, Torres A, Niederman MS, Rello J (2013) EU-VAP Study Investigators: Potentially resistant microorganisms in intubated patients with hospital-acquired pneumonia: the interaction of ecology, shock and risk factors. Intensive Care Med 39:672–681

The manufacturer's authorised representative in the EU is Springer Nature Customer Service Centre GmbH, Europaplatz 3, 69115 Heidelberg, Germany. If you have any concerns regarding our products, please contact ProductSafety@springernature.com

Printed and bound by CPI Group (UK) Ltd, Croydon, CR0 4YY
12/08/2026
02194528-0001